PROGRESS IN CLINICAL AND BIOLOGICAL RESEARCH

Series Editors

Nathan Back   Vincent P. Eijsvoogel   Kurt Hirschhorn   Sidney Udenfriend
George J. Brewer   Robert Grover   Seymour S. Kety   Jonathan W. Uhr

Please contact publisher for information about previous titles in this series.

THE MAILLARD REACTION IN AGING, DIABETES, AND NUTRITION

THE MAILLARD REACTION IN AGING, DIABETES, AND NUTRITION

Proceedings of an NIH Conference on the Maillard Reaction in Aging, Diabetes, and Nutrition Held in Bethesda, Maryland, September 22–23, 1988

Editors

John W. Baynes
Department of Chemistry
University of South Carolina
Columbia, South Carolina

Vincent M. Monnier
Institute of Pathology
Case Western Reserve University
Cleveland, Ohio

ALAN R. LISS, INC. • NEW YORK

Address all Inquiries to the Publisher
Alan R. Liss, Inc., 41 East 11th Street, New York, NY 10003

```
Library of Congress Cataloging-in-Publication Data

NIH Conference on the Maillard Reaction in Aging,
    Diabetes, and Nutrition (1988 : Bethesda, Md.)
    The Maillard reaction in aging, diabetes, and
nutrition.

    (Progress in clinical and biological research ;
v. 304)
    Includes bibliographies and index.
    1. Maillard reaction--Physiological effect--
Congresses.  2. Diabetes--Pathophysiology--Congresses.
3. Aging--Physiological aspects--Congresses.
4. Nutrition--Congresses.  5. Proteins--Metabolism--
Congresses.  6. Diabetes--Complications and
sequelae--Etiology--Congresses.  I. Baynes, John W.
II. Monnier, Vincent M.  III. Title.  IV. Series.
[DNLM: 1. Aging--congresses.  2. Diabetes Mellitus--
congresses.  3. Maillard Reaction--congresses.
4. Nutrition--congresses.  W1 PR66BE v. 304 /
WT 104 N691m 1988]
RB171.N54  1988    616.07          89-2561
ISBN 0-8451-5154-1
```

We thank the publishers for permission to reproduce the following material.
Marcel Dekker, Inc.: Figure 4, Njoroge and Monnier.
Biochemistry, copyright 1988 American Chemical Society: Figures 1, 2, Walton et al.
The Journal of Experimental Medicine, by copyright permission of The Rockefeller University Press: Figure 1, Bitensky et al.
Biochemical Journal, copyright 1988 The Biochemical Society, London: Figures 1, 2, 3, Table 2, Scheme, Wolff et al.
American Institute of Nutrition: Table 1, Oste.
American Chemical Society: Figures 1, 2, 3, Table 2, Oste.
Japanese Cancer Association: Figures 1, 2, Weisburger and Jones.

Contents

Contributors

Edathara C. Abraham, Department of Cell and Molecular Biology, Medical College of Georgia, Augusta, GA 30912–2100 [123]

Mahtab U. Ahmed, Department of Chemistry, University of South Carolina, Columbia, SC 29208; present address: Department of Chemistry, University of Dhaka, Dhaka, Bangladesh [43]

Naseem H. Ansari, Department of Human Biological Chemistry & Genetics, University of Texas Medical Branch, Galveston, TX 77550 [171]

Katsura Arai, Department of Biochemistry, Osaka University Medical School, Osaka 530, Japan [277]

Shigeaki Baba, Second Department of Internal Medicine, Kobe University School of Medicine, Kobe 650, Japan [69]

Allen J. Bailey, AFRC Institute of Food Research—Bristol, Bristol BS18 7DY, England [109]

Zainab A. Bascal, Toxicology Laboratory, University College London, London WC1E 6JJ, England [259]

John W. Baynes, Department of Chemistry and School of Medicine, University of South Carolina, Columbia, SC 29208 [xv,xxi,43,391]

Jakob Beck, Institut für Pharmazie und Lebensmittelchemie, Universität München, 8000 München 2, Federal Republic of Germany [23]

Aruni Bhatnagar, Department of Human Biological Chemistry & Genetics, University of Texas Medical Branch, Galveston, TX 77550 [171]

Mark W. Bitensky, Life Sciences and Physics Divisions, Los Alamos National Laboratory, Los Alamos, NM 87545 [185]

Michael Brownlee, Department of Medicine and Diabetes Research Center, Albert Einstein College of Medicine, Bronx, NY 10461 and Laboratory of Medical Biochemistry, The Rockefeller University, New York, NY 10021 [205,235]

Anthony Cerami, Laboratory of Medical Biochemistry, The Rockefeller University, New York, NY 10021 [205,291]

The numbers in brackets are the opening page numbers of the contributors' articles.

xi

Ballabh Das, Department of Human Biological Chemistry & Genetics, University of Texas Medical Branch, Galveston, TX 77550 [171]

John A. Dunn, Department of Chemistry, University of South Carolina, Columbia, SC 29208 [43]

Sabine Estendorfer, Institut für Pharmazie und Lebensmittelchemie, Universität München, 8000 München 2, Federal Republic of Germany [23]

Paul-André Finot, Nestec Ltd., Nestlé Research Centre, CH–1000 Lausanne 26, Switzerland [343]

Carolyn I. Fisher, Department of Chemistry, University of South Carolina, Columbia, SC 29208 [43]

Diane E. Furniss, Nestec Ltd., Nestlé Research Centre, CH–1000 Lausanne 26, Switzerland [343]

Greg Hair, Department of Human Biological Chemistry & Genetics, University of Texas Medical Branch, Galveston, TX 77550 [171]

Fumitaka Hayase, Department of Agricultural Chemistry, The University of Tokyo, Tokyo 113, Japan [69]

Bernhard Huber, Institut für Pharmazie und Lebensmittelchemie, Universität München, 8000 München 2, Federal Republic of Germany [23]

Clifford J. Hull, Department of Chemistry, University of South Carolina, Columbia, SC 29208 [43]

James V. Hunt, Toxicology Laboratory, University College London, London WC1E 6JJ, England [259]

Susumu Iizuka, Kucchan Kousei Hospital, Kucchan 057, Hokkaido, Japan [277]

R. Conrad Jones, American Health Foundation, Valhalla, NY 10595 [377]

Amar Kaanane, Department of Food Science and Nutrition, University of Minnesota, St. Paul, MN 55108; present address: Department of Food Science, Hassan II Institute of Agronomy and Veterinary Medicine, Rabat, Morocco [301]

Hiromichi Kato, Department of Agricultural Chemistry, The University of Tokyo, Tokyo 113, Japan [69]

M.J. Christine Kent, AFRC Institute of Food Research—Bristol, Bristol BS18 7DY, England [109]

Noriaki Kinoshita, Department of Biochemistry, Osaka University Medical School, Osaka 530, Japan [277]

Theodore Koschinsky, Department of Medicine, University of California, San Diego, La Jolla, CA 92093; present address: Diabetes-Forschungsinstitut, Universität Düsseldorf—Klinische Abteilung, 4000 Düsseldorf, Federal Republic of Germany [219]

Anjaneyulu Kowluru, Life Sciences Division, Los Alamos National Laboratory, Los Alamos, NM 87545 [185]

Renu A. Kowluru, Life Sciences Division, Los Alamos National Laboratory, Los Alamos, NM 87545 [185]

Theodore P. Labuza, Department of Food Science and Nutrition, University of Minnesota, St. Paul, MN 55108 [301]

Franz Ledl, Institut für Pharmazie und Lebensmittelchemie, Universität München, 8000 München 2, Federal Republic of Germany; present address: Institut für Lebensmittelchemie und Analytische Chemie, Universität Stuttgart, 7000 Stuttgart 80, Federal Republic of Germany [23]

Annette T. Lee, Laboratory of Medical Biochemistry, The Rockefeller University, New York, NY 10021 [291]

Siqi Liu, Department of Human Biological Chemistry & Genetics, University of Texas Medical Branch, Galveston, TX 77550 [171]

John D. McPherson, Department of Biochemistry, Queen's University, Kingston, Ontario, Canada K7L 3N6 [163]

Richard A. Miller, Department of Pathology, Boston University School of Medicine, Boston, MA 02118 [249]

Vincent M. Monnier, Institute of Pathology, School of Medicine, Case Western Reserve University, Cleveland, OH 44106 [xv,xxi,1,85,391]

Takafumi Naito, Department of Orthopedics, Sapporo Medical College, Sapporo 010, Japan [277]

F. George Njoroge, Institute of Pathology, School of Medicine, Case Western Reserve University, Cleveland, OH 44106; present address: Organic Chemical Research, Schering–Plough Corp., Bloomfield, NJ 07003 [85]

Munetada Oimomi, Second Department of Internal Medicine, Kobe University School of Medicine, Kobe 650, Japan [69]

Helga Osiander, Institut für Pharmazie und Lebensmittelchemie, Universität München, 8000 München 2, Federal Republic of Germany [23]

Rickard Öste, Department of Nutrition, Chemical Center, University of Lund, 22100 Lund, Sweden [329]

Jeffrey S. Patrick, Department of Chemistry, University of South Carolina, Columbia, SC 29208 [43]

Ronald E. Perry, Department of Cell and Molecular Biology, Medical College of Georgia, Augusta, GA 30912–2100 [123]

Manfred Sengl, Institut für Pharmazie und Lebensmittelchemie, Universität München, 8000 München 2, Federal Republic of Germany [23]

Theodor Severin, Institut für Pharmazie und Lebensmittelchemie, Universität München, 8000 München 2, Federal Republic of Germany [23]

Takayuki Shibamoto, Department of Environmental Toxicology, University of California, Davis, Davis, CA 95616 [359]

Brian H. Shilton, Department of Biochemistry, Queen's University, Kingston, Ontario, Canada K7L 3N6 [163]

Dong Bum Shin, Department of Agricultural Chemistry, The University of Tokyo, Tokyo 113, Japan; present address: Department of Biochemistry, University of Missouri, Columbia, MO 65211 [69]

Satish K. Srivastava, Department of Human Biological Chemistry & Genetics, University of Texas Medical Branch, Galveston, TX 77550 [171]

Gerardo Suarez, Department of Biochemistry, New York Medical College, Valhalla, NY 10595 **[141]**

Mruthinti S. Swamy, Department of Cell and Molecular Biology, Medical College of Georgia, Augusta, GA 30912–2100 **[123]**

Naoyuki Taniguchi, Department of Biochemistry, Osaka University Medical School, Osaka 530, Japan **[277]**

Suzanne R. Thorpe, Department of Chemistry, University of South Carolina, Columbia, SC 29208 **[43]**

Masamichi Usui, Department of Orthopedics, Sapporo Medical College, Sapporo 010, Japan **[277]**

Helen Vlassara, Laboratory of Medical Biochemistry, The Rockefeller University, New York, NY 10021 **[205]**

Donald J. Walton, Department of Biochemistry, Queen's University, Kingston, Ontario, Canada K7L 3N6 **[163]**

Nancy G. Watkins, Department of Chemistry, University of South Carolina, Columbia, SC 29208 **[43]**

John H. Weisburger, American Health Foundation, Valhalla, NY 10595 **[377]**

Joseph L. Witztum, Department of Medicine, University of California, San Diego, La Jolla, CA 92093 **[219]**

Simon P. Wolff, Toxicology Laboratory, University College London, London WC1E 6JJ, England **[259]**

Preface

In 1912, Louis Camille Maillard at the Sorbonne reported that aqueous solutions of reducing sugars turned progressively yellow-brown when heated or when stored under physiological conditions. His prediction that the reaction could occur in vivo and perhaps explain the increased excretion of amino acids in diabetes went unnoticed at the time. Instead, for the next half-century, progress in understanding Maillard's reaction was largely restricted to the realm of food science and technology. Through this research the Maillard reaction has come to be recognized as a mixed blessing; a powerful tool for improving the flavor, taste, consistency, and overall appeal of foods, and yet at the same time a potential cause of losses in nutritional value and a source of toxic products and genotoxic agents. The thrust in food research has been on manipulation of Maillard reaction chemistry in order to improve the quality of food products. Major efforts have been directed at understanding the mechanisms involved in flavor enhancement and deterioration in processed and stored foods, as well as at the physiological and toxicological impact of browned foods on the organism. An essential element of these studies has been the development of sophisticated analytical methods for qualitative and quantitative analysis of the changes in food composition at all stages in its preparation. That effort continues unabated today in the food industry, contributing to improvements in the production and quality of such diverse products as breakfast foods, colas, caramel, chocolates, soy sauce, beer, infant formulas, and solutions for parenteral nutrition; anywhere, in fact, where the Maillard reaction can effect wanted or unwanted changes in product quality.

In contrast to the steady progress toward understanding the chemistry and significance of the Maillard reaction in food systems in vitro, for more than 50 years after Maillard's original paper there was negligible interest in studies on this reaction in physiological systems in vivo. This period of inattention ended with the discovery of nonenzymatically glycosylated (glycated) hemoglobins, followed by evidence that glycation of hemoglobin was increased in diabetes. Measurements of glycated hemoglobin are now widely used as an index of glycemia in diabetes. When glycation was detected as a common posttranslational modification of other proteins in vivo, it was quickly recognized that increased glycation could be involved in the pathogenesis of diabetic complications. Since glycation was known as an early step in the Maillard reaction, the realization that long-lived proteins become browned, fluorescent, and insoluble with age and at an accelerated rate in diabetes suggested that later stages of the Maillard reaction might proceed in vivo and contribute to some of the pathophysiology associated with both aging and diabetes.

The implications of this hypothesis on the role of the Maillard reaction in aging and diabetes are as complex as the reaction itself. The test of the hypothesis will require major advances in understanding the chemistry of the reaction, as well as the development of methods for assessing the progress and biological effects of the reaction in vivo. Progress toward these goals will require an interdisciplinary effort on the part of scientists with a wide range of expertise and talents.

Based on this premise, a conference was convened on September 22–23, 1988, at the National Institutes of Health in Bethesda, Maryland, with the aim of summarizing current knowledge of the Maillard reaction as it pertains to the biochemistry and biology of aging, diabetes, and nutrition. In contrast to the first three international symposia [1–3] on the Maillard reaction, which placed greater emphasis on food technological and toxicological aspects of the reaction, this conference focuses on the "endogenous" aspects of the Maillard reaction. Because research on the role of the Maillard reaction in vivo is still in its infancy and much of the essential data are yet to be gathered, it was felt to be premature to debate the question of whether the pathology of age- and diabetes-related phenomena can be better explained by the Maillard reaction than by other mechanisms. Thus, in planning the conference and its proceedings, particular attention was paid to the presentation and development of hypotheses, guidelines, concepts, and preliminary observations which may serve as a basis for future studies on the Maillard reaction in vivo.

The Maillard Reaction in Aging, Diabetes, and Nutrition begins with an introductory chapter presenting a critical analysis of current evidence and hypothesized mechanisms for the role of the Maillard reaction in the pathophysiology of aging and diabetes. There follow five major sections dealing with various aspects of the Maillard reaction. The first section introduces the chemistry of the Maillard reaction through studies in model systems under physiological conditions. The second includes recent results on the effects of glycation on the properties of structural proteins, such as collagen and lens crystallins. Three chapters in this section also deal with recent evidence for interplay between the Maillard reaction and the sorbitol pathway in the alteration of tissue proteins in diabetes. Evidence is presented for glycation and browning of proteins by fructose and for effects of glycation on the kinetic properties of aldose reductase. These papers add a new dimension to the long-standing controversy on the relative roles of the Maillard reaction and the sorbitol pathway in the development of pathophysiology in diabetes; they suggest instead that the two mechanisms may be united at the molecular level. The third section of the book addresses the clinical significance of effects of glycation and Maillard reactions on the recognition and turnover of plasma proteins and lipoproteins. Also included are recent studies on the macrophage receptor for Advanced Glycosylation Endproducts (AGE) in proteins and a chapter on recent efforts at pharmacological modulation of the Maillard reaction. The fourth section is devoted to cellular aging and the interface between Maillard- and oxidation-mediated damage to macromolecules. It includes a discussion of recently described autoxidative pathways of glycation of protein, effects of glycation on the antioxidative enzyme, superoxide dismutase, and the potential role of the Maillard reaction in the aging of T-cells and DNA. The final section of the book bridges the borderline between endogenous and exogenous Maillard reactions. The five chapters in this section treat the Maillard reaction from a food science perspective, dealing with the effects of Maillard products on the metabolism and nutritional value of foods, and concluding with chapters on the genotoxicity of Maillard products.

The broad scope of this book reflects both the breadth of and recent growth in interest in the Maillard reaction in physiological systems. We are convinced that further studies on this reaction are essential to the understanding of aging and diabetes, and hope that the text presents this message clearly and mirrors our own enthusiasm as well as that of the many participants in the conference.

We wish to express our appreciation to Dr. Margo Cohen and Dr. Milton Feather for their assistance in chairing sessions, and to the speakers and participants for their contributions to the success of this conference. Special thanks go also to the National Institute on Aging (NIA) and the Diabetes Branch of the National Institute of Diabetes, Digestive and Kidney Disease (NIDDK) for their sponsorship of the conference. We also thank these agencies and our industrial sponsors for their generous financial support. We particularly acknowledge the personal efforts of Dr. Ann Sorenson and Dr. Huber Warner from the NIA, and Dr. Elaine Collier and Dr. Robert Silverman from the Diabetes Branch of NIDDK. Also, we thank those who worked behind the scenes, especially Ms. Mollie Hilty at the NIA and Ms. Tonya Marshall at Case Western Reserve University.

REFERENCES

1. Eriksson C (ed) (1981) *The Maillard Reaction in Foods*. Prog Food Nutr Sci vol 5, Oxford: Pergamon Press.
2. Waller G, Feather MS (eds) (1983) *Maillard Reactions in Food and Nutrition*. American Chemical Society Symposium Series, vol 215, Washington DC: American Chemical Society.
3. Fujimaki M, Namiki A, Kato H (eds) (1986) *Amino-carbonyl Reactions in Food and Biological Systems*. Dev Food Sci, vol 13, Amsterdam: Elsevier.

John W. Baynes
Vincent M. Monnier

Acknowledgments

The Organizing Committee thanks the following corporate sponsors for their generous support: Ajinomoto Co., Inc.; Alcon Laboratories, Inc.; The Coca-Cola Company; Lilly Research Laboratories; Mead-Johnson & Co.; Miles Inc.; Nestlé Enterprises, Inc.; The NutraSweet Company; Quaker Oats Co.; Roche Diagnostic Systems; Sethness Caramel Color; Squibb-Novo, Inc.; The Upjohn Co.

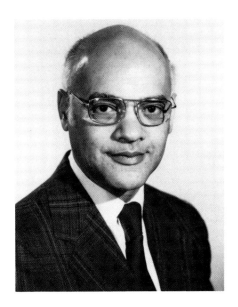

To John E. Hodge on the occasion of his 75th birthday

Dedication

There is no published, comprehensive history of research on the Maillard reaction. Writing such a book would indeed be a complex task, for the history is widely distributed among disciplines and journals in academic, industrial, and government laboratories throughout the world. It is safe to say, however, that no history would be complete without reference to the fundamental contributions of John E. Hodge throughout his career of 40 years at the U.S. Department of Agriculture's Northern Regional Research Center in Peoria, Illinois. We were fortunate at this conference to have John Hodge as the keynote speaker at our dinner.

John Edward Hodge was born in Kansas City, Kansas, on October 12, 1914. He earned his B.A. (Cum Laude, Phi Beta Kappa, 1936) and M.A. (1940) from the University of Kansas, and was Professor of Chemistry at Western University in Quindaro, Kansas from 1939 to 1941. He joined the USDA Northern Regional Research Center in 1941, received a Department of Agriculture Superior Service Award in 1953, two Research Team Awards (1955, 1960), and retired as Supervisory Research Chemist in 1980. During his career he served as a Grant Officer in the USDA (1962–1975), and consultant to the National Research Council (1964–1980) and the National Academy of Sciences (1970–1980). He also served as a member of the Editorial Advisory Board of the journal, Carbohydrate Research (1965–1975), and is a past Chairman of the Division of Carbohydrate Chemistry of the American Chemical Society (1964) and of the Carbohydrate Division of the American Association of Cereal Chemists (1971).

His research focused on the complex chemistry of intermediates in the Maillard reaction, including the glycosylamines, Amadori compounds, and reductones; the relationship between structure and flavor; the chemical mechanisms of browning reactions and methods for controlling the browning and deterioration of foods via the Maillard reaction. In his distinguished career he authored more than 70 papers and 10 book chapters, edited one book on the "Physiological Effects of Food Carbohydrates" (1975), and obtained nine patents. His classic 1953 paper, "Dehydrated Foods: Chemistry of Browning Reactions in Model Systems," was identified as a "Citation Classic" in 1979 [J Ag Food Chem 1:928–943 (1953), cited in Current Contents: March 19, 1979; p. 12]. The entire article was reproduced as an example of a model review article in *Scientific Thinking and Scientific Writing* by M.S. Peterson (Reinhold Publishing, New York, 1961). His Scheme for the Maillard reaction in that paper in 1953 remains a guidepost for continuing research, and is frequently referenced and reproduced today.

Since 1980 John Hodge has continued to work as a consultant to the grain processing and brewing industries. He has been active in community activities, serving as the Secretary to the Mayor's Commission for Senior Citizens and Member of the Advisory Board for the Central Illinois Agency for Aging in Peoria. He is an Adjunct Professor of Chemistry at Bradley University in Peoria.

We thank John E. Hodge for joining us at the NIH Conference on the Maillard Reaction in Aging, Diabetes, and Nutrition. It is an honor to dedicate this book to him in recognition of his many rigorous and creative contributions to research on the Maillard reaction and for the inspiration he has given to us all.

John W. Baynes
Vincent M. Monnier

The Maillard Reaction in Aging,
Diabetes, and Nutrition, pages 1–22
© 1989 Alan R. Liss, Inc.

TOWARD A MAILLARD REACTION THEORY OF AGING

VINCENT M. MONNIER. Institute of Pathology, School of
Medicine, Case Western Reserve University, Cleveland,
Ohio 44106

ABSTRACT: The inescapable chronic exposure of cellular and
extracellular matrix molecules to reducing sugars which can initiate
the Maillard reaction in vivo suggests that the fundamental aging
process might be mediated by the Maillard reaction. An attempt
to explain aging on the basis of the Maillard reaction, however,
raises a number of conceptual questions. These questions are
formulated below as a basis for a theory of aging based on the
Maillard reaction.

INTRODUCTION AND HISTORICAL DEVELOPMENT

Ling (1908), in England, first postulated that the color changes
occurring during the brewing process may stem from reactions
occurring between sugars and proteins. It was Louis Camille Maillard,
however, who in 1912 carried out the first experiment in which he
heated 1 part of glycine with 4 parts of glucose in water (Maillard,
1912). After 10 min, the liquid turned yellow, then rapidly deep-
brown. Formation of CO_2 was noted. Presence of oxygen, nitrogen,
hydrogen or vacuum did not affect the reaction. Maillard repeated the
same reaction with sarcosine, alanine, valine, leucine, tyrosine and
glutamic acid and found that alanine was the most active amino acid.
He also reacted glycine with a variety of saccharides and noted that
xylose and arabinose reacted "instantaneously", that fructose, galactose,
glucose and mannose reacted "fairly rapidly" and that lactose and
maltose reacted "slowly". In contrast, saccharose reacted "not at all for
several hours". He noted that "the reaction occurred with such facility
that one was surprised it had not been discovered earlier and already
studied in great detail." Maillard cautioned that this reaction might
lead to "profound analytical errors in chemical biology" and
hypothesized that the reaction might be of relevance to a variety of
areas in science such as geology ("combustible minerals", fossilization),
agronomy (peat, humus, etc.), plant physiology (alkaloids) and

medicine. He postulated the reaction he had discovered would be of relevance to diabetes. In particular, he hypothesized that sugars could be destroying amino acids, thus explaining in part their increased excretion in diabetes. Maillard went even as far as suggesting the possible therapeutic use of amino acids in diabetic subjects for a "better utilization of sugars".

In essence, most of Maillard's predictions have proven to be correct. The Maillard reaction is now under active investigation in geological and agricultural science, particularly what concerns polymerization reactions involving xylose and other sugars in the formation of melanoidins contained in humus (Benzing-Purdie, 1983). The reaction is also of major interest to food and nutrition science, whereby the goal is to maximize food flavor through heat-induced Maillard reaction without, however, impairing nutritive value or creating carcinogenic compounds. Examples of industrial applications include production of caramel, cola, coffee, brewed products and infant formulas.

In the medical field, the concept that reducing sugars might damage amino acids has proven correct in many ways. Manufacturers of solutions for total parenteral nutrition have long realized that solutions of amino acids and glucose should not be autoclaved or stored together. The prediction that the reaction would be of potential importance to diabetes has been confirmed in recent years by the bulk of the literature on the nonenzymatic glycosylation reaction which initiates the Maillard reaction in vivo. A more detailed discussion of the chemistry of the reaction will be provided later. Contrary to Maillard's thinking, however, it is now well established that the urinary loss of amino acids in diabetes results primarily from decreased cellular uptake of amino acids and increased protein catabolism rather than from the Maillard reaction itself. Nevertheless, some reports indicate preferential loss of glycated proteins in the urine (Kowluru, et al., 1987).

Finally, Maillard's speculation that amino acids might be used for a "better utilization of sugars" has been echoed by the proposition that aminoguanidine might be useful in preventing crosslinking and other deleterious processes resulting from the advanced Maillard reaction (Brownlee et al., 1986).

Thus, Maillard realized immediately the broad implications of his discovery, most of which have led to major developments over the years. However, his proposition that the reaction would be of importance to diabetes was forgotten in the years following his discovery. The major reason for this development can be undoubtedly attributed to the fact that elucidation of the cause rather than the consequence of elevated glycemia in diabetes was a research priority at the beginning of the century. This culminated in the discovery of insulin 10 years after Maillard's landmark paper (Banting and Best, 1922).

Evidence for the occurrence of the Maillard reaction in vivo came indirectly, primarily through the study of minor hemoglobins which had been found elevated in diabetes (Trivelli et al., 1971). The use of borohydride reduction made it possible to both label the Amadori product which is formed in the early stage of the reaction and to isolate it via acid hydrolysis for purpose of quantitation (Bookchin and Gallop, 1968, Stevens et al. 1978). It also became apparent that the formation of Amadori products occurred through nonenzymatic attachment of glucose to proteins, thus leading to the concept of "nonenzymatic glycosylation" and the investigation of its potential role in diabetic complications (Cerami and Koenig, 1978: Cerami et al. , 1979). These developments have already been reviewed several times in the past and the reader is referred to previous reviews (Bunn 1981;Brownlee et al., 1984; Kennedy and Baynes, 1984).

Although the Maillard reaction was not studied in vivo in the 60 years following Maillard's discovery, substantial progress was achieved in the meantime in understanding its chemistry in relationship to food science. In essence, the concept evolved that food proteins that are stored or processed in the presence of reducing sugars undergo an aging process characterized by nonenzymatic browning and crosslinking which leads to impaired biological availability (Hodge 1953; Eriksson, 1981). The realization that similar changes were observed in long-lived proteins such as lens crystallins and collagen that could be duplicated by incubating the protein with hexoses, greatly catalyzed the interest in the potential role of Maillard reaction in the aging process (Monnier and Cerami, 1981, 1983).

Four observations of fundamental importance offer a strong rationale for implicating the Maillard reaction in the basic aging process. 1) The most definitive age-related changes occur in non-renewable tissues, 2) many of these changes are accelerated by diabetes 3) the same changes as well as many age-related diseases are retarded by food restriction 4) both diabetes and food restriction act on glycemia and may affect the intracellular level of reducing sugars, all of which can engage in Maillard-type reactions. Evidence in support of these statements is presented below and emerging issues with attempting to explain age-related phenomena on the basis of the Maillard reaction will be addressed.

AGE-RELATED CHANGES IN NON-RENEWABLE TISSUES

As pointed out by Kohn and Schnider (1982) the most dramatic age-related changes occur in non-renewable tissues. Human lens crystallins, for example, do not turn over. They become progressively less soluble and acquire with age protein-bound yellow chromophores and fluorophores (Pirie, 1968). During cataract formation, the pigmentation process may dramatically increase in the nucleus which is the old part of lens or it may involve the entire lens as in brunescent cataracts. Such changes are usually accompanied by the formation of non-disulfide covalent crosslinks. One possible functional consequence of age-related postsynthetic modification of crystallins by the Maillard reaction is the linear loss of accommodation with advancing age.

Collagen-rich tissues are particularly prone to the aging process. With age, there is a loss of elasticity in skin, arteries, lungs and joints (Kohn and Monnier, 1987). Collagen in these tissues, as well as throughout the body becomes less soluble, less digestible by collagenase, less expandable, and more resistant to heat denaturation with advancing age (Schnider and Kohn, 1982). Furthermore, as in the human lens, fluorescent and yellow chromophores accumulate in collagen which may represent Maillard-derived crosslinks (Monnier et al., 1984). Some of the possible physiological consequences resulting from increased collagen crosslinking include decreased ability of immune cells to penetrate tissue and fight infections, increased blood pressure due to stiffened arteries, decreased vital capacity, emphysema and decreased joint mobility.

Whereas there is little evidence that stem cells such as bone marrow cells lose their ability to divide in aging (Kohn, 1982), definite losses of functional capacity have been observed in T-cells, many of which are very long-lived "memory" cells (Makinodan and Kay, 1980; Abet et al. 1980). Changes include decreased mitogenic response to PHA and Con A, decreased IL-2 production, decreased IL-2 response, and increased tendency of lymphocytes to cell cycle arrest. There is also a decrease in natural killer cell activity (Weindruch et al., 1983). The global impairment of the aging immune system is thought to explain the increased susceptibility to infections, cancers and autoimmune diseases in aging (Weindruch et al., 1983; Jung et al. 1982)

As for collagen and lens crystallins, it is likely that long-lived T-cells as well as fibroblasts which are resting cells could be prime targets of the Maillard reaction. Thus, in-depth study of the Maillard reaction in these tissues is expected to provide important insight into their mechanism of aging and perhaps clues to the fundamental aging process.

DIABETES ACCELERATES AGE-RELATED PROCESSES

If the Maillard reaction is expected to explain basic age-related phenomena, a prerequisite would be that diseases and conditions associated with hyperglycemia would also accelerate the onset and the magnitude of the symptoms of the aging syndrome. In effect, the observation that subjects with diabetes show signs of accelerated aging has been known for many years and reiterated several times by Kohn (1983). Cataracts, for example occur on the average 10-15 years earlier in diabetes and lens opacities are early predictors of death in diabetic subjects (Podgor et al., 1985). Atherosclerosis, myocardial infarction and strokes are more frequent in younger diabetic subjects than in age-matched nondiabetic controls (Kannel and McGee, 1979). Arteries and joints are prematurely stiff (Pillsbury et al. 1974; Grgic et al. 1975), elasticity of the lungs and vital capacity are prematurely decreased (Schuyler et al., 1976) whereas the susceptibility to infections is increased in diabetes (Rayfield et al. 1982). Hypertension is more prevalent among diabetic subjects who also have accelerated bone loss and osteoarthritis at a younger age (Waine et al., 1961).

At the microscopic and submicroscopic levels, capillary basement membranes thicken at a higher rate (Kilo et al. 1972), fluorophores in lens (Bleeker et al. 1986), dura mater (Monnier et al., 1984), skin (Monnier et al., 1986) and cartilage (Monnier, unpublished) accumulate more rapidly, and collagen is more resistant to collagenase digestion than in subjects without diabetes (Hamlin et al., 1975). Although no increased rate of cancers has been reported in diabetes, impaired T-cell function was observed, particularly in subjects with insulin-dependent diabetes (Zier et al. 1984).

Thus, the acceleration of age-related processes by diabetes offers a strong rationale for linking them to the Maillard reaction.

FOOD RESTRICTION RETARDS AGE-RELATED PROCESSES

Experimental food restriction is one of the prime tools for investigation of fundamental mechanisms of aging since it is the only intervention that is known to prolong maximal life-span (Masoro et al., 1982). There is increasing evidence to support the notion that the beneficial effect of food restriction expresses itself ubiquitously, i.e., by acting on the fundamental aging rate. Thus, food restriction in rodents is effective in retarding the aging of the immune system, as evidenced by decreased rate of autoimmune phenomena and malignancies (Weindruch et al., 1979). It also retards the onset of nephrosis, osteoporosis (Kalu et al., 1984) and the onset of degenerative disease of the musculoskeletal system (Berg and Simms, 1960). At the cellular and molecular level, food restriction retards the loss of gamma-crystallins from the lens (Leveille et al., 1984), decreases the rate of tendon collagen crosslinking (Everitt, 1971), retards the loss of natural killer cell activity and preserves T-cell response to mitogens (Weindruch et al.,1982b, 1983). Food restriction may also retard aging of brain functions as evidenced by, for example, improved learning in food restricted vs ad libitum fed mice (Idrobo et al., 1987; Ingram et al., 1987).

Thus, food restriction is the corollary to diabetes when it comes to evaluate mechanisms and interventions that affect the aging rate of the entire organism. Whereby diabetes leads to hyperglycemia, food restriction is expected to induce a drop in mean glycemia, as well as in the level of glycolytic intermediate that can initiate the Maillard reaction. In support of this concept is the recent demonstration that food-restricted Fisher 344 rats had significantly lower level of glycosylated hemoglobin than those of ad libitum fed animals (Masoro et al., 1989).

CURRENT UNDERSTANDING OF THE MAILLARD REACTION IN LIGHT OF THE AGING PROCESS

A number of issues need to be addressed should one attempt to explain age-related phenomena on the basis of the Maillard reaction. In the following we will use a simplified scheme of the overall Maillard

Reaction as it is currently understood (Fig.1), and address specific points as we progress from the early to the late stages of the reaction. The choice of this approach is dictated by the fact that each step of the reaction might be involved in the pathology of aging by a different mechanism.

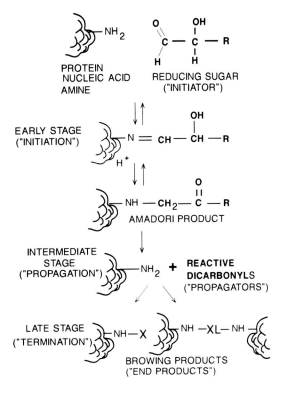

Fig. 1. General Scheme of the Maillard Reaction.

In essence, the Maillard reaction is initiated by the nonenzymatic condensation of a sugar aldehyde or ketone with a free amino group and is assumed to proceed via a Schiff base. This stage of the reaction is fully reversible but acid catalysis favors the Amadori rearrangement which leads to a fairly stable ketoamine compound called the Amadori product. This early stage of the reaction is referred to as nonenzymatic glycosylation or more accurately "glycation" (Roth et al., 1983). The Amadori product is then degraded into a variety of carbonyl compounds, the predominance of which depends on reaction conditions. The compounds have α-dicarbonyl groups which make them much more reactive than the sugar from which they are derived. Therefore, they act as propagators of the reaction.

Most of the propagators of the Maillard reaction are deoxyglucosones and sugar fragmentation products. In vitro, these carbonyl compounds react again with free amino groups to form a variety of UV active, often fluorescent adducts and crosslinks. These products are thermodynamically stable and are expected to accumulate onto long-lived biological molecules. Their formation would effectively terminate the Maillard reaction in vivo. In vitro, however, polymerization occurs leading to deep brown solutions rich in insoluble polymers called melanoidins.

a) Targets of the Maillard Reaction

As a general rule, all molecules that have free amino groups, whether these are proteins, nucleic acids or low molecular weight amines can be the target of reducing sugars and help initiate the reaction in vivo. The evidence to suggest that the initial stage of the Maillard reaction proceeds in vivo is very strong. It is based on the demonstration of glucose-derived Amadori products in cellular and extracellular proteins throughout the body and their occurrence in elevated amounts in diabetes (for reviews see Monnier and Cerami, 1983; Kennedy and Baynes, 1984; Brownlee et al. 1984).

Whereas the presence of a free amino group is a prerequisite for initiation of the Maillard reaction, target groups of the advanced reaction might also include the functional residues of arginine, histidine, tyrosine, and tryptophan, depending on reaction conditions (Reynolds et al., 1985). Serine and threonine could also be modified by forming ether bridges with hydroxymethyl-pyrrole carboxaldehyde groups (Olsson et al., 1981). If the target groups are crucial for maintenance of proper molecular function, their modification either by early or advanced products of the Maillard reaction is expected to have deleterious effect. Examples include impaired ligand binding, conformational changes, change in charge, solubility, enzyme inactivation. From a logical viewpoint, short-lived molecules such as those from plasma are expected to be modified predominantly by early products of the Maillard reaction whereas long-lived molecules like lens crystallins, collagen, DNA in long-lived cells are expected to accumulate predominantly and irreversibly advanced products of the Maillard reaction.

Obviously, fundamental aspects that will need to be addressed in relationship to the aging process are whether some key cellular or extracellular molecules are preferential targets of the Maillard reaction and whether the extent of their modification is sufficient to explain impaired tissue function in aging.

b) Reducing Sugars as Initiators of the Maillard Reaction

In principle, all reducing sugars whether aldose or ketoses can initiate the Maillard reaction in vivo. By and large, this concept can be enlarged to include molecules related to sugars like ascorbate (Hodge 1953; Orwerth et al., 1988). Table I provides an overview of the carbohydrates that might be implicated in the reaction.

Table I. INITIATORS OF THE MAILLARD REACTION IN VIVO

ALDOSES	KETOSES	OTHERS
Glucose	Fructose	Ascorbate
Glucose-6-P	Fructose-6-P	Hexosamines
Mannose	Fructose 1-P	Sedoheptulose
Mannose 6-P	Fructose 1,6-P	
Galactose		
Ribose	Ribulose	
Ribose 5-P	Ribulose 5-P	
2-Deoxy-ribose		
Xylose	Xylulose	
Arabinose	Xylulose 5-P	
Erythrose		
Erythrose 4-P		
Glyceraldehyde	Dihydroxyacetone	
Glyceraldehyde-3 P	Dihydroxyacetone-P	

Because glucose is the most abundant sugar and because it is elevated in diabetes, most studies so far have focused on this sugar. A number of observations concerning the biology of glucose are worth considering. First, it is one of the most tightly regulated blood metabolites in the non-diabetic individual (Ciba-Geigy: tables on blood metabolites, 1972). Neither hypoglycemic nor hyperglycemic deviations from euglycemia are tolerated, suggesting that not only hypoglycemia, but also hyperglycemia might be deleterious to body functions. Thus, glucose can be considered a toxin, whereby chronic exposure of the organism to this sugar is expected to damage long-lived molecules via the Maillard reaction even in euglycemic subjects. The second important observation is that glucose is one of the slowest reacting sugars in terms of nonenzymatic attachment of proteins. This led Bunn & Higgins (1981) to postulate an evolutionary significance for the fact that glucose emerged as the major carrier of energy from cell to cell in vertebrates. Third, if a hypothesis of aging is to be based on glucose as the major culprit (Cerami, 1985), one of the conceptual difficulties to solve is the observation that average glycemia does not correlate with species longevity. In effect, average glycemia is overall the same in mammalian species and reaches very high values in some birds, e.g., parakeets, the longevity of which is similar to that of humans (Fowler, 1984; Altman and Kirmayer, 1976). This, by itself, would not make a glucose theory of aging impossible should one be able to demonstrate that the ability to prevent or remove molecules and cells damaged by glucose (Vlassara et al. 1985, 1986) is inversely related to species longevity. Finally, although the bulk of the studies so far have focused on glucose, recent evidence suggests that fructose (Suarez et al. 1988; McPherson et al. 1988) and pentoses are much more potent Maillard reactants than glucose (Bunn and Higgins, 1981) and might thus play a significant role in diabetes and age-related processes. Although extracellular concentration of these sugars is much lower than that of glucose, their high reactivity makes them strong candidates for mediation of molecular damage to long-lived molecules (Table II). Evidence for implication of ribose in protein crosslinking in aging is discussed below.

Table II. RELATIVE REACTIVITY OF SELECTED REDUCING SUGARS

Reducing Sugar	Rate of Schiff base formation with protein[1]	Overall reaction rate as in browning[2]
2-Deoxy-D-Ribose	---	217
D-Ribose	16.6	129
2-Deoxy-D-glucose	---	26
D-Arabinose	---	16.4
D-Fructose	7.5	---
D-Xylose	4.8	7
D-Galactose	4.6	4.6
D-Mannose	5.3	3
D-Glucose	1	1

[1]Bunn & Higgins, Science 213, 222 (1981)
[2]Overend et al., J. Chem. Soc., 3490 (1981)

c) The Amadori Product

There is a dual biological significance to the Amadori product what concerns the Maillard reaction cascade. The Amadori product of glucose is relatively stable and thus represents a stop in the propensity of the sugar aldehyde to crosslink molecules. In effect, a side reaction may occur, called the Namiki pathway (Namiki 1975), in which the initial condensation product may lead directly to browning while by-passing the Amadori product. However, there is no evidence yet that the Namiki pathway can occur under physiological conditions. On the other hand, the Amadori product is the parent compound of the advanced Maillard reaction (Hodge & Rist, 1953) and kinetic data indicate that the latter is generally considered a zero order reaction respective to concentration of glucose and amine (Labuza and Saltmarch, 1981). That means that it is expected to be strongly dependent on the concentration of the Amadori product. In that context, the relevant observation is that mean plasma concentration of Amadori products by fructosamine assay is about 2.5 mM in euglycemic subjects and can reach 6.0 mM in diabetes (Lim and Staley, 1985). Thus, in view of the fact that Amadori products are much more reactive than glucose in the initiation of the advanced Maillard reaction, the total concentration of circulating glucose-derived Amadori products is by no means trivial.

Although the plasma concentration of Amadori product in species with various longevities remains to be established, it is not expected to correlate inversely with longevity since there is a priori no reason for the Amadori product to brown faster in short vs long-lived species. However, modulation of plasma and cellular level of Amadori product could take place via oxidative C2-C4 fragmentation in presence of metal catalyst (Ahmed et al. 1986). The fragment remaining attached to the protein residue is a carboxymethyl group linked to a lysyl residues. Carboxymethyl-lysine was found to accumulate in aging lens crystallins suggesting the presence of an oxidative process in the aging human lens (Ahmed et al, 1986). It would be of interest to investigate whether the accumulation or excretion rate of carboxymethyl-lysine is inversely related to species longevity. A positive finding could be taken as evidence that the oxidation rate of tissues is a life-span limiting process by formation of free radicals (Harman, 1956).

Another mechanisms by which level of Amadori products could be controlled, is via receptor mediated uptake or by turnover of immune complexes. There is presently no evidence for the presence of specific receptors for Amadori products. However, molecules or cells incubated with glucose are preferentially taken up by macrophages (Vlassara et al. 1985, 1986, 1987), endothelial cells (Williams et al., 1981) or excreted (Kowluru et al. 1987). The presence of autoantibodies to glycated proteins has been detected in some subjects (Witztum et al., 1984) and may have a regulatory role for the removal of glycated molecules. However, increased removal rate of glycated LDL has not been observed in animals immunized against the borohydride reduced glycated protein (Witztum et al., 1983).

In summary, unless an unlikely inverse relationship between level of Amadori product and species longevity is uncovered, Amadori products by themselves are not expected to be life-span determining factors.

d) Deoxyglucosones as Propagators of the Maillard Reaction

Although it is conceivable that the Amadori product might undergo further addition reactions to e.g., glucosyl pyrroles (Farmar et al., 1988), current evidence suggests that the bulk of advanced Maillard

Table III. PROPAGATORS OF THE MAILLARD REACTION

CH_3	H	CH_2OH	R
|	|	|	|
C = O	C = O	C = O	C = O
|	|	|	|
C = O	C = O	C = O	C (O, OH)
|	|	|	|
C(H, OH)	CH_2	CH_2	R
|	|	|	
R	C (H, OH)	R	
	|		
	R		
1-deoxy osone	3-deoxy osone	4-deoxy osone	fragmentation products and free radicals

reaction products result from degradation and fragmentation of Amadori products (Ledl et al. 1986). As noted above, deoxyglucosones propagate the reaction by forming chromophores and fluorescent adducts and crosslinks involving amino groups. These "propagators" of the Maillard reaction are listed in Table III.

From experiments in vitro it has been established that the formation of 3-deoxyglucosone (3-DG) is generally favored at lower, pH, whereas that of 1-deoxyglucosone (1-DG) is favored at neutral pH (Feather, 1981). Nevertheless, experiments that were conducted with glucose at 37°C and at neutral pH revealed that pyrrole compounds derived from 3-DG were quantitatively more important than those derived from 1-DG (Njoroge et al. 1987). Further interest in 3-DG comes from experiments by Kato (1960, 1962) and other investigators (Shin et al., 1988) who have demonstrated that 3-DG has the ability to form crosslinks.

As pointed out above, the fact that mean glycemia is overall identical in short versus long-lived mammalian species makes it difficult to conceive a theory of aging based on glycemia or plasma level of Amadori product alone. If, however, plasma and cellular propagators of the Maillard reaction are metabolized, the rate of molecular damage by the advanced Maillard reaction could be under genetic control and thus inversely related to species longevity. Preliminary evidence in effect suggests that 3-deoxyglucosone can be metabolized by liver enzymes (Hata et al. 1988). It is thus possible that in contrast to short-lived animal species, longevous species would have more efficient or higher levels of enzymes for detoxification of the α-dicarbonyl compounds that propagate the Maillard reaction in vivo.

An alternative or additional potential anti-Maillard mechanism is suggested by the work with aminoguanidine which was found to inhibit crosslinking and formation of fluorescent compounds in the extracellular matrix of diabetic animals and during Maillard reaction in vitro (Brownlee et al. 1986). Based on this concept, it is conceivable that cellular and extracellular free amino acids and bioorganic amines like taurine, creatine, guanidino-acetic acid and spermidine-type compounds could trap and inactivate deoxysones, thus preventing damage to essential molecules. In that context it is of interest to note that urine contains a large variety of fluorescent molecules (Sell and Monnier, unpublished) which may represent the reaction product of deoxyosones trapped by low molecular weight amines. Assay of some of these advanced products of the Maillard reaction in the urine of mammals with various longevities might provide important information to test the Maillard reaction theory of aging.

e) End Products of the Maillard Reaction

Once formed, the end products of the Maillard reaction signal the irreversibility which is inherent to the aging process. These molecules are generally stable, and unless the entire molecule on which they form is turned over, the molecular lesion is irreversible. However, a potential mechanism for removal of molecules and cells modified by the advanced Maillard reaction may exist. As noted above, Vlassara et al. (1985, 1987) observed that molecules and cells modified by advanced glycosylation end products were preferentially taken up by macrophages. The uptake appears to be mediated by a specific receptor. Of interest, is these authors' proposition that increased challenge of macrophages by Maillard proteins, as in diabetes, may induce the release of cytokines like IL-1 and TNF which might mediate some of the vascular lesions observed in diabetes (Vlassara et al., 1988).

Until recently, evidence for occurrence of the advanced Maillard reaction in long-lived molecules has been largely based on the presence of fluorescence that can be duplicated by incubation of proteins with glucose (Monnier et al, 1984, 1986). Borohydride reducible as well as fluorescent products that co-chromatograph with similar molecules isolated from glucose-incubated proteins have been detected in lens and collagen (Monnier and Cerami, 1983; Oimomi et al. 1988a, 1988b). Further studies on the nature of the fluorophores which accumulate in aging human collagen revealed the presence of two major fluorophores with excitation-emission maxima at 335/385 nm and 360/460 nm respectively (Sell and Monnier, 1989). Complete structure elucidation of one of the fluorophores indicates presence of a lysyl-arginine crosslink involving, surprisingly, a pentose in an imidazo [4,5b] pyridinium ring (Sell and Monnier, submitted). The pentose is most likely ribose which is released during cell death and ribonucleotide turnover. The newly discovered molecule was named pentosidine. The fact that the guanido group of arginine is involved in the heterocyclic ring suggests that a similar reaction between single-stranded DNA and arginine-rich histones or other proteins may occur in long-lived cells like the peripheral T-cells. If such a mechanism is involved in limiting life-span, one would expect an inverse relationship between accumulation rate of pentosidine in long-lived tissue and maximum life span of mammals. The emergence of ribose as a potent crosslinking agent in vivo raises major new questions concerning the aging process.

CONCLUSION

The Maillard reaction offers an attractive new concept for the explanation of many of the wear-and-tear phenomena that have been to date only partially and unsatisfactorily explained on the basis of other aging theories. It should be pointed out, however, that the newness of this concept is relative for two reasons. First, many of the biological consequences of the Maillard reaction are expected to result from increased crosslinking, and a role for crosslinking in aging was already postulated in 1965 by Bjorksten in 1942. Second, after this article was written, the author came across the article by Bensusan (1965) who had already postulated that the Maillard reaction would explain collagen crosslinking in vivo, long before glucose-derived Amadori were discovered in biological tissues. Thus, should a Maillard reaction theory of aging ever prove to be correct, these authors will deserve credit for their intuition. The availability of anti-Maillard compounds as well as specific probes for the propagators and the end products of the Maillard reaction will be necessary to investigate rigorously the validity of the Maillard reaction theory of aging.

ACKNOWLEGEMENTS

This work was supported by grants AG 05601 and AG 06927 from the National Institute on Aging and grant EY 07099 from the National Eye Institute.

REFERENCES

Abet T, Morimoto C, Toguchi T, Kiyotaki M and Homma M (1980). The cellular basis of impaired T lymphocyte function in the elderly. J Am Ger Soc 28:265-271.

Ahmed MU, Thorpe SR, Baynes JW (1986). Identification of N^ϵ-carboxymethyllysine a degradation product of fructoselysine in glycated protein. J Biol Chem 261:4889-4894.

Altman RB, Kirmayer AH (1976). Diabetes mellitus in the avian species. J Am Anim Hosp Assoc 12:531 .

Banting FG and Best CH (1922). The internal secretion of the pancreas. J Lab Clin Med VII, 5:256-271.

Bensusan HB (1965). A novel hypothesis for the mechanism of crosslinking in collagen. In "Structure and Function of Connective and Skeletal Tissue" Harkness RD, Partridge SM, Tristiam GR, Eds. Butterworth, London 42-46.

Benzing-Purdie L, Ripmeester JA (1983). Melanoidines and soil organic matter; evidence of strong similarities revealed by ^{13}C CP-MAS NMR. Soil Sci Soc Am J 47:56-61.

Berg BN, Simms HS (1960). Nutrition and longevity in the rat. II. Longevity and onset of disease with different levels of food intake. J Nutr 75:25

Bjorksten J, Champion WJ (1942). Mechanical influence upon tanning. J Am Chem Soc 64:868-869.

Bjorksten J (1958). A common molecular basis for the aging syndrome. J Am Geriatrics Soc 6:740-748.

Bleeker JC, vanBest JA, Vrij L, van der Velde EA, Oosterhuis JA (1986). Autofluorescence of the lens in diabetic and healthy subjects by fluoremetry. Inv Opth Vis Sci 27:791-794.

Bookchin RM, Gallop PM (1968). Structure of hemoglobin A_{1c}: Nature of the N-terminal beta chain blocking group. Biochim. Biophys Res Comm 32:86-93.

Brownlee M, Vlassara H, Kooney A, Ulrich P and Cerami A (1986). Aminoguanidine prevents diabetes-induced arterial wall protein cross-linking. Science 232:1629-1632.

Brownlee M, Vlassara H, Cerami A (1984). Nonenzymatic glycosylation and the pathogenesis of diabetic complications. Am Int Med 101:527-537.

Brownlee M, Cerami A, Vlassara H (1988). Advanced glycosylation endproducts in tissue and the biochemical basis of diabetic complications. N Engl J Med 318:1315-1321.

Bunn HF (1981). Nonenzymatic glycosylation of protein: relevance to diabetes. Am J Med 70:325-330.

Bunn HF, Higgins PJ (1981). Reaction of monosaccharides with proteins: possible evolutionary significance. Science 213:222-224.

Caliero E, Maiello M, Boeri D, Roy S, Lorenzi M (1988). Increased expression of basement membrane components in human endothelials cells cultured in high glucose. J Clin Inv 82: 735-738.

Cerami A, Koenig RJ (1978). Hemoglobin A_{1c} as a model for the development of the sequelae of diabetes mellitus. Biochem Sci April:73-75.

Cerami A, Stevens VJ, Monnier VM (1979). Role of nonenzymatic glycosylation in the development of the sequelae of diabetes. Metabolism 28:431-437.

Cerami A. (1985) Hypothesis: glucose as a mediator of aging. J Am Ger Soc 33:626-634.

Ciba-Geigy SA (1972). Scientific tables, 7th, french edition, data on mean values and 95% confidence interval of blood metabolites. 611-622.

Eriksson C (1981) Ed. Maillard Reactions in Food. Prog Fd & Nutr Sci 5:1-501 Pergamon Press, Oxford.

Everitt AV, Seedsman NJ and Jones F (1980). The effects of hypophysectomy and continous food restriction, begun at ages 70 and 400 days, on collagen aging, proteinuria, incidence of pathology and longevity in the male rat. Mech Aging Dev 12: 161-172.

Everitt AV, (1971). Food intake, growth and the ageing of collagen in rat tail tendon. Geront 17:98-104.

Farmar JG, Ulrich PC, Cerami A (1988). Novel pyrroles from sulfite-inhibited Maillard reactions. Insight into the mechanism of inhibition. J Org Chem 53: 2346-2349.

Feather MS (1981). Amine assisted sugar dehydration reactions. In "Maillard Reactions in Food", Eriksson C. Ed. Prog Fd Nutr Sci 5:37-46, Pergamon Press, Oxford.

Fowler ME, Ed. (1986). Zoo and wild animal medicine. W.B. Saunders Co. Philadelphia, p 272-276.

Fujimaki M, Namiki M, Kato H, Eds. (1986). Amino-carbonyl reactions in food and biological systems. Dev Fd Sci 13: 1-583,Elsevier, Amsterdam.

Grgic A, Rosenbloom AL, Weber FT, Giordana B (1975). Joint contracture in childhood diabetes. N Engl J Med 292: 372-376.

Hamlin CR, Kohn RR, Luschin JH (1975). Apparent accelerated aging of human collagen in diabetes mellitus. Diabetes 24:902-904.

Harman D (1956). Aging: a theory based on free radical and radiation chemistry J Gerontol 11: 298-300.

Hata F, Igaki N, Nakamichi T, Masuda S, Nishimoto S, Oimomi M, Baba S, Kato H (1988). Suppresive effect of α-ketoaldehyde dehydrogenase on the advanced process of the Maillard reaction. Diab Res Clin Pract 5:5413.

Hodge JE, Rist CE (1953). The Amadori rearrangement under new conditions and its significance for non-enzymatic browning reactions. J Amer Chem Soc 1953 75:316-322.

Hodge JE (1953). Chemistry of browning reactions in model systems. J Agric Food Chem 1:928-943.

Holehan AM and Merry BJ (1986). The experimental manipulation of aging by diet. Biol Rev 61:329-368.

Idrobo F, Nandy K, Mostofsky DI, Blatt L, Nandy L (1987). Dietary restriction: effects on radial maze learning and lipofuscin pigment deposition in the hippocampus and frontal cortex. Arch Gerontol Geriatr 6:355-362.

Ingram DK, Weindruch R, Spangler EL, Freeman JR and Walford RL (1987). Dietary restriction benefits learning and motor performance of aged mice. J Geront 42:78-81.

Jung KL, Pallandino MA, Calvano S, Mark DA, Good RA and Fernandes G (1982). Clin Imm Immunopath 25: 295-301.

Kalu DN, Hardin RR, Cockerham R, Yu BP, Norting BK and Egan JW (1984). Lifelong food restriction prevents senile osteopenia and hyperparathyroidism in F344 rats.

Kannel WB, McGee DL (1979). Diabetes and cardiovascular disease: The Framingham Study. JAMA 241:2035-38.

Kato H (1962). Chemical studies on amino-carbonyl reaction: Part I Isolation of 3-deoxypentosone and 3-deoxyhexosones formed by browning degradation of N-glycosides. Agr Biol Chem (Tokyo) 26:187-191.

Kato H (1960). Studies on browning reactions between sugars and amino compounds. Isolation and characterization of new carbonyl compounds, 3-deoxyosones formed from N-glycosides and their significance for browning reaction. Agric Biol Chem (Tokyo) 24:1-12.

Kennedy L, Baynes JW (1984). Nonenzymatic glycosylation and the chronic complications of diabetes: an overview. Diabetologia 26:93-98.

Kilo C, Volger N, Williamson JR (1972). Muscle capillary basement membrane changes related to aging and to diabetes mellitus. Diabetes 21:881-905.

Koenig RJ, Cerami A (1975). Synthesis of hemoglobin A_{Ic} in normal and diabetic mice: potential model of basement membrane thickening. Proc Natl Acad Sci USA 72:3687-3691.

Kohn RR (1982). Evidence against cellular aging theories. In "Testing the Theories of Aging". Adelman RC and Roth GS, Eds. CRC Press, Boca Raton FL, 221-231.

Kohn RR and Monnier VM (1987). Normal aging and its parameters. In. Swift C.G. (Ed.) "Clinical Pharmacology in the Elderly", Marcel Dekker, Inc. New York 3-30.

Kohn RR and Schnider SL (1982). Glucosylation of human collagen. Diabetes 31 (Suppl. 3):47-51.

Kohn RR (1983). Effects of age and diabetes mellitus on cyanogen bromide digestion of human duran mater collagen. Conn Tissue Res 11:169-173.

Kowluru A, Kowluru R, Bitensky MW, Corwin EJ, Solomon SS and Johnson JD (1987). Suggested mechanism for the selective excretion of glucosylated albumin. J Exp Med 166:1259-1279.

Ledl F, Fritsch G, Hiebl J, Parchmayr O, Severin T (1985). Degradation of Maillard products. In "Amino-carbonyl reactions in food and biological systems" Fujimaki M, Namiki M, Kato H, Eds. Elsevier, Amsterdam, Dev Fd Sci 13:173-182.

Leveille PJ, Weindruch R, Walford RL, Bok D and Horwitz J. Dietary restriction retards age-related loss of gamma crystallins in the mouse lens. Science 224:1247-1249.

Lim YS, Staley MJ (1985) Measurement of plasma fructosamine evaluated for monitoring diabetes. Clin Chem 31:731-733.

Ling AR and Malting J (1908). J Inst Brew 14:494-521.

Maeda H, Gleiser CA, Masoro EJ, Murata I, McMahan CA and Yu BP (1985). Nutritional influences on aging of Fischer 344 rats: II Pathology. J Geront 40: 671-688.

Maillard LC (1912) Action des acides aminés sur les sucres; formation des melanoidines par voie methodique. C R Acad Sci 154:66-68.

Makinodan T and Kay MMB (1980). Age influence on the immune system. Adv Immun 29:287-329.

Mark DA, Alonso DR, Tack-Goldmank., Tzvi Thaler H, Tremoli E, Weksler B and Weksler ME (1984). Effects of nutrition on disease and life span. Am J Pathol 117:125-131.

Masoro EJ, Yu BP, Bertrand HA (1982). Action of food restriction in delaying the aging process. Proc Natl Acad Sci 79:4239-4241.

Masoro EJ, Katz MS, McMahan CA (1989). Evidence for glycation hypothesis of aging from the food restricted model. J Gerontol Bio Sci 44:B20-22.

McPherson JD, Shilton B, Walton DJ (1988). Role of fructose in glycation and crosslinking of proteins. Biochemistry 27:1901-1907.

Melby EC, Altman NH, Eds. (1974) Handbook of Laboratory Animal Science Volume II. 366.

Monnier VM, Cerami A (1981) Nonenzymatic browning in vivo:possible process for aging of long-lived proteins. Science 211:491-493.

Monnier VM, Cerami A (1983). Nonenzymatic glycosylation and browning of proteins in vivo. In "The Maillard Reaction in Foods and Nutrition", Waller GR and Feather MS. Eds, American Chemical Society, Symposium Series 215:431-449.

Monnier VM, Kohn RR, Cerami A (1984). Accelerated age-related browning of human collagen in diabetes mellitus. Proc Natl Acad USA 81:583-587.

Monnier VM, Vishwanath V, Frank KE, Elmets CA, Dauchot P, Kohn RR (1986). Relation between complications of Type I diabetes mellitus and collagen-linked fluorescence. N Engl J Med 314:403-408.

Namiki M, Hayashi T (1975). Development of novel free radicals during amino-carbonyl reaction of sugars with amino acids. J Agric Food Chem 23:487-491.

Njoroge FG, Sayre LM, Monnier VM (1987a). Detection of D-glucose-derived pyrrole compounds during Maillard reaction under physiological conditions. Carbohydr Res 167:211-220.

Oimomi M, Maeda Y, Hata F, Kitamura Y, Matsumoto S, Baba S, Iga T, Yamamoto M (1988). Glycation of cataractous lens in non-diabetic senile subjects and in diabetic patients. Exp Eye Res 46:415-420.

Olsson K, Pernemalm A, Theander O (1981). Reaction products and mechanism in some simple model systems. In "Maillard Reactions in Food", Eriksson C, Ed. Prog. Fd. Nutr Sci 5:81-91. Pergamon Press, Oxford, 47-56.

Ortwerth BJ, Feather MS, Olesen PR (1988). The precipitation and crosslinking of lens crystallins by ascorbic acid. Exp Eye Res 47:155-168.

Overend WG, Peacoke AR, Smith JB (1961). J Chem Soc 3487-3492.

Pillsbury HC, Hung W, Kyle MC, Freis ED (1974). Arterial pulse waves and velocity and systolic time intervals in diabetic children. Am Heart J 87:783-90.

Pirie A (1968). Color and solubility of the protein of human cataract. Invest Opthalmol 7:634-50.

Podgor MJ, Cassel GH and Kannel WB (1985). Lens changes and survival in a population-based study. N Eng J Med 313:1430-1444.

Rayfield EJ, Ault MJ, Keusch GT, Brother MJ, Nechemias C, Smith H (1982). Infection and diabetes: the case for glucose control. Am J Med 72:439-450.

Roth M (1983) "Glycated hemoglobin, not "glycosylated" or "glucosylated", Letter to the editor. Clin Chem 29:1991

Reynolds TM (1965). Chemistry of Nonenzymatic Browning II. Adv Food Res 14:167-283.

Schnider SL and Kohn RR (1982). Effects of age and diabetes mellitus on the solubility of collagen from human skin, tracheal cartilage and dura mater. Exp Gerontol 17:185-194.

Schuyler MR, Niewoehner DE, Inkley SR, Kohn RR (2976). Abnormal lung elasticity in juvenile diabetes mellitus. Am Rev Repir Dis 113:37-41.

Sell DR, Monnier VM (1989). Isolation, purification and partial characterization of fluorophores from aging human extracellular matrix. Conn Tissue Res: in press.

Sell DR, Monnier VM (submitted). Structure elucidation of a crosslink from aging human extracellular matrix. Implication of ribose in the aging process.

Shin DB, Hayase F, Kato H (1988). Polymerization of proteins caused by reaction with sugars and the formation of 3-deoxyglucosone under physiological conditions. Agric Biol Chem 52:1451-1458.

Stevens VJ, Rouzer CA, Monnier VM, Cerami A (1978). Diabetic cataract formation: potential role of glycosylation of lens crystallins. Proc Natl Acad Sci (USA) 75:2918-22.

Suarez G, Rajaram R, Bheyan KC, Oronsky AL and Goidl JA (1988). Administration of aldose reductase inhibitor induces a decrease of collagen fluorescence in diabetic rats. J Clin Inv 82:624-627.

Trivelli LA, Ranney HM and Hont-Tien L (1971) Hemoglobin components in patients with diabetes mellitus. N Engl J Med 284:353-357.

Vlassara H, Brownlee M, Cerami A (1985). High affinity-receptor-mediated uptake and degradation of glucose-modified proteins: a potential mechanism for the removal of senescent macromolecules. Proc Natl Acad Sci USA 2:5588-92.

Vlassara H, Brownlee M, Cerami A (1986). Novel macrophage receptor for glucose-modifed proteins is distinct from previously described scavenger receptors. J Exp Med 164:1301-9.

Vlassara H, Valinksy J, Brownlee M, Cerami C, Nishimoto S, Cerami A (1987). Advanced glycosylation endproducts on erythrocyte cell surface induced receptor-mediated phagocytosis by macrophages. A model for turnover of aging cells. J Exp Med 166:539-549.

Vlassara H, Brownlee M, Manogue K, Pasagian (1988). Science 240:1546-1549.

Waine H, Nevinny D, Rosenthal J, Joffe IB (1961). Association of osteoarthritis and diabetes mellitus. Tufts Folia Med 7:13-19.

Weindruch RH, Kristie JA, Cheney KE and Walford RL (1979). Influence of controlled dietary restriction on immunologic function and aging. Fed Proc 38: 2007-2016.

Weindruch RH, Kristie JA, Naeim F, Mullen BG, Walford RL (1982b). Influence of weaning-initiated dietary restriction on responses to T cell mitogens and on splenic T cell mitogens and on splenic T cell levels in a long-lived F_1-hybrid mouse strain. Exper Gerontol 49-64.

Weindruch R and Walford RL (1982). Dietary restriction in mice beginning at 1 year of age: Effect on life-span and spontaneous cancer incidence. Science 215:1415-1417.

Weindruch R, Devens BH, Raff HV and Walford RL. (1983). Influence of dietary restriction and aging on natural killer cell activity in mice. J Imm 130: 993-996.

Williams SK, Devenny JJ, Bitensky MW (1981). Micropinocytic ingestion of glycosylated albumin by isolated microvessels: possible role in pathogenesis of diabetic microangiopathy. Proc Natl Acad Sci USA 78:2392-2397.

Witztum JL, Steinbrecher UP, Kesaniemi YA, Fisher M. (1984). Autoantibodies to glucosylated proteins in the plasma of patients with diabetes mellitus. Proc Natl Acad Sci USA 81:3204-3208.

Zier KS, Leo MM, Spielman RS, Baker L (1984). Decreased synthesis of interleukin II (IL-2) in insulin-dependent diabetes mellitus. Diabetes 33:552-555.

The Maillard Reaction in Aging,
Diabetes, and Nutrition, pages 23–42
© 1989 Alan R. Liss, Inc.

CHEMICAL PATHWAYS OF THE MAILLARD REACTION

Franz Ledl, Jakob Beck, Manfred Sengl,
Helga Osiander, Sabine Estendorfer,
Theodor Severin and Bernhard Huber

Institut für Lebensmittelchemie und
Analytische Chemie der Universität Stuttgart, Pfaffenwaldring 55, 7ooo Stuttgart
80 (F.L.) and Institut für Pharmazie und
Lebensmittelchemie der Universität München, Sophienstr. 10, 8000 München 2, FRG

ABSTRACT. From reaction mixtures of reducing sugars with primary and secondary
amines many heterocyclic and carbocyclic
compounds have been separated. From the
structures of these substances together
with the knowledge about reactive intermediates some degradation pathways can
be proposed. Caused by the nature of the
sugar (pentose, mono- or disaccharide)
and the amine (primary or secondary)
differences in the pathways are observed.
An attempt is made to present some reactions with emphasis to the Maillard
reaction in mammalians.

INTRODUCTION

The degradation of reducing sugars in food is
usually induced by heat, but changes also take
place after long-time storage at room temperature.
Amino acids and proteins help to accelerate the
reactions and influence the product formation.
Sugar-amine interactions are termed non-enzymatic
browning, or Maillard reaction. In food, major
changes can be attributed to the formation of aro-

matic and flavouring ingredients, browning products, high molecular compounds (melanoidins), stabilizing and mutagenic substances and loss of nutritive value.

The Maillard reaction also takes place in the human body. The point is made by catchwords such as "Saccharification with increasing age" or "Aging - a baking oven process". The increased glucose concentration in the blood of diabetics means that it may be possible to detect the formation of higher concentrations of Maillard products in their bodies. Investigations are still necessary to find out to what extent the changes observed during aging and in diabetics can be ascribed to the Maillard reaction.

Normally degraded in foodstuffs are the reducing monosaccharides glucose and fructose, the disaccharides maltose and lactose, and in some cases the reducing pentoses. The reaction partners are amino acids and in proteins the ε-amino group of lysine. In the mammalian organism it is mainly glucose and proteins that take part in the Maillard reaction.

EARLY STAGE OF THE MAILLARD REACTION

It can be assumed that in the Maillard reaction the amine reacts with the sugar both as a nucleophile and a base (in the scheme glucose has been chosen as the example, and the structures are shown open-chained for simplification). As the nucleophile the amine attacks the carbonyl function of the sugar, and after water elimination and eno- lisation an aminoketose of type 1 is formed (Paul- sen and Pflughaupt, 1980). It has been possible to detect compounds of the general structure 1 in heated, long stored and dried foodstuffs (Ciner- Doruk and Eichner, 1979), and in the human body (Baynes et al., Boissel et al., Monnier et al., 1986).

If the ϵ-amino group of lysine reacts in this way the essential amino acid is no more available to the organism (Mauron, 1981). The result is then a reduction in the nutritive value of food and feedstuffs. In the case of aminoketoses in the mammalian organism there has been observed an oxi- dative cleavage to carboxymethyllysine 3 (Ahmed et al., 1985). The proof of amine-containing C3 fis- sion products in the Maillard reaction would in- dicate a retro-aldol reaction to 1-amino-3-hydroxy- acetone derivates 2. Such low-molecular fragments are very reactive and accelerate the browning and cross-linking reactions. Similar reactions of the aldose or of the imine produce C2 products (Hayashi and Namiki, 1986).

$$
\begin{array}{ccc}
HN- & HN- & NH- \\
| & | & | \\
H_2C & H_2C & CH_2 \\
| & | & | \\
C=O & C=O & COOH \\
| & | & \\
H_2C-OH & HO-CH & \underline{\underline{3}} \\
& | & \\
\underline{\underline{2}} & HC-OH & \\
& | & \\
& HC-OH & \\
& | & \\
& H_2C-OH & \\
\\
HC=O & \underline{\underline{1}} & COOH \\
| & & | \\
HC-OH & & HC-OH \\
| & & | \\
H_2C-OH & & HC-OH \\
& & | \\
& & H_2C-OH
\end{array}
$$

The reaction of an aminoketose with an addi- tional molecule of glucose and amine was assumed for the formation of the so-called FFI 4 (Pongor et al., 1984). The results of further experiments have indeed indicated that the FFI is a product that is created during the preparation and separation process (Huber et al., Njoroge et al., 1988).

Aminoketoses are converted more or less quickly to the deoxyosones 5 (Anet, Kato, 1960) and 6 (Beck et al., 1988) depending on the conditions of the reaction. The very reactive deoxyosones are then formed from the reactive reducing sugar with amino ketoses as intermediates. There is no bondage between the amine and the deoxyosones of type 5 and 6. This could be important for

the Maillard reaction in mammals, because a meta-
bolisation and/or removal of deoxyosones is conceivable, before a new reaction with amine groups
of the lysine side chains takes place. The aminoketoses of disaccharides are transformed in the
same way (Beck, 1988). A glucosyl or galactosyl
group is bonded over the oxygen atom on C4 of the
sugar chain, depending on whether maltose or lactose is taking part. In addition with the disaccharides it is evident that their aminoketoses are
also converted to 1-amino-1,4-dideoxyosones of
structure 7 (Beck, 1988). However, there is still
no proof of this degradation path in the case of
monosaccharides, which could be of interest for
in-vivo reactions.

Amines can also accelerate the transformation
of sugars in the pH range of 4-7 without aminoketoses being formed. Besides the conversion to
deoxyosones of structure 5 there is observed the
formation of the deoxyosone 8, accompanied by isomerisation of the aldose to a ketose, which can
produce the 2-aminoaldose 9 under amine attack.
2-Aminoaldoses are not very stable and rearrange
into aminoketoses amongst others (Heyns et al.,
1967). There are indications that aminoaldoses are
formed in vivo (Walton et al., 1988).

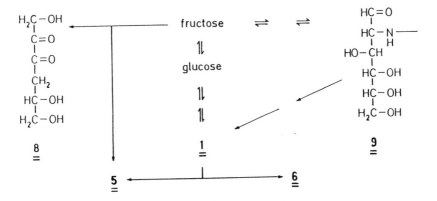

Deoxyosones are important intermediate products of the Maillard reaction. Ring formation,
enolisation, dehydration and condensations and
C-C fission reactions lead to numerous more or less

characteristic compounds.

DEGRADATION OF THE 3-DEOXYOSONES

Cyclisation of the 3-deoxyosone 5 and dehydration lead to the hydroxymethylfurfural 10
(Hodge, 1955), in the presence of primary amines
the formation of 10 is suppressed in favour of the
pyrrolaldehyde 11 (Jurch and Tatum, 1970) and of
the pyridiniumbetaine 12 (Pachmayr et al., 1985).

Proteins react with the $\mathcal{E}$-amino groups of the
lysine side chains to the appropriate product.
After heating a protein in the presence of glucose
one finds, for example, after dialysis and hydrolysis the pyrrole derivative 11a in the HPLC chromatogram   between the amino acids phenylalanine and

tryptophane if the hydrolysate is eluted over a reversed phase column with triethylammonium form-ate (Sengl, 1988). From the structures of the di-merisation products 13 and 14 it is revealed that secondary reactions can easily occur via the hy-droxymethyl group in the pyrroles of type 11 (Olsson et al., 1977), which can lead to cross-linkages in proteins.

The structures of the pyrroles 15 and 16 in-dicate that 3-deoxyosones take part in the forma-tion of these compounds (Njoroge et al., 1987, Farmar et al., 1988, Severin und Krönig, 1973). The mobility of the hydroxyl groups in the vicinity of the pyrrol ring can easily cause secondary re-actions in the substances 15 and 16. In reaction mixtures of glucose and fructose with primary ami-nes one finds after periodate treatment the expec-

ted formylpyrroles 19 and 20 and also the substances 17 and 18, an indication that other condensation reactions take place with the participation of deoxyosones (Krönig, 1974).

3-Deoxyosones possess a reactive methylene
group and condensation reactions with carbonyl
compounds can be observed. As an example is indicated the yellow ß-pyranone 21, whose isolation is
achieved after stabilisation of the semi-acetal
function. In aqueous systems rearrangement and
further condensation lead to furanone 22 (Ledl et
al., 1983).

The degradation of 3-deoxyosones in the presence of secondary amines naturally does not proceed as with the primary amines. The formation of
carbocyclic compounds is observed to a large degree. Both in the structure of the maltoxazine 23
(Tressl et al., 1982), an ingredient of beer, and
in that of the coloured pentose product 24 (Ledl
et al., 1983) the cyclopentenone ring could be derived from the 3-deoxyosone.

The formation of the metasaccharinic acid lactone 25 from the 3-deoxyosone will not be dealt with further here. There are results that a reaction comparable to the benzilic acid rearrangement does not happen (Beck, 1988). It is interesting that the lactone 26 is created likewise from the 3-deoxyosone (Sengl, 1988). Lactone 26 and formaldehyde can be produced via an α-diketo cleavage. Further experiments will have to be carried out in order to achieve clarity on this type of reaction.

If amino acids are involved in the Maillard reaction the Strecker degradation with the 3-deoxyosones leads to the formation of the pyrrole 27 and of the pyridine 28 (Nyhammar et al., 1983). It has not yet been fully clarified whether with aliphatic amines, for example those of the lysine side chain, as with the decarboxylation of amino acids, there is the splitting off of a proton forming a formyl group (Namiki et al., 1986).

DEGRADATION OF 1-DEOXYOSONES

A whole series of characteristic Maillard products is formed from 1-deoxyosones. Cyclisation and water elimination lead to the hydroxyfuranones of type 29. The pentose product 29a (Severin and Seilmeier, 1967), and above all the 5-methylpentose compound 29b (Hodge et al., 1963), are important flavour substances, or react to form interesting sulphur-containing aroma compounds (Ouweland and Peer, 1975). 29a participates in the browning of pentoses; compound 24 is the extractable main product from the reaction with secondary amines (Ledl et al., 1983) and in the presence of primary amines the condensation product 30 is produced (Krönig and Severin, 1973). In addition to the cyclisation to the hydroxyfuranone 29c (Hiebl et al., 1987) the formation of a 6-ring compound is

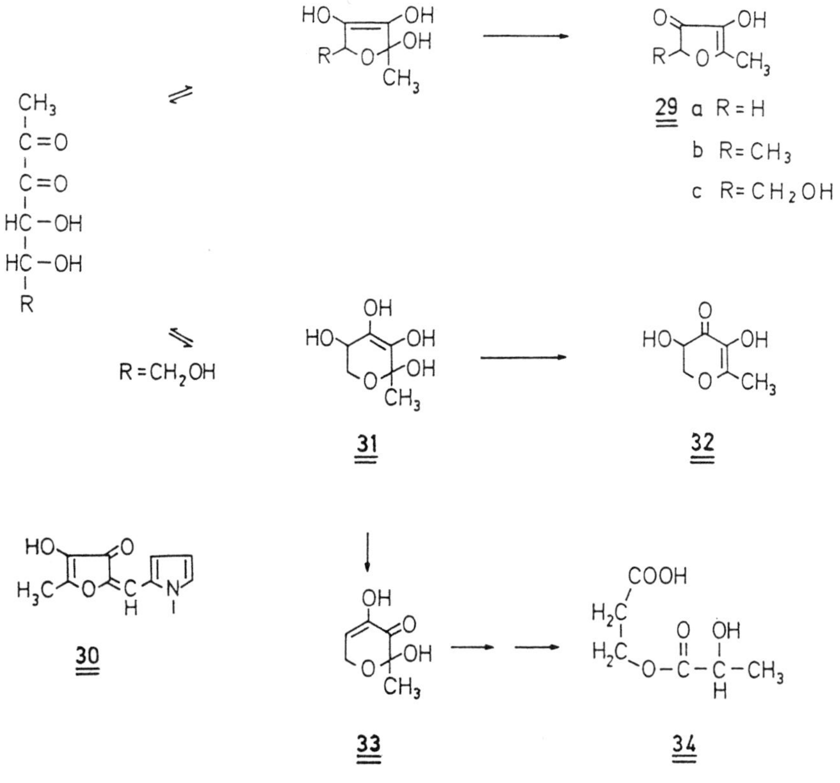

29 a R = H
b R = CH₃
c R = CH₂OH

31

32

30

33

34

possible with hexoses. The dihydropyranone 32
(Severin and Seilmeier, 1968, Mills et al., 1970)
can be found in just about all heated foodstuffs
(Ledl et al., 1976, Ledl, 1987). The gas chromatographic determination of 32 can be easily performed and therefore this compound is very suitable for proving a Maillard reaction in foodstuffs.
The significance of 32 during the in-vivo reaction of glucose and proteins is difficult to estimate. 32 reacts with amines only under somewhat
more drastic conditions.

The elimination of water from the endiol 31
causes not only the dihydropyranone 32, the ß-
pyranone 33 is also formed. This substance is moreover not stable, by a rearrangement the ester 34
is obtained (Sengl, 1988), after its hydrolysis
lactic acid and ß-hydroxypropionic acid are detectable. The isomerisation of 31 to the ketone 35
leads firstly to ß-diketo cleavages forming C3 and
C4 products (Mills et al., 1970, Ledl and Severin,
1979), or acetic acid and glyceric acid, and secondly water elimination produces the hydroxyfuranone 37 (Hodge et al., 1963), which can exist
in various tautomeric forms.

The isomeric compounds 29c, 32 and 37 are still not stable end products. Substance 37 is very easily involved in secondary reactions with primary and secondary amines, followed by furanone 29c. With secondary amines one obtains the so-called aminohexose reductones of type 36 (Weygand et al., 1958). The primary amines replace in the hydroxyfuranone 37 the ring oxygen with formation of the pyrrolinone reductones of type 38 (Ledl and Fritsch, 1984). The pyrrolinones possess anti-oxidative and fluorescent properties and dimerize easily. This makes them very interesting as possible decomposition products in the Maillard reaction in mammals, because one sometimes observes here a strong fluorescence with the proteins in question. Disaccharides are also broken down to amino reductones of the structures 36 and 38, while the glucosyl or galactosyl group is bonded by the enolic oxygen (Ledl, 1984).

From reaction mixtures of proline and sugars, a number of substances can be isolated, which can be associated with various classes of structures. An important role in product formation could be the stabilisation of the pyrrolinium cation 39 created after the Strecker degradation of the proline. Reduction, proton elimination, ring opening, ring extension and nucleophilic additions lead among others to the substances 40 - 44 with different ring shapes (Tressl et al., 1986). Compound 40 (Pabst et al., 1985) and also the bitter substance 41 (Pabst et al., 1984) derived from a roasted mixture of proline and sugars, can be assigned as 1-deoxyosone products.

The degradation of 1-deoxyosones from disaccharides is partly different from that of the monosaccharides. Thus, the endiol 45 cannot produce the dihydropyranone 32, the splitting of the hydroxyl group on the C5 atom leads to the ß-pyranone 46, a reactive intermediate product (Ledl et al., 1986). After ring contraction and water elimination the galactosyl (Hodge and Nelson, 1961) or glucosylisomaltol 48 (Goodwin, 1983) is obtained. The formation of maltol 49 with pyrylium compounds as intermediates is conceivable. In the presence of primary amines the pyridinium betaine 47 can be isolated (Ledl et al., 1988) , which easily rearranges to form the pyridone 50 (Severin and Loidl, 1976). The compound 50 is also accessible from maltol 48 or the isomaltol derivatives 48. The interaction of the ß-pyranone 46 with secondary amines leads to the substances 51 and 52, among others.

In the case of 1-deoxyosones it may be possible for the α-diketo cleavage to take place, just like the 3-deoxyosones. The proof of the erythronic acid lactone 53 would indicate this (Sengl,

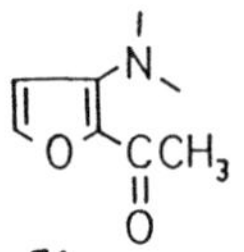

51 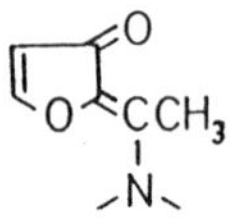   **52** 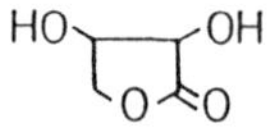   **53**

1988). It is still not certain whether the formation of acetic acid amides can likewise be explained by the same reaction type (Hayase and Kato, 1985).

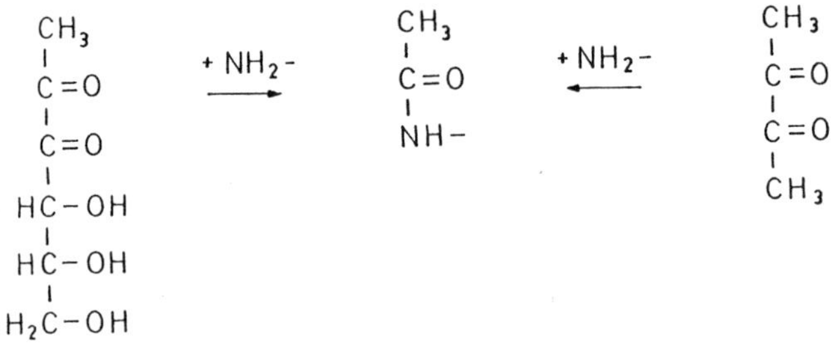

The activated methyl group causes the 1-de-
oxyosones to condense with carbonyl compounds and
thus producing the formation of the coloured products 54 and 55 (Ledl and Severin, 1982). The extractable coloured main product from the reaction
mixture of hexose with secondary amines has the
structure 56 (Ledl et al., 1983). The formation
path has not yet been fully clarified, possible is
a retroaldol reaction of 29c with splitting of

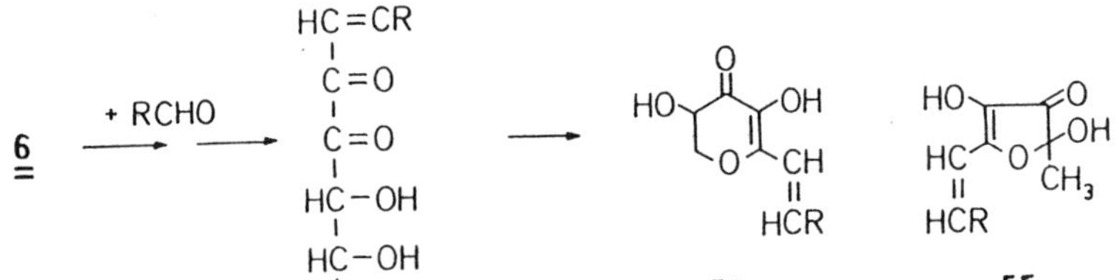

54   **55**

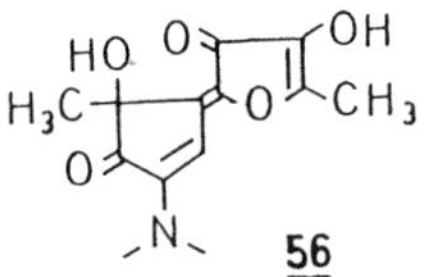

56

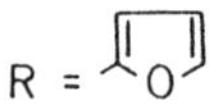

$R = $

formaldehyde, in which case the condensation with the aminocyclopentenone results in the compound 56.

DEGRADATION OF 4-DEOXYOSONES

The hydroxyacetylfuran 57 is taken to be the decomposition product of the 4-deoxyosone of type 8. In the presence of primary amines the formation of the furan can be completely suppressed and then the corresponding pyrrole 58 (Jurch and Tatum, 1970), or the pyridinium betaine 59 (Pachmayr et al., 1985) are obtained.

There is still very little known about the 1-amino-1,4-dideoxyosones of structure 7 and their significance for the Maillard reaction. The furane 60 can be separated as a secondary product from reaction mixtures of disaccharides with secondary amines (Beck et al., 1988). The stability of this compound is pH dependent. There is still no proof about the formation of the corresponding furane with primary amines. It is known, for example, that furanes of the type 60 easily rearrange to FFI 4 in the presence of ammonia.

CONCLUSION

The term Maillard reaction includes a number of sugar degradation reactions with participation of amines. Maillard products are absorbed daily in more or less large quantities in food, and they influence the functionality of proteins having a higher biological half-life in the mammalian organism. It is therefore of great interest to know as much as possible of the structures and properties of such compounds. Although we already know of some reaction pathways, this however is just the top of the iceberg, and the Maillard reaction still remains a challenge to medicine and the food chemistry.

REFERENCES

Ahmed MU, Thorpe SR, Baynes J (1985). Identification of N-carboxymethyllysine, a modified amino acid formed by decomposition of fructoselysine in glycated proteins. Fed Proc 44:1621.

Anet EFLJ (1960). Degradation of carbohydrates I. Isolation of 3-deoxyosones. Aust J Chem 13:396-403.

Baynes JW, Ahmed MU, Fisher CI, Hull CJ, Lehmann TA, Watkins NG, Thorpe SR (1986). Studies on glycation of proteins and Maillard reaction of glycated proteins under physiological conditions. In Fujimaki M, Namiki M, Kato H (eds): "Amino-carbonyl reactions in food and biological systems," Tokyo, Amsterdam, Oxford, New York, Toronto: Kodansha Elsevier, pp 421-431 and literature cited herein.

Beck J (1988). Untersuchungen zur Anfangsphase des aminkatalysierten Zuckerabbaus. Dissertation University of Munich.

Beck J, Ledl F, Severin T (1988). Formation of 1-deoxy-D-erythro-2,3-hexodiulose from Amadori compounds. Carbohydr Res 178:240-243.

Beck J, Ledl F, Severin T (1988). Formation of glucosyl-deoxyosones from Amadori compounds of maltose. Z Lebensm Unters Forsch 187: in press.

Boissel JP, Kasper T, Bunn HF (1986). Protein crosslinking during in vitro non-enzymatic glycation. In see Baynes et al., 1986, pp 433-438 and literature cited herein.

Ciner-Doruk M, Eichner K (1979). Bildung und Stabilität von Amadori-Verbindungen in wasserarmen Lebensmitteln. Z Lebensm Unters Forsch 168:9-20 and literature cited herein.

Farmar JG, Ulrich PC, Cerami A (1988). Novel

pyrroles from sulfite-inhibited Maillard reactions: Insight into the mechanism of inhibition. J Org Chem 53:2346-2349.

Goodwin JC (1983). Isolation of 3-O-α-D-gluco- and 3-O-ß-D-galacto-pyranosyloxy-2-furyl methyl ketones form nonenzymic browning of maltose and lactose with secondary amino acids. Carbohydr Res 115:281-287.

Hayase F, Kato H (1985). Maillard reaction products from D-glucose and butylamine. Agric Biol Chem 49:467-473.

Hayashi T, Namiki M (1986). Role of sugar fragmentation in the Maillard reaction. In see Baynes et al, 1986, pp 29-38.

Heyns K, Müller G, Paulsen H (1967). Quantitative Untersuchungen der Reaktionen von Hexosen mit Aminosäuren. Ann 703:202-214.

Hiebl J, Ledl F, Severin T (1987). Isolation of a 4-hydroxy-2-(hydroxymethyl)-5-methyl-3(2H)-furanone from sugar amino acid reaction mixtures. J Agric Food Chem 35:990-993.

Hodge JE (1955). The Amadori rearrangement. Advances in Carbohydrate Chem 10:169-205.

Hodge JE, Nelson EC (1961). Preparation and properties of galactosylisomaltol and isomaltol. Cereal Chem 38:207-221.

Hodge JE, Fisher BE, Nelson EC (1963). Dicarbonyls, reductones and heterocyclics produced by reaction of reducing sugars with secondary amine salts. Proc Am Soc Brew Chem 84-85.

Huber B, Ledl F, Severin T, Stangl A, Pfleiderer G (1988). Formation of 2-(2-furoyl)-4(5)-(2-furyl)-1H-imidazole in the Maillard reaction. Carbohydr Res 181: in press.

Jurch GR, Tatum JH (1970). Degradation of D-glucose with acetic acid and methylamine. Carbohydr Res 15:233-239.

Kato H (1960). Studies on browning reactions between sugars and amino acids. V. Isolation and characterisation of new carbonyl compounds, 3-deoxyosones formed from N-glycosides and their significance for browning reaction. Bull Agr Chem Soc Japan 24:1-12.

Krönig U (1974). Umsetzung von reduzierenden Zuckern mit Alkylaminen als Beitrag zur Kenntnis der Maillard-Reaktion. Dissertation University of Munich.

Krönig U, Severin T (1973). Formation of pyrrole derivatives from pentoses and alkylammonium salts. Chem Mikrobiol Technol Lebensm 2:49-51.

Ledl F (1984). Formation of amino reductones from disaccharides. Z Lebensm Unters Forsch 179: 381-384.

Ledl F (1987). Analytik flüchtiger Zuckerabbau-produkte. Lebensmittelchem Gerichtl Chem 41: 83-87.

Ledl F, Severin T (1979). Formation of aminore-ductones from glucose and primary amines. Z Lebensm Unters Forsch 169:173-175.

Ledl F, Severin T (1982). Formation of coloured compounds from hexoses. Z Lebensm Unters Forsch 175:262-265.

Ledl F, Fritsch G (1984). Formation of pyrroli-none reductones by heating hexoses with amino acids. Z Lebensm Unters Forsch 178:41-44.

Ledl F, Schnell W, Severin T (1976). Proof of 2,3-dihydro-3,5-dihydroxy-6-methyl-4H-pyran-4-one in foods. Z Lebensm Unters Forsch 160: 367-370.

Ledl F, Hiebl J, Severin T (1983). Formation of coloured ß-pyranones from hexoses and pentoses. Z Lebensm Unters Forsch 177:353-355.

Ledl F, Ellrich G, Klostermeyer H (1986). Proof and identification of a new Maillard compound in heated milk. Z Lebensm Unters Forsch 182: 19-24.

Ledl F, Krönig U, Severin T, Lotter H (1983). Isolation of N-containing coloured products. Z Lebensm Unters Forsch 177:267-270

Ledl F, Osiander H, Pachmayr O, Severin T (1988). Formation of maltosine, a product of the Maillard reaction with a pyridone structure. Z Lebensm Unters Forsch 187: in press.

Mauron J (1981). The Maillard reaction in food, a critical review from the nutritional stand-point. In Eriksson C (ed): "Maillard reactions in food," Oxford, New York, Paris, Toronto, Frankfurt, Sydney: Pergamon Press pp 5-35.

Mills FD, Baker BG, Hodge JE (1970). Thermal de-gradation of 1-deoxy-1-piperidino-D-fructose. Carbohydr Res 15:205-213.

Mills FD, Weisleder D, Hodge JE (1970). 2,3-Dihydro-3,5-dihydroxy-6-methyl-4H-pyran-4-one, a novel nonenzymatic browning product. Tetrahedron Lett 1243-1246.

Monnier VM (1986). The paradoxical effects of the Maillard reaction in vivo: Impaired maturation and accelerated aging of collagen. In see Baynes et al., 1986, pp 459-474 and literature cited herein.

Namiki M, Terao A, Ueda S, Hayashi T (1986). Deamination of lysine in protein by reaction with oxidized ascorbic acid or active carbonyl compounds produced by Maillard reaction. In see Baynes et al., 1986, pp 105-114.

Njoroge FG, Sayre LM, Monnier VM (1987). Detection of D-glucose-derived pyrrole compounds during Maillard reaction under physiological conditions. Carbohydr Res 167:211-220.

Njoroge FG, Fernandes AA, Monnier VM (1988). Mechanism of formation of the putative advanced glycosilation endproduct and protein crosslink 2-(2-furoyl)-4(5)-(2-furanyl)-1H-imidazole (FFI). Pers. Com.

Nyhammar T, Olsson K, Pernemalm PA (1983). On the formation of 2-acylpyrroles and 3-pyridinols in the Maillard reaction through Strecker degradation. Acta Chem Scand B 37:879-889.

Olsson K, Pernemalm PA, Popoff T, Theander O (1977). Reaction of D-glucose and methylamine in slightly acidic, aqueous solution. Acta Chem Scand B 31:469-474.

Ouweland GAM, Peer HG (1975). Components contributing to beef flavour: Volatile compounds produced by the reaction of 4-hydroxy-5-methyl-3(2H)-furanone and its thio analogue with hydrogen sulfide. J Agric Food Chem 23:501-505.

Pabst HME, Ledl F, Belitz H-D (1984). Bitter compounds obtained by heating proline and sucrose. Z Lebensm Unters Forsch 178:356-360.

Pabst HME, Ledl F, Belitz H-D (1985). Bitter compounds obtained by heating sucrose, maltose and proline. Z Lebensm Unters Forsch 181:386-390.

Pachmayr O, Ledl F, Severin T (1985). Formation of 1-alkyl-3-oxypyridiniumbetaines from sugars. Z Lebensm Unters Forsch 182:294-297.

Paulsen H, Pflughaupt KW (1980). Glycosylamines. In Pigman W, Horton D (eds): "Carbohydrates IB,"

New York, London, Toronto, Sydney, San Francisco: Academic press, pp 881-927.

Pongor S, Ulrich PC, Bencsath FA, Cerami A (1984). Aging of proteins: Isolation and identification of a fluorescent chromophore from the reaction of polypeptides with glucose. Proc Natl Acad Sci USA 81:1684-1688.

Sengl M (1988). Identifizierung niedermolekularer, polarer Zuckerumwandlungsprodukte sowie Nachweis eines proteingebundenen Produkts aus der Spätphase der Maillard-Reaktion. Dissertation University of Munich.

Severin T, Seilmeier W (1967). Umwandlung von Pentosen unter dem Einfluß von Aminacetaten. Z Lebensm Unters Forsch 134:230-232.

Severin T, Seilmeier W (1968). Umwandlung von Glucose unter dem Einfluß von Methylammoniumacetat. Z Lebensm Forsch 137:4-6.

Severin T, Krönig U (1973). Condensation of xylose with methylammoniumacetate. Z Lebensm Unters Forsch 152:42-46.

Severin T, Loidl A (1976). Formation of pyridone derivatives from maltose and lactose. Z Lebensm Unters Forsch 161:119-124.

Tressl R, Helak B, Rewicki D (1982). Malzoxazin, eine tricyclische Verbindung aus Gerstenmalz. Helv Chim Acta 65:483-489.

Tressl R, Helak B, Martin N, Rewicki D (1986). Formation of proline specific Maillard products. In see Baynes et al., 1986, pp 235-244.

Walton DJ, McPherson JD, Shilton BH (1988). Evidence for nonenzymatic fructosylation of human ocular lens proteins in vivo. XIVth International Carbohydrate Symposium, Stockholm, Sweden.

Weygand F, Simon H, Bitterlich W, Hodge JE, Fisher BE (1958). Structure of piperidinohexose-reductone. Tetrahedron 6:123-138.

The Maillard Reaction in Aging,
Diabetes, and Nutrition, pages 43–67
© 1989 Alan R. Liss, Inc.

THE AMADORI PRODUCT ON PROTEIN: STRUCTURE AND REACTIONS

John W. Baynes. Nancy G. Watkins, Carolyn I. Fisher,
Clifford J. Hull, Jeffrey S. Patrick, Mahtab U.
Ahmed, John A. Dunn and Suzanne R.Thorpe.

Department of Chemistry and School of Medicine
University of South Carolina, Columbia, SC 29208

ABSTRACT. The Amadori Rearrangement Product is
the first stable adduct formed during glycation
(nonenzymatic glycosylation) of protein. This
review deals with the structure of the Amadori
adduct on protein, factors affecting the kinetics
and specificity of glycation of protein, measurements of the extent of glycation of proteins *in
vivo*, and the possible significance of glycation
itself, versus post-glycation reactions, in the
development of pathophysiology in diabetes.

STRUCTURE OF THE AMADORI PRODUCT ON PROTEIN

After the initial formation of a labile Schiff base
between reducing sugar and amino groups on protein, the
Amadori Rearrangement yields a stable, ketoamine adduct to
the protein. The Amadori adduct is stabilized by equili-
bration of the linear ketoamine structure into several
cyclic, hemiketal conformations in solution (Neglia et al.
1983, 1985). As shown in Fig. 1, the conformational
distribution for the Amadori compound formed between
glucose and amino groups in the protein, RNase, is similar
to the distribution observed for the model compound, N^{α}-
formyl-N^{ε}-fructoselysine (fFL). Although the chemical
shift of the anomeric carbon of the Amadori adduct is
affected by the pK_a of the amino group, the conformation
of the sugar does not appear to be sensitive to the pK_a of
the amino group or the local environment of the protein

since the anomeric distributions are similar at each of
the different types of amino groups in RNase. The
similarity in conformations of the model compound and
Amadori adducts on protein infers similar reactivity,
although reactions on protein would be affected by
adjacent functional groups either within the protein
molecule or accessible via intermolecular reactions.

EFFECT OF PROTEIN STRUCTURE ON SPECIFICITY OF GLYCATION

That some amino groups in protein are more reactive
with glucose than others has been recognized since the
original reports that glucose reacted primarily with the
β-chain terminal valine residues of HbA$_{Ic}$. The NMR
spectrum in Fig. 1B indicates that not all amino groups in
RNase are equally reactive with glucose, i.e., N^α-Lys-1 and
N^ϵ-Lys-41 are more reactive than the average peripheral
lysine residue in the protein. Table 1 lists a number of
factors which are known or are likely to affect the site
specificity of glycation of proteins.

The low pK_a α-amino group of proteins, by virtue of
its greater nucleophilicity, should be the most reactive
site for the initial formation of Schiff base adducts, but
other factors appear to be more important in determining
the eventual distribution of Amadori adducts on protein.
Thus, the α- and β-chain terminal valine residues of hemoglobin (Hb) have similar pK_as, while the observed ratio of
β- to α-chain valine glycation of Hb *in vivo* is about 10
(Shapiro et al., 1980). Similarly, RNase and lysozyme
(LZM) have amino-terminal lysine residues with similar
pK_as, however, compared to RNase, the α-amino group of LZM
is relatively unreactive toward glycation (Hull, 1986).
The relative reactivity of the α- and ϵ-amino groups of
Lys-1 also varies from 3:2 in RNase (Watkins et al., 1985)
to 1:4 in LZM (Hull, 1986). One possible explanation for
this difference is the involvement of the α-amino group in
LZM in a hydrogen bond to Thr-40, which partially shields
this functional group from solvent. Another factor to
consider is the specific reactivity of different amino
groups in each of the two steps of the glycation process,
i.e., forming the Schiff base and undergoing the Amadori
rearrangement. For example, while the α-amino group of
RNase accounts for about 70% of the Schiff base adduct
formed on the protein in 0.2 M phosphate buffer at pH 7.4,

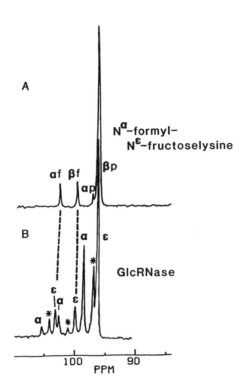

Figure 1.(A) ^{13}C-NMR spectrum of the anomeric region of
the Amadori compound, N^{α}-formyl-N^{ε}-fructoselysine (fFL).
The spectrum was acquired in 0.2 M phosphate buffer, pH
7.4. Resonances are assigned to the α- and β-furanose and
β-pryanose conformers.
(B) ^{13}C-NMR spectrum of the anomeric region of Amadori
adducts to RNase. RNase was glycated with [2-^{13}C]glucose
(1 mol Glc/mol RNase) to label the anomeric carbon of the
Amadori adduct. The complex spectrum was interpreted as
the sum of three sets of resonances, i.e., Amadori adducts
to ε-amino groups of peripheral lysine residues, $pK_a \sim 10.5$
(ε), the ε-amino group of active site Lys-41, $pK_a \sim 8.8$ (*) and
the α-amino group of Lys-1, $pK_a \sim 7.5$ (α). In each set, three
resonances are observed in approximately the same
distribution as seen in fFL (Neglia et al., 1985).

TABLE 1. Factors Affecting Kinetics and Sites of Glycation
          of Protein

---

1. General Structural Effects
    - pK$_a$ of amino group
    - vicinal side-chain functional groups

2. Ligand Binding Sites
    - binding sites for buffer ions
        - phosphate, bicarbonate
    - allosteric and active sites
        - diphosphoglycerate
        - phosphorlyated intermediates
    - binding sites for other anionic ligands
        - glycosoaminoglycans
        - fatty acids
    - others ligands ?
        - cationic ligands
        - pharmacological agents

3. Long Range Interactions
    - ligand-induced allosteric effects
    - salt bridges and hydrogen bonding

---

it accounts for less than 20% of the final distribution of
Amadori adducts to the protein (Watkins et al., 1985). To
account for the difference between the initial distribution of Schiff base and the final distribution of Amadori
adducts to Lys-1 of RNase, the rate of the Amadori
rearrangement at the ε-amino group must be about 4 times
that at the α-amino group. Similar differences were
observed in the reactivities of other amino groups in
RNase, with a range of at least 10-fold in the rate of the
Amadori rearrangement at the ε-amino groups of different
lysine residues. Thus, the distribution of Amadori
adducts on a protein is determined by both the equilibrium
distribution of Schiff base adducts, as well as the
specific rate of the Amadori rearrangement at each site.

Vicinal acidic or basic amino acid residues are known
to modulate the reactivity of lysine residues in protein
with glucose. Thus, in studies on the glycation of lysine
residues in Hb, Bunn and colleagues (Bunn et al., 1979;

Shapiro et al., 1980) noted that the more reactive lysines in Hb were located adjacent to acidic amino acids in the primary or three-dimensional structure of the protein. This suggested that properly oriented, vicinal carboxylate groups might catalyze the Amadori rearrangement on specific lysine residues. Watkins et al. (1985,1987) later observed that two of the reactive amino group in RNase, Lys-1 and Lys-37, were also located adjacent to acidic amino acids in its primary sequence. Lysines in Lys-Lys sequences also appear to be favored sites for glycation of protein, based on studies with Hb (Shapiro et al., 1980), human albumin (HSA) (Garlick and Mazer, 1983) and LZM (Hull, 1986). This observation was extended by Iberg and Fluckiger (1987) who noted that reactive lysine residues in albumin were located in Lys-Lys, Lys-His, Lys-Lys-Lys and Lys-His-Lys sequences, or were near disulfide bridges which could place lysine amino groups in apposition to other functional groups at a distance in the primary structure of the protein. They proposed that local acid-base catalysis of the Amadori rearrangement by vicinal histidine and lysine residues was a major determinant of the specificity of glycation of proteins.

EFFECT OF BUFFERING IONS AND BOUND LIGANDS ON THE KINETICS AND SPECIFICITY OF GLYCATION OF PROTEIN

Watkins et al. (1987) observed that the rates of both glycation and inactivation of RNase by glucose were more rapid in phosphate than in organic amine buffers, such as TAPSO and MOPS. Further studies showed that the kinetics of modification of RNase were dependent on the phosphate concentration in the buffer and that the specificity of modification of RNase was significantly different in phosphate versus TAPSO buffer. The enchanced inactivation of RNase in phosphate was the result of phosphate-dependent catalysis of glycation of lysine residues in or near the active site of RNase, particularly the active site lysine, Lys-41. Similar kinetic enhancements were observed with arsenate and bicarbonate (Table 2), suggesting a general effect of anionic buffers on both the kinetics and sites of glycation of proteins. Further, the phosphate effect was not limited to RNase since, compared to TAPSO, phosphate also stimulated the rate of glycation of cytochrome c, HSA, LZM and Hb (Watkins et al., 1987). The sites of glycation of LZM were also different in phosphate,

TABLE 2. Effect of Buffers on Kinetics of Glycation of
RNase

Buffer	mol Glc/mol RNase[*]
Expt. 1	
0.2 M TAPSO	0.33
0.2 M Phosphate	1.02
0.2 M TAPSO + 0.2 M Phosphate	1.01
0.2 M TAPSO + 0.2 M Arsenate	1.56
0.2 M TAPSO + 0.2 M NaCl	0.29
Expt. 2	
0.2 M TAPSO	0.40
Ham's F-10 Medium (14 mM HCO_3^-, 2 mM P_i)	0.58
Ham's F-10 + 0.2 M Phosphate	1.41
Ham's F-10 + 0.2 M Bicarbonate	1.46

[*]RNase (25 mg/ml) was incubated with 0.4 M [6-^{3}H] glucose
(0.25 Ci/mol) at pH 7.4 for 3 days at 37°C. Schiff base
adducts were discharged in acid (Bissé et al., 1982), and
incorporation of glucose was estimated from the specific
radioactivity of the protein (Watkins et al., 1987).

compared to TAPSO buffer. The overall effect of phosphate
on glycation of LZM was to enhance the reactivity of all
amino groups in the protein, but rate enhancements by
phosphate varied by as much as 5-fold among the different
amino groups (Hull, 1986).

The biological significance of these observations with
RNase and LZM was evaluated in studies on the effect of
phosphate on the specificity of glycation of Hb. As with
RNase, the rate of glycation of Hb was ~2-fold greater in
phosphate than in TAPSO buffer (Watkins et al., 1987). In
0.2 M TAPSO, however, glycation of amino terminal valine
residues was hardly detectable, the ratio of valine:lysine
glycation in the protein being ≤1:16. This ratio was
increased to 1:8 in 0.2 M phosphate and 1:5 in 0.2 M TAPSO
containing 10 mM 2,3-diphosphoglycerate (DPG) (Watkins et
al., 1987). The latter ratio approaches the 1:3 ratio
observed with Hb glycated *in vivo* (Bunn et al., 1979). The
remaining difference between glycation *in vitro* and *in vivo* may

result from effects of oxygen saturation or other environmental variables which cannot be duplicated in the *in vitro* incubations. These effects of phosphate and DPG on glycation of Hb provide a reasonable explanation for differences in glycation of lysine residues in Hb *in vivo* vs. *in vitro* (Shapiro et al., 1980), i.e., they probably result from differences between the *in vitro* buffer system and the *milieu interieur* of the erythrocyte. Others have also shown that the kinetics of formation of HbA$_{Ic}$ in erythrocytes is affected by physiologically relevant changes in the concentration of DPG and partial pressure of O$_2$ and CO$_2$, as well as pH (Smith et al., 1982; Lowrey et al., 1985). These ligands may also affect the specificity of glycation of lysine residues in Hb *in vivo*.

Similarities between the active site of RNase and the allosteric site of Hb, suggest that in both cases the catalytic effect of the phosphate or organic phosphates is mediated by binding of the buffer anion or ligand to a cationic pocket, formed by an array of basic amino acid residues in the protein (Watkins et al., 1987). The bound phosphate then exerts local catalysis of the Amadori rearrangement on active and allosteric site lysine residues. These observations suggest that the preferential glycation of lysine residues in basic sequences or regions of other proteins, including HSA (Iberg and Fluckiger, 1986), may be determined by the binding of buffering species, rather than by direct catalysis by the functional groups of vicinal basic amino acid residues. Certainly, the available data indicate that biological buffers (phosphate and bicarbonate) and endogenous ligands can exert significant effects on the rate and specificity of glycation of proteins *in vivo*. The possibility that other types of ligands, such as phosphorylated metabolic intermediates, fatty acids and glycosaminoglycans (Table 1) may also influence the pattern of glycation of proteins remains to be explored in greater detail. With different proteins the ligands may serve either to protect or enhance the rate of glycation of specific lysine residues.

CAUTIONS REGARDING GLYCATION OF PROTEINS *IN VITRO*

From the above discussion, it is apparent that rates and sites of glycation of proteins measured *in vitro* may vary greatly among laboratories because of differences in

buffer species and concentration. Under these circumstances, it cannot be assumed that proteins glycated *in vitro*
are equivalent to naturally glycated proteins. Ideally,
experiments *in vitro* should be carried out in the appropriate
physiological milieu with all its component metabolites,
as opposed to the commonly used physiological buffers,
bicarbonate or phosphate-buffered saline. Because of the
inconvenience of maintaining a partial pressure of CO_2
over the reaction mixture, the bicarbonate system has been
rarely used in studies on glycation of protein. Phosphate-
buffered saline is most commonly used, but in dilute
concentration, 10-25 mM phosphate, the buffering power is
often inadequate to maintain pH in concentrated glucose-
protein reaction systems. Thus, many researchers have
used 0.2-0.5 M phosphate buffer to maintain pH control.
In these instances the high phosphate concentration
undoubtedly affects the rate and pattern of glycation of
the protein under study. A more suitable experimental
design might be to use dilute protein solutions in 10-20
mM phosphate buffer, which approximates the total bicarbonate and phosphate concentration *in vivo*. In critical
studies on the effects of glycation on protein structure
and function, it is obviously important to establish that
the sites of modification of the protein *in vitro* are
equivalent to those modified *in vivo*.

Table 3 summarizes a number of factors which must be
considered in experiments on the effects of glycation on
protein structure and function. Foremost among these is
the need to focus on effects of glycation to extents which
are likely to be attained *in vivo*. Parallel control experiments with polyols (sorbitol) are also essential to
exclude artifacts such as proteolysis and aggregation of
the protein during prolonged incubation. A polyol rather
than a buffer control is especially important when high
concentrations of sugar are used since hydrogen bonding
interactions with the sugar may affect the stability of
the protein during prolonged incubation. These controls
notwithstanding, it is still possible that damaging
effects of glucose may not be the result of glycation
alone. Thus, glucose, especially in phosphate and
bicarbonate salts containing a trace of metal ions and
exposed to air, can initiate oxidative, free radical
damage to the protein independent of (or subsequent to)
glycation. This oxidative damage can be detected by
analysis for carboxymethyllysine (CML) formed on oxidation

TABLE 3. Design and Evaluation of *in vitro* Experiments on Glycation of Protein

---

1. Selection of Glycation Reaction Conditions
   - maintenance of physiological pH
   - choice of buffer and concentration
   - inhibition (or assessment) of oxidative damage

2. Control Experiments
   - parallel incubation with polyol
   - measurement of proteolysis and aggregation
   - comparative analysis of sites of glycation
     of the protein *in vitro* and *in vivo*

3. Interpreting Effects of Glycation of Protein
   - (patho)physiological levels of glycation
   - kinetic analysis to distinguish
     - effects of glycation vs. browning
     - effects of labile vs. stable glycation
   - relevance to pathophysiology
   - reserve capacity of physiological system

---

of the Amadori adduct to lysine residues (Ahmed et al., 1986, 1988). The appearance of CML provides evidence of exposure of the protein to oxidative stress and this may compromise the interpretation of experiments since it may not be possible to distinguish effects of glycation versus oxidation of the protein. This may be a more serious problem with lipoproteins since glucose may also induce oxidation of lipids, formation of lipid peroxides and malondialdehyde and then a cascade of chemical modifications of the protein not directly dependent on glucose. Recent work of Wolff and Dean (1987) and Hicks et al. (1988) suggests that the Amadori adduct itself may also catalyze oxidative modifications of proteins and associated lipids, however, the physiological significance of these oxidative reactions, compared to direct effects of glycation, is not known. To control the oxidation reactions, experiments can be conducted under nitrogen using chelex-treated buffers with a trace of a strong redox metal chelator, such as diethylenetriaminepenta-acetic acid (DTPA, DETAPAC). Finally, even with these precautions, the interpretation of experiments on the effects of glycation may be compromised by the occurrence of browning reactions during the course of the glycation reactions, particularly during prolonged incubations. Thus, the kinetics of changes in the properties of the protein should be compared with the kinetics of glycation and development of Maillard type fluorescence in order to establish that there is a direct temporal relationship between glycation and altered structure or function. A lag phase in the appearance of functional alterations may suggest that browning or oxidation reactions, rather than glycation alone, are responsible for changes in the properties of the protein. The observations may still be relevant, however, if there is evidence for these types of changes in the protein in diabetes or aging *in vivo*.

KINETICS AND RATES OF GLYCATION OF PROTEIN *IN VIVO*.

There has been only one direct study on the kinetics of glycation of a protein *in vivo*, that by Bunn et al. (1976) on formation of human HbA$_{Ic}$ following infusion of ^{59}Fe-transferrin. The rate of formation of HbA$_{Ic}$ *in vivo*, i.e., glycation of the β-terminal valine residue, was 0.018%/mM Glc/day, which was consistent with the mean level of HbA$_{Ic}$ in normal blood. In subsequent studies on glycation of Hb *in vitro* (Higgins and Bunn, 1981), the observed rate of formation of HbA$_{Ic}$ was 0.009%/mM Glc/day, or approximately one-half the *in vivo* rate. In retrospect, the faster reaction *in vivo* probably resulted from the presence of DPG and other effectors in the erythrocyte milieu (Watkins et al., 1987). Bunn et al. (1979) also reported that Hb glycated *in vivo* contains ~2.5 times as many glucose adducts to lysine as to valine residues, indicating that the rate of glycation of Hb at lysine residues was ~0.045% GlcHbA$_O$/mM Glc/day. Baynes et al. (1984) studied the rate of glycation of HSA *in vitro*, and concluded that the rate of glycation of HSA was ~0.21% GlcHSA/mM Glc/day, consistent with the extent of glycation of HSA and its biological half-life *in vivo*. After adjusting for the difference in lysine content of the proteins (22 per αβ-dimer in Hb and 57 in HSA), the rates of glycation of lysine residues in Hb and HSA are ~0.0008% and 0.0037%/mM Glc/day, respectively. Thus, the rate of glycation of lysines in HSA is, on average, ~4-5 times as fast as glycation of those in Hb. A wide range in rates of glycation of plasma proteins was also reported by Schleicher and Wieland (1986), and the rates of glycation of HSA, γ-globulin, fibrin, HDL and LDL *in vitro* in 5 mM phosphate buffer were in good agreement with the extent of glycation of the proteins and their plasma half-lives *in vivo*.

REVERSAL OF THE AMADORI REARRANGEMENT

Tables 4 and 5 summarize published information on the extent of glycation of various proteins in human blood and other tissues. Where possible original data have been normalized to mol Glc/mol Lys in the protein. Of interest, as shown in the first columns of data, most proteins contain, on average, less than 1 mol Glc/mol protein, and the extent of glycation of lysine residues in long-lived extracellular matrix proteins (Table 5) does not differ greatly from that of the shorter-lived blood proteins (Table 4). This observation argues either that the extracellular matrix proteins are glycated much more slowly than blood proteins or that glycation is a revers-ible process. Regarding a possible differential in rates of glycation of soluble and matrix proteins, there is little experimental data to support this point. Schleicher and Wieland (1986) have shown in fact that the rate of glycation of glomerular basement membrane proteins *in vitro* is not significantly different from that of plasma proteins per mg protein. It could be argued that the rate of glycation of these proteins in situ might be suppressed by interactions among the various components of the extracellular matrix, however steady changes in glycation of collagen and basement membrane proteins occur within weeks to months after the onset of diabetes or galactosemia in experimental animals. Thus, these long-lived proteins do not appear to be protected from reaction with glucose.

Since the formation of the Schiff base and Amadori adduct to proteins is the result of a series of equilibrium reactions, reversibility of these reactions should be measurable. This has been clearly documented in studies on the reaction of glyceraldehyde, with Hb (Acharya and Sussman, 1984), in which about 20% of the glyceraldehyde was released after incubation of (2-oxo-3-hydroxypropyl)-Hb in phosphate buffered saline, pH 7.4, for ~1 day at 37°C. The rate of the reverse reaction, like that of the forward reaction, was sensitive to pH and buffer species. The rates of reversal of glycation of valine

TABLE 4. Glycation of Lysine Residues in Human Blood Proteins *in vivo*[a]

Protein	mol Glc / mol Lys	mol Glc / mol Protein	nmol Glc / mg Protein	Meth[b]	Ref[c]
Albumin	0.004	0.24	<u>3.6</u>	Fur	1,2
	0.005	<u>0.29</u>	4.3	BT4⁻	3
	0.002	<u>0.12</u>	1.8	BT4⁻	4
	0.007	<u>0.43</u>	6.4	HPLC	5
	0.009	<u>0.49</u>	7.3	IO4⁻	5
	0.006	<u>0.37</u>	5.5	IO4⁻	6
	0.004	<u>0.24</u>	3.6	BT4⁻	6
Fibrin(ogen)	0.014	2.9	<u>0.86</u>	Fur	2
	0.005	<u>0.95</u>	0.27	Fur	7
g-Globulin	—	~0.3	<u>1.6</u>	Fur	2
HDL	—	—	<u>1.8</u>	Fur	2
LDL (Apo B)	0.0016	0.31	<u>1.2</u>	Fur	2
Whole Serum	—	—	<u>~3.3</u>	Fur	7
Hemoglobin[d]	0.003	0.06	<u>2.0</u>	Fur	2
	0.002	<u>0.04</u>	1.2	HPLC	5
RBC membrane	—	—	<u>2.0</u>	Fur	8

[a] Data from studies using chemical analyses with synthetic standards. Average values are shown where a range is given. Underlined values are in the chemical units originally reported by authors; others are calculated from this value using published data.

[b] Methods: Fur, measurement of furosine released by acid hydrolysis of unreduced protein; BT4⁻, reduction of protein with NaB3H4, followed by hydrolysis and isolation of radioactive hexitollysines by ion exchange or affinity chromatography; HPLC, measurement of nonradioactive hexitollysine by reversed phase HPLC of fluorescent derivatives; IO4⁻, oxidation of protein with periodate followed by measurement of formaldehyde by the Hantsch Reaction (9).

[c] References: (1) Schleicher and Wieland, 1981; (2) Schleicher and Wieland, 1986; (3) Baynes et al., 1984; (4) Garlick, 1986; (5) Walton and McPherson, 1986; (6) Olufemi et al., 1987; (7) Wieland et al., 1983; (8) Schleicher et al., 1981; (9) Gallop et al., 1981.

[d] Data for Hb are expressed per mol αβ-dimer.

Table 5. Extent of Glycation of Proteins in Human Tissues[a]

Protein	$\frac{\text{mol Glc}}{\text{mol Lys}}$	$\frac{\text{mol Glc}}{\text{mol Protein}}$	$\frac{\text{nmol Glc}}{\text{mg Protein}}$	Meth[b]	Ref[c]
Lens	0.004-0.03 0.002	0.009-0.057[d] –	0.45-2.85[e] 0.76	BT4- Fur	1 2
Glomerular Base Memb	0.0035 0.0076	– –	0.8 1.6	Fur BT4-	3 4
Skin Collagen			3.7	BT4-	5
Osteocalcin	-	0-0.16[f]		BT4-	6

a Data based on dry weight of tissue or protein, using chemical analyses with synthetic standards. Underlined values are in the chemical units originally reported by authors; others are calculated from this value using published data.
b Methods: See Table 4, Footnote b.
c References: (1) Garlick et al., 1984; (2) Unpublished observations;(3) Schleicher and Wieland, 1986; (4) Garlick et al., 1988; (5) Vishwanath et al., 1986; (6) Gundberg et al., 1986.
d The conversion from nmol Glc/mg protein to mol Glc/mol protein in Ref. 1 was based on $M_r=20,000$ and 2 mol Lys/mol protein for α-crystallin.
e An age-dependent increase in glycation was reported.
f Glycation of amino terminal Tyr; no Lys in osteocalcin.

and lysine residues in Hb also differed significantly, suggesting local effects of the protein environment on the reverse reaction. With glucose, the apparent rate of the reverse reaction would be decreased because of stabiliza- tion of the ketoamine adduct as the cyclic hemiketal. With any sugar, however, the products of the reverse reaction should include both of the C-2 epimers of the original sugar, since the ketoamine is achiral at the C-2 carbonyl. Thus, both glucose and mannose should be recovered on reversal of the Amadori rearrangement from proteins glycated with glucose. Ahmed et al. (1986, 1988)

have shown that mannose and glucose are recovered, along
with lysine, among the products of decomposition of fFL at
physiological pH and temperature. It should be noted,
however, that other products were also formed during this
reaction, including CML and browning products, so that the
mere release of radioactive sugar from protein or disappearance of the Amadori compound is not sufficient evidence for reversal of the Amadori rearrangement. However,
based on the yield of lysine and comparable total yields
of mannose and glucose, the half-life of fFL in 0.2 M
phosphate, pH 7.4, at 37°C could be estimated to be about
1 week. While the reverse reaction, like the forward
reaction, would be slower at physiological phosphate
concentration, similarities in the structure of fFL and
the Amadori adducts on protein argue that the reverse
reaction on protein would be a biologically relevant
reaction, especially for longer-lived proteins.

Products formed on reversal of the Amadori rearrangement from glycated protein have not yet been characterized. However, Bunn et al. (1976) observed that the rate
of accumulation of HbA_{Ic} declined with the age of the red
cell in vivo and concluded that their kinetic data were most
consistent with a reaction which was "slightly" reversible. In later studies in vitro, Mortensen and Christophersen
(1983) showed that HbA_{Ic} reverted to a protein with
electrophoretic properties of HbA_0 at a first order rate,
with a half-life of about 5 d. Using a kinetic model
which included reversibility of HbA_{Ic} formation, Mortensen
et al. (1984) were able to demonstrate that their predictions regarding levels and rates of change in HbA_{Ic} in
response to changes in glycemic control were in close
agreement with clinical experience. There is also indirect evidence for reversal of the Amadori rearrangement
on other proteins. Studies with glycated HSA in vitro
(Baynes et al., 1984) suggest a minimum half-life of 3
weeks for the reverse reaction in 0.2 M phosphate, based
on release of radioactivity from protein glycated with
$[6-^3H]$-glucose. Schleicher and Wieland (1986) estimated a
half-life of at least 2 months for the Amadori adduct to
HSA, based on loss of fructoselysine (as furosine) from
the protein in 5 mM phosphate. In studies on glycated LZM
(Hull, 1986) in which the Amadori adduct was measured as
hexitollysine by amino acid analysis, its half-life was
about 1 week in 0.2 M phosphate. In none of these
studies, however, were the products released from the

protein characterized; thus, these are minimal estimates of the half-life of the Amadori compound on protein since some of the loss of Amadori adduct could result from sugar fragmentation, dehydration or browning reactions. While there is clearly a need for additional study, the concentration of Amadori adduct on long-lived protein is probably at a steady state with respect to plasma glucose concentration. This steady state may be somewhat removed from the equilibrium of the glycation reaction, depending on the rate of post-glycation reactions, but the reverse reaction is likely to have an important role in limiting the extent of glycation of structural proteins *in vivo*.

RELATIONSHIP BETWEEN GLYCATION AND AGING

With reversibility of the Amadori rearrangement, the extent of glycation of long-lived proteins in tissues should eventually attain a steady state level in equilibrium with respect to ambient glucose concentration and other processes including oxidation, browning reactions and turnover of the protein. That a steady state does exist is indicated by two recent studies from our laboratory (Fig. 2) which indicate that the extent of glycation of human lens protein remains essentially constant between ages 5 and 80. Recent data on glycation of lens proteins in the rat (Swamy and Abraham, 1987: Perry et al., 1987) also show little change with age in mature animals. While our results are at odds with earlier studies reporting an age-dependent increase in glycation of bovine (Chiou et al., 1981) and human (Garlick et al., 1984) lenses, sample sizes in the earlier studies were smaller and the trends with age modest. Similarly, despite earlier evidence for increased glycation of human skin and tendon collagens with age (Kohn and Schnider, 1982), Vishwanath et al. (1986) and Garlick et al. (1988) have recently reported that they find no increase in glycation of human skin or basement membrane collagens with age. In this case the discrepancy probably results from differences in assay methodology. The earlier conclusions were based on thiobarbituric acid (TBA) assay which is sensitive to interference by enzymatically bound sugars (Schleicher and Wieland, 1981) and possibly lysine oxidase derived aldehyde and ketoamine crosslinks in collagen. In contrast, the more recent work made use of specific NaB^{3}H$_4$-reduction and affinity or ion exchange chromato-

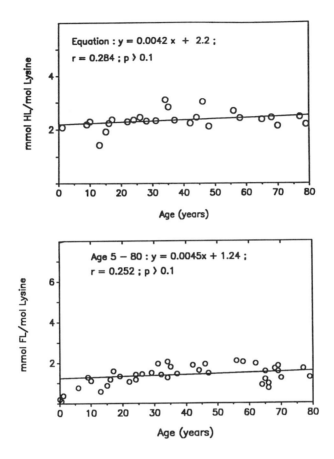

Figure 2. Relationship between age and glycation of lens proteins. (Top) Glycation was measured by reduction of lens proteins with [3H]NaBH₄, hydrolysis of the protein and quantitation of [3H]hexitollysines by phenylboronate (PBA) affinity chromatography (Bottom) Glycation was measured by analysis for furosine, following hydrolysis of unreduced protein, using selected ion monitoring GC/MS. Both assays were standardized by addition of known amounts of fFL. Both studies indicate that glycation does not increase significantly with age in the adult lens. The quantitative difference between the assays may be attributed to small amounts of nonspecifically bound radioactivity and the detection of fructose adducts using the affinity chromatographic procedure.

graphic assay procedures. Oimomi et al. (1986) have
reported age-related increases in glycation of rat aorta
and sciatic nerve protein with age, however in this case
the assays appear to have been done on total tissue
protein, so that age-dependent changes in tissue protein
composition and turnover cannot be excluded as a source of
an apparent increase in glycation. It should also be
noted, however, that Schleicher and Wieland (1986)
detected only a slight, if significant, increase in
glycation of aorta protein with age and attributed this
change to a decline in glucose tolerance with age.
Similarly, while several groups have reported increased
glycation of blood proteins with age, Kabadi (1988)
observed no increase in glycation of plasma proteins with
age in healthy, normoglycemic subjects. Overall, we
conclude from these studies that the extent of glycation
of proteins begins to approach a steady state early in
life and that, in the absence of compromised glucose
tolerance or changes in tissue protein composition or
turnover, there is little evidence of significant
age-dependent increases in glycation of proteins.

RELEVANCE OF GLYCATION TO THE PATHOPHYSIOLOGY OF DIABETES

There are a number of considerations beyond the extent
of glycation of a protein that need to be addressed before
concluding that increased glycation of a protein in
diabetes (or aging) is of any pathophysiological significance. Among these are the adaptability and reserve
capacity of physiological systems, which can attenuate
effects of glycation. One classic example of adaptation
is the observation that despite evidence for altered
oxygen binding by glycated hemoglobins (McDonald et al.,
1979), whole blood oxygen saturation curves are not
altered in diabetes (Samaja et al., 1982; Roberts et al.,
1984). Similarly, while glycation of albumin affects its
tryptophan fluorescence, indicating underlying structural
changes, and alters the binding of bilirubin and parinaric
acid (Shaklai et al., 1984), salicylate (Mereisch et al.,
1981) and sulfonylureas (Tsuchiya et al., 1984), there is
no evidence indicating that increased glycation of albumin
in diabetes has any impact on its metabolism or on drug
pharmacokinetics. Binding and transport of palmitate
appear to be unaffected by glycation of albumin to extents
observed *in vivo* (Murtiashaw and Winterhalter, 1986), and

even when functions are affected, the concentration of unglycated albumin present in blood appears to be adequate to assume the biological functions of the protein.

Other studies suggest that glycation is not likely to affect the function or recognition of several plasma proteins, including transferrin and α_2-macroglobulin (Ney et al., 1985), fibrinogen (Ney et al., 1985; McVerry et al., 1981), and immunoglobulins (Morin et al., 1987). The situation with lipoproteins is less clear. Extensive glycation, especially in the presence of NaBH$_3$CN, is known to affect the recognition and catabolism of lipoproteins (Gonen et al., 1981; Witztum et al., 1982; Sasaki and Cottam, 1982; Steinbrecher et al., 1983). There is also evidence that glycation of LDL to extents observed in diabetes retards the catabolism of the protein via the Brown and Goldstein pathway (Steinbrecher and Witztum, 1984). Lyons et al. (1987) have also shown a good correlation between glycation of LDL *in vivo* and enhancement of cholesterol synthesis in macrophages by LDL isolated from diabetic patients. At higher extents of glycation, but probably exceeding that which would be attained even in diabetes, Lopes-Virella et al. (1988) observed enhanced uptake of LDL and accumulation of cholesterol ester by human macrophages in tissue culture. However, Schleicher et al. (1985) reported that glycation of LDL to extents comparable to those seen in diabetes had no effect on its catabolism by human fibroblasts in tissue culture or the cholesterol content and cholesterol esterification in human monocyte-derived macrophages. Overall, while there is some evidence for a relationship between glycation and altered metabolism of diabetic lipoproteins by either the LDL-receptor (Steinbrecher and Witztum, 1984) or scavenger (Lopes-Virella et al., 1988) pathways, it is possible that other factors, including lipid peroxidation (Yagi, 1982), triglyceride content or insulin-dependent effects on lipoprotein and lipid metabolism may be more relevant to the alterations in lipoprotein metabolism and development of vascular disease in diabetes. In other work, Furcht and colleagues (Tarsio et al., 1985, 1988) have shown that glycation of fibronectin and laminin significantly affects their interaction with heparin and collagen, suggesting a possible mechanism for basement membrane alterations in diabetes. These effects were observable at levels of glycation which would be observed in diabetes, although comparative studies between fibronectin isolated from normal and diabetic blood were not presented. However, even with the functional alterations in the properties of these glycated proteins, protein turnover and the availability of adequate amounts of unglycated protein may be sufficient to counter effects of their increased glycation in diabetes.

While the above discussion has been somewhat negative regarding the contribution of glycation alone to the pathophysiology of diabetes, Ceriello et al. (1987) have presented evidence that glycation of antithrombin III (ATIII) may contribute to the hypercoagulable state associated with diabetes. Brownlee et al. (1984) had observed that glycation of ATIII interfered with its inhibitory activity toward thrombin, and in recent work Ceriello et al. (1987) have shown an inverse correlation between transient changes in blood glucose and ATIII activity. These observations suggest that it is the labile Schiff base adduct to ATIII, rather than the permanent modification via the Amadori rearrangement, which decreases the activity of ATIII during hyperglycemia. Alterations in ATIII activity during periods of transient hyperglycemia could be one of several factors contributing to increased coagulability and the development of vascular disease in diabetes. It should be recognized that during episodic hyperglycemia, the amount of labile Schiff base adduct on a protein may exceed that of the stable Amadori adduct. Indeed, the amount of labile adduct to Hb, measured as pre-HbA$_{Ic}$, can be a source of major errors and fluctuations in HbA$_{Ic}$ when using mini-column cation exchange chromatographic assays (Goldstein et al., 1984). With Hb, the pre-HbA$_{Ic}$ fraction accounts for as much as 20% of total glycated Hb during postprandial hyperglycemia, and this fraction should be larger for shorter-lived proteins which have less time for accumulation of the Amadori adduct. While the physiological system may be able to adjust to long-term shifts in protein function induced by stable glycation, it may prove less effective in dealing with transient changes induced by labile glycation. In general, the role of transient glycation in the development of complications in diabetes deserves much more attention as a possible source of chronic disease.

SUMMARY STATEMENT

The Amadori product on protein is a steady state intermediate which can revert to free sugar and protein or participate in subsequent oxidation and browning reactions of the protein. There is limited evidence that increased glycation alone is of any pathological consequence in aging or diabetes, however subsequent reactions of the Amadori adduct on protein and accumulation of the products of these reactions may alter the structure and function of long-lived proteins and contribute to the pathophysiology of aging and diabetes.

Abbreviations used: CML, N^ε-carboxymethyllysine; DPG, 2,3-diphosphoglycerate; fFL, N^α-formyl-N^ε-fructoselysine; Hb, hemoglobin; HSA, human serum albumin; LZM, hen egg white lysozyme; PBA, phenylboronic acid; RNase, bovine pancreatic ribonuclease A.

REFERENCES

Acharya AS, Sussman LG (1984). The reversibility of the ketoamine linkages of aldoses with proteins. J Biol Chem 259:4372-4378.

Ahmed MU, Dunn JA, Walla MD, Thorpe SR, Baynes JW (1988). Oxidative degradation of glucose adducts to protein: formation of 3-(N^ε-lysino)-lactic acid from model compounds and glycated proteins. J Biol Chem 263:8816-8821.

Ahmed MU, Thorpe, SR, Baynes, JW (1986). Identification of carboxymethyllysine as a degradation product of fructoselysine in glycated protein. J Biol Chem 261:4889-4994.

Baynes JW, Thorpe SR, Murtiashaw MH (1984). Nonenzymatic glycosylation of lysine residues in albumin. Meth Enzymol 106:88-98.

Bissé E, Berger W, Flückiger R (1982). Quantitation of glycosylated hemoglobin: elimination of labile glycohemoglobin during sample hemolysis at pH 5. Diabetes 31:630-634.

Brownlee M, Vlassara H, Cerami A (1984). Inhibition of heparincatalyzed human antithrombin III activity by nonenzymatic glycosylation: possible role in fibrin deposition in diabetes. Diabetes 33:532-535.

Bunn HF, Higgins PJ (1981). Reaction of monosaccharides

with protein: possible evolutionary significance. Science 231:222-224.

Bunn HF, Haney DN, Kamin S, Gabbay KH, Gallop PM (1976). Biosynthesis of human hemoglobin A_{Ic}: slow glycosylation of hemoglobin *in vivo*. J Clin Invest 57:1652-1659.

Bunn HF, Shapiro R, McManus MJ, Garrick L, McDonald MJ, Gallop PJ, Gabbay KH (1979). Structural heterogeneity of human hemoglobin A due to nonenzymatic glycosylation. J Biol Chem 254:3892-3898.

Burton HS, McWeeney DJ (1963). Nonenzymatic browning reactions: consideration of sugar stability. Nature 197:266-268.

Ceriello A, Giugliano D, Quatraro A, Stante A, Concoli G, Dello Russo P, D'onofrio F (1987). Daily rapid blood glucose variations may condition antithrombin III biological activity but not its plasma concentration in insulin-dependent diabetes: a possible role for labile nonenzymatic glycation. Diab & Metab 13:16-19.

Chiou SH, Chylack LT Jr., Tung WH, Bunn HF (1981). Nonenzymatic glycosylation of bovine lens crystallins: effect of aging. J Biol Chem 256:5176-5180.

Gallop PM, Flückiger R, Hannehen A, Minninsohn MM, Gabbay KH (1981). Chemical quantitation of hemoglobin glycosylation: fluorometric detection of formaldehyde released upon periodate oxidation of glycoglobin. Anal Biochem 117:427-433.

Garlick R L (1986). Measurement of nonenzymatic glycation of hemoglobin, serum albumin, lens crystallin, and glomerular basement membrane protein. In Methods in Diabetes Research Vol. II: Clinical Methods (Clarke WL, Lawner J, Pohl SL, eds.) John Wiley and Sons, NY, pp. 521-532.

Garlick RL, Bunn HF, Spiro RG (1988). Nonenzymatic glycation of basement membranes from human glomeruli and bovine sources. Diabetes 37:1144-1150.

Garlick RL, Mazer JS (1983). The principal site of nonenzymatic glycosylation of human serum albumin *in vivo*. J Biol Chem 258:6142-6146.

Garlick RL, Mazer JS, Chylack LT Jr, Tung WH, Bunn HF (1984). Nonenzymatic glycation of human lens crystallin: effect of aging and diabetes mellitus. J Clin Invest 74:1742-1749.

Gillery P, Monboisse JC, Maquart FX, Borel JP (1988). Glycation of proteins as a source of superoxide. Diab & Metab 14:25-30.

Goldstein DE, Wiedmeyer HM, England JE, Little RR, Parker

KM (1983). Recent advances in glycosylated hemoglobin meaurements. CRC Crit. Rev. Clin Lab Sci 21:187-228.

Gonen B, Baenziger J, Schonfeld G, Jacobson D, Farrar P (1981). Nonenzymatic glycosylation of low density lipoproteins *in vivo*. Diabetes 30:875-878.

Gundberg CM, Anderson M, Dickson I, Gallop PM (1986). Glycated osteocalcin in human and bovine bone: the effect of age. J Biol Chem 261:14557-14561.

Hicks M, Delbridge L, Yue DK, Reeve TS (1988). Catalysis of lipid peroxidation by glucose and glycosylated collagen. Biochem Biophys Res Commun 291:649-655.

Higgins PJ, Bunn HF (1981). Kinetic analysis of nonenzymatic glycosylation of hemoglobin. J Biol Chem 256:5204-5208.

Hull CJ (1986). Studies on Glycation and Maillard Reactions of Protein. Ph.D. Thesis, Univ.of South Carolina.

Iberg N, Fluckiger R (1986). Nonenzymatic glycosylation of albumin *in vivo*: identification of multiple glycosylated sites. J Biol Chem 261:13542-13545.

Kabadi UM (1988). Glycosylation of proteins: lack of influence of aging. Diabetes Care 11:429-432.

Kohn RL, Schnider SL (1982). Glucosylation of human collagen. Diabetes 31 (Suppl 3):47-51.

Lopes-Virella MF, Klein RL, Lyons TJ, Stevenson HC, Witztum JL (1988). Glycosylation of low-density lipoprotein enhances cholesteryl ester synthesis in human monocyte derived macrophages. Diabetes 37:550-557.

Lowrey CH, Lyness SJ, Soeldner JS (1985). The effect of hemoglobin ligands on the kinetics of human hemoglobin A$_{Ic}$ formation. J Biol Chem 260:11611-11618.

Lutjens A, te Velde AA, van der Veen EA, Meer JVD (1985). Glycosylation of human fibrinogen *in vivo*. Diabetologia 28:87-89.

Lyons TJ, Klein RL, Baynes JW, Stevenson HC, Lopes-Virella MF (1987). Stimulation of cholesterol ester synthesis in human monocyte-derived macrophages by low-density lipoproteins from Type I (insulin-dependent) diabetic patients: the influence of non-enzymatic glycosylation of low-density lipoproteins. Diabetologia 30:916-923.

McDonald MJ, Bleichman M, Bunn H F, Noble RW (1979). Functional properties of glycosylated minor components of adult hemoglobin. J Biol Chem 254:702-707.

McVerry VA, Thorpe S, Gaffney JP, Huehns ER (1981). Nonenzymatic glucosylation of fibrinogen. Hemostasis 10:261-270.

Mereish KA, Rosenberg H, Cobby J (1982). Glucosylated

albumin and its influence on salicylate binding.
J Pharmaceut Sci 71:235-238.

Morin G, Austin GE, Burkhalter A (1987). Nonenzymatic
glycation of immunoglobulins does not impair antigen-
antibody binding. Clin Chem. 33:692-694.

Mortensen HB, Christophersen C (1983). Glucosylation of
human haemoglobin A in red blood cells studied *in vitro*:
kinetics of the formation and dissociation of hemoglobin
A_{Ic}. Clin Chim Acta 134:317-326.

Mortensen HB, Volund A, Christophersen C (1984).
Glucosylation of human hemoglobin A: dynamic variation in
HbA_{Ic} described by a biokinetic model. Clin Chim Acta
136:75-81.

Murtiashaw MH, Winterhalter KH (1986). Nonenzymatic
glycation of human albumin does not alter its palmitate
binding. Diabetoglogia 29:366-370.

Neglia CI, Cohen HJ, Garber AR, Ellis PD, Thorpe SR,
Baynes JW (1983). ^{13}C-NMR investigation of nonenzymatic
glucosylation of protein: model studies using RNase A.
J Biol Chem 258:14279-14283.

Neglia CI, Cohen HJ, Garber AR, Thorpe SR, Baynes JW
(1985). Characterization of glycated proteins by ^{13}C NMR
spectroscopy: identification of specific sites of protein
modification by glucose. J Biol Chem 260:5406-5410.

Ney KA, Pasqua JJ, Colley KA, Guthrow EA, Pizzo SG (1985).
In vitro preparation of nonenzymatically glucosylated human
transferrin, a_2-macroglobulin, and fibrinogen with
preservation of function. Diabetes 34:462-470.

Oimomi M, Kitamura Y, Nishimoto S, Matsumoto S, Hatanaka
H, Baba S (1986). Age-related acceleration of glycation
of tissue proteins in rats. J Gerontol 41:695-698.

Olufemi S, Talwar D, Robb DA (1987). The relative extent
of glycation of haemoglobin and albumin. Clin Chim Acta
163:125-136.

Ortwerth BJ, Olesen PR (1988). Glutathione inhibits the
glycation and crosslinking of lens protein by ascorbate.
Exp Eye Res, in press.

Perry RE, Swamy MS, Abraham EC (1987). Progressive changes
in lens crystallin glycation and high-molecular weight
aggregate formation leading to cataract development in
streptozotocin-diabetic rats. Exp Eye Res 44:269-282.

Roberts AP, Story CJ, Ryall, R.G. (1984). Erythrocyte
2,3-bisphosphoglycerate concentrations and haemoglobin
glycosylation in normoxic Type I (insulin-dependent)
diabetes mellitus. Diabetologia 26:389-391.

Samaja, M, Melotti D, Carenini A, Pozza G (1982).

Glycosylated haemoglobins and the oxygen affinity of whole blood. Diabetologia 23:399-402.

Sasaki J, Cottam, GL (1982). Glycosylation of human LDL and its metabolism in human skin fibroblasts. Biochem Biophys Res Commun 104:977-983.

Schleicher E, Deufel T, Wieland OH (1981). Nonenzymatic glycosylation of human serum lipoproteins, FEBS Let 129:1-4.

Schleicher E, Olgemoeller B, Schoen J, Duerst T, Wieland OH (1985). Limited nonenzymatic glucosylation of low-density lipoprotein does not alter its catabolism in tissue culture. Biochim Biophys Acta 846:226-233.

Schleicher E, Scheller L, Wieland OH (1981). Quantitation of lysine-bound glucose of normal and diabetic erythrocyte membrane by HPLC analysis of furosine. Biochem Biophys Res Commun 99:1011-1019.

Schleicher E, Wieland OH (1981). Specific quantitation by HPLC of protein (lysine) bound glucose in human serum albumin and other glycosylated proteins. J Clin Chem Clin Biochem 19:81-87.

Schleicher E, Wieland OH (1986). Kinetic analysis of glycation as a tool for assessing the half-life of proteins. Biochim Biophys Acta 884:199-205.

Shaklai N, Garlick RL, Bunn HF (1984). Nonenzymatic glycosylation of human serum albumin alters its conformation and function. J Biol Chem 259:3812-3817.

Shapiro R, McManus MJ, Zalut C, Bunn HF (1980). Sites of nonenzymatic glycosylation of human hemoglobin A. J Biol Chem 255:3120-3127.

Smith RJ, Koenig RJ, Binnerts A, Soeldner JS, Aoki TT (1982). Regulation of hemoglobin A_Ic formation in human erythrocytes $in vitro$: effects of physiological factors other than glucose. J Clin Invest 69:1164-1168.

Steinbrecher UP, Witztum JL (1984). Glucosylation of low density lipoproteins to an extent comparable to that seen in diabetes slows their catabolism. Diabetes 33:130-134.

Steinbrecher UP, Witztum JL, Kesaniemi YA, Elam RL (1983). Comparison of glucosylated low density lipoprotein with methylated or cyclohexanedione-treated low density lipoprotein in the measurement of receptor-independent low density lipoprotein catabolism. J Clin Invest 71:960-964.

Swamy MS, Abraham EC (1987). Lens protein composition, glycation and high molecular weight aggregation in aging rats. Invest Opthalmol Vis Sci 28:1693-1701.

Tarsio JF, Reger LA, Furcht LT (1988). Molecular mechanisms in basement membrane complications in diabetes: Alterations in heparin, laminin, and Type IV collagen association. Diabetes 37:532-539.

Tarsio JF, Widness B, Rhode TD, Rupp WM, Buchwald H, Furcht LT (1985). Nonenzymatic glycation of fibronectin and alterations in the molecular association of cell matrix and basement membrane components in diabetes mellitus. Diabetes 34:477-484.

Tsuchiya S, Sakurai T, Sekiguchi SI (1984). Nonenzymatic glucosylation of human serum albumin and its influence on binding capacity of sulfonylureas. Biochem Pharmacol 33:2967-2971.

Vishwanath V, Frank KE, Elmets CA, Dauchot PJ, Monnier VM (1986). Glycation of skin collagen in Type 1 diabetes mellitus: correlation with long-term complications. Diabetes 35: 916-921.

Walton DJ, McPherson JD (1988). Non-enzymic glycation of proteins: analysis of N-(1-deoxyhexitol-1-yl) amino acids by high-performance liquid chromatography. Carbohyd Res 153:285-293.

Watkins NG, Neglia CI, Dyer DG, Thorpe SR, Baynes JW (1987). Effect of phosphate on the kinetics and specificity of glycation of proteins. J Biol Chem 262:7207-7212.

Watkins NG, Thorpe SR, Baynes JW (1985). Glycation of amino groups in protein: studies on the specificity of modification of RNase A by glucose. J Biol Chem 260:10629-10636.

Wieland OH, Dolhofer R, Schleicher E, Reindl R, Vogt B (1983). Non-enzymatic glucosylation of proteins and possible pathophysiological consequences. In Structural Carbohydrates in the Liver (Popper H, Reutter W, Kottgen E, Gudat F, eds) MTP Press Ltd., Boston, MA, pp 517-526.

Witztum JL, Fisher M, Pietro T, Steinbrecher UP, Elam RL (1982). Nonenzymatic glucosylation of high-density lipoprotein accelerates its catabolism in guinea pigs. Diabetes 31:1029-1032.

Wolff SP, Dean RT (1987). Glucose autoxidation and protein modification: potential role of autoxidative glycosylation in diabetes. Biochem J 245:243-250.

Yagi K (1982). Assay of serum lipid peroxide level and its clinical significance. In Lipid Peroxides in Biology and Medicine (Yagi K, ed) Academic Press, NY, pp 223-242.

The Maillard Reaction in Aging,
Diabetes, and Nutrition, pages 69–84
© 1989 Alan R. Liss, Inc.

3-DEOXYGLUCOSONE, AN INTERMEDIATE PRODUCT OF THE MAILLARD
REACTION

Hiromichi Kato, Fumitaka Hayase, Dong Bum Shin,
Munetada Oimomi and Shigeaki Baba

Department of Agricultural Chemistry (H.K., F.H.,
D.B.S.), The University of Tokyo, Tokyo 113, and
Second Department of Internal Medicine (M.O., S.B.),
Kobe University School of Medicine, Kobe 650, Japan

ABSTRACT. The Maillard reactions between proteins
and glucose or fructose, in 0.2M phosphate buffer
(pH 7.4) at 37°C, were investigated and the following results were obtained: 1) 3-deoxyglucosone
(3DG) is formed as the major carbonyl intermediate;
2) fructose has a higher reactivity than glucose
and 3DG is formed also from fructose without involvement of amino groups; 3) 3DG is a crosslinker
responsible for polymerization of proteins; 4) 3DG
is involved in the formation of a fluorescent
advanced-stage product named "Peak L_1" in vitro
and in vivo.

INTRODUCTION

3-Deoxyglycosones had been postulated as an intermediate in the formation of furfurals from reducing sugars by
the action of acid (Wolfrom et al., 1948). In 1960, two
workers independently reported the isolation of 3-deoxy-
glycosones under the condition of the Maillard reaction.
Kato (1960) isolated 3-deoxyglucosone (3DG, 3-deoxy-D-
erythro-hexosulose), 3-deoxygalactosone (3-deoxy-D-threo-
hexosulose) and 3-deoxypentosone (3-deoxypentosulose) as
their bis-2,4-dinitrophenylhydrazones from the degradation
mixture of N-butyl-glycosylamine acetates at 55°C and proposed that 3-deoxyglycosones are the major intermediates in
the browning reaction. Anet (1960) elucidated that di-D-
fructoseglycine [1,1'-(carboxymethylamino)bis(1-deoxy-D-

fructose] is readily decomposed to 3DG and D-fructoseglycine
(1-deoxy-1-glycino-D-fructose),the Amadori compound, at pH
5.5 at 100°C, and similarly, di-D-tagatoseglycine [1,1'-
(carboxymethylamino)-bis(1-deoxy-D-tagatose)] gives 3-deoxy-
galactosone and D-tagatoseglycine (1-deoxy-1-glycino-D-taga-
tose). Scheme 1 shows three kinds of 3-deoxyglycosones and
their proposed formation pathway, in which 1,2-eneaminol of
Amadori compound is dehydrated to protonated Schiff base of
the enol of 3-deoxyglycosone (Anet, 1960; Kato, 1960; Reynolds, 1963).

Kato et al. (1961) detected 3DG in some traditional
fermented foods such as miso and soy sauce, which was distributed from 3mg/100g (light-colored product) to 40mg/100g
(dark-colored product). Several 2-oxoaldehydes such as 3DG,
3-deoxypentosone, glucosone, xylosone in addition to methyl-
glyoxal were detected in calf and rabbit livers as their
bis-2,4-dinitrophenylhydrazones (Kato et al., 1970).

However, the formation of active carbonyl intermediates
such as 3DG in the Maillard reaction between proteins and
reducing sugars is not obvious, although the formation of
Amadori rearrangement products has been demonstrated in many
proteins in vivo (Monnier and Cerami, 1983). In a previous
paper, Cho et al. (1985) described the mechanism of glucose-
induced polymerization of lysozyme, which was stored with
glucose in the solid state at 75% relative humidity at 50°C,
and postulated that 3DG is the major crosslinker. In this
paper, we examine the formation of 3DG under the physiological condition and discuss the role of 3DG in the protein-
involving Maillard reaction in vitro and in vivo.

RESULTS AND DISCUSSION

1) Reaction of Lysozyme with Various Sugars

At first, we examined the reaction with various sugars
using lysozyme as a model protein. Lysozyme (10mg/ml) was
incubated with glucose, fructose, galactose, mannose, xylose
or ribose (200mM) in 0.2M sodium phosphate buffer (pH 7.4)
at 37°C for 28 days. Table 1 indicates the degree of polymerization and the damage to lysine and arginine residues of
lysozyme incubated with sugars. The degree of polymerization of lysozyme by the pentoses was higher than that by the
hexoses except for fructose. Fructose showed a high polyme-

Scheme 1.

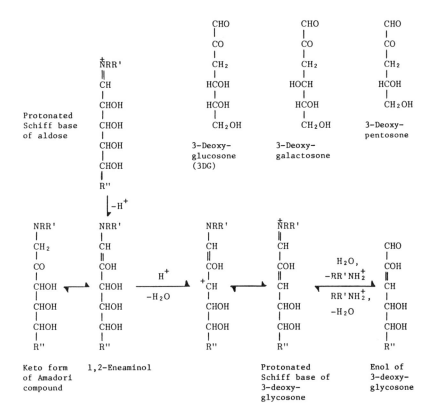

$R = -CH_2CH_2CH_2CH_3$ or $-CH_2COOH$
$R' = -H$ or -1-deoxyketose
$R'' = -H$ or $-CH_2OH$

rization rate similar to that in the case of the pentoses.
It is suggested that the reactivity of a reducing sugar depends on the extent to which it exists in the carbonyl form
(Bunn and Higgins, 1981). The impairment of amino acid residues was observed for lysine and arginine residues, but
none of the other amino acid residues were impaired (tryptophan residues were not analyzed in this experiment). The
decrease in lysine residues of lysozyme incubated with the
pentoses was greater than that incubated with the hexoses.
In the case of the reaction of lysozyme with fructose, despite of high degree of polymerization, the loss of lysine

residues was not so much. Fructose, xylose and ribose, however, caused the loss of arginine residues much more than the case of glucose.

TABLE 1. Polymerization and remaining amounts of lysine and arginine residues of lysozyme after incubation with sugars in 0.2M phosphate buffer (pH 7.4) at 37°C for 28 days (Shin et al., 1988). Electrophoresis was conducted as described by Weber and Osborn (1969) using 10% slab gels. The rate of polymerization of the incubated proteins was determined by scanning the stained protein bands with a densitometer. After incubation, the proteins were hydrolyzed with 6N HCl in evacuated tubes at 110°C for 24 hours. Amino acid analysis of the hydrolysates was performed with a Hitachi Amino Acid Analyzer 835 (Okitani et al., 1984).

Sugar	−	Glc	Fru	Gal	Man	Xyl	Rib
Polymerization(%)*	1	6	40	13	12	38	44
Lys(%)**	100	74	83	87	81	59	37
Arg(%)**	100	96	85	88	93	84	64

   * The degree of polymerization of lysozyme is expressed
     as the percentage of oligomers and polymers.
  ** The remaining amounts of lysine and arginine residues
     are expressed as percentages compared to that in the
     case of the control incubated without sugar. The amino
     acid residues in the control remained unchanged.

Fructose is an important food component and is produced from glucose through the polyol pathway. Then, we examined the Maillard reaction of proteins induced by fructose in comparison with that by glucose.

2) Reaction of Various Proteins with Glucose or Fructose

Table 2 shows tha polymerization and the remaining amounts of lysine and arginine residues of lysozyme, ribonuclease A (RNase A), ovalbumin (OVA) and bovine serum albumin (BSA) incubated with glucose or fructose under the same condition to that of Table 1. Lysozyme and RNase A were polymerized in the presence of fructose or glucose, although the rate of the former was much higher than that for the latter. On the other hand, OVA and BSA were not polymerized in the presence of glucose, in spite of the impairment of lysine and arginine residues. These results propose that intramolecular crosslinks were formed instead of intermolecular ones, because of anionic intermolecular repulsion by predominant carboxyl anions in these albumin molecules.

TABLE 2. Polymerization and remaining amounts of lysine and arginine residues of lysozyme, RNase A, OVA and BSA after incubation with glucose or fructose at 37°C for 28 days (Shin et al., 1988).

	Lysozyme		RNase A		OVA		BSA	
	Glc	Fru	Glc	Fru	Glc	Fru	Glc	Fru
Polymerization(%)*	6	40	7	17	0	2	0	15
Lys(%)*	74	83	73	93	92	79	84	81
Arg(%)*	96	85	89	89	96	88	85	72

* The degree of polymerization and the remaining amounts of amino acids are expressed as in Table 1. Amino acid residues of the proteins incubated without sugars remained unchanged.

It is of interest that the rates of the decreases in lysine and arginine residues were different each other. In the case of the reactions with glucose, lysine residues decreased at a higher rate than arginine residues, but in the case of fructose, the decreases in arginine and lysine residues were almost the same. Furthermore, a strong relationship is considered between the polymerization and the decrease in arginine residues (Tables 1 and 2). The marked polymerization of lysozyme incubated with fructose may depend on the abundance of arginine residues in this protein.

3) Formation of 3DG in the Reaction of Proteins with Glucose or Fructose

In order to elucidate the mechanism of the polymerization of proteins, we analyzed the carbonyl compounds in the low molecular weight fractions separated from the reaction mixtures of proteins incubated with glucose or fructose by centrifugation at 5000×g for 30 min in a microconcentrator (Centricon 10, Amicon). Thin layer chromatography (TLC) of 2,4-dinitrophenylhydrazones of each low molecular weight fraction indicated that 3DG was the major carbonyl intermediate, as seen in Fig. 1. Field desorption mass spectrometry of the fraction assigned to 3DG showed that the base peak was at 523 ($M^+ + 1$), being identical to bis-2,4-dinitrophenylhydrazone of 3DG (Shin et al., 1988).

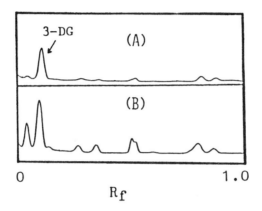

Figure 1. TLC of 2,4-dinitrophenylhydrazones of low molecular weight fractions obtained from lysozyme incubated with glucose (A) and fructose (B) in 0.2M phosphate buffer (pH 7.4) at 37°C for 28 days (Shin et al., 1988). TLC was performed on silica gel 60F plates (Merck) using a mixture of benzene-ethyl acetate-pyridine-acetic acid, 95:5:5:3, as developer. The developed plates were scanned as to the absorbance at 440nm with a Toyo DMU-33C Densitometer.

The amount of 3DG, which was produced on each reaction system, was quantified by comparing the band area on the TLC plate with that of standard 3DG prepared according to the method of Kato et al. (1987a). Figure 2 shows the amount of 3DG in the low molecular weight fractions derived from the reaction mixtures of proteins with glucose or fructose. 3DG formed in the reaction mixture of proteins with fructose was approximately 1.3-2.0 times as much as in the case of the protein-glucose reaction. The largest quantity of 3DG was formed in the BSA-fructose reaction.

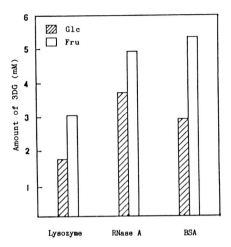

Figure 2. Amounts of 3DG in the low molecular weight fractions obtained from lysozyme, RNase A and BSA incubated with
glucose or fructose at 37°C for 28 days (Shin et al., 1988).

4) Mechanisms Proposed for Polymerization of Proteins
   Incubated with Glucose or Fructose

    Cho et al. (1985) have postulated that 3DG is generated
on the reaction between ε-amino groups of lysine residues of
proteins and glucose at 50°C under 75% relative humidity,
and that it causes crosslinking of protein molecules with
impairment of arginine, lysine and tryptophan residues. The
results of the protein-glucose reaction in Fig. 2 also propose that ε-amino groups of lysine residues act as genera-
tors of 3DG and arginine residues act as attackers of 3DG.

    On the other hand, in the case of the protein-fructose
reaction, the relationship of the formation of 3DG and the
polymerization of proteins was quite different (Fig. 2). It
is well known that fructose reacts with amino compounds in
the early stage of the Maillard reaction, followed by rearrangement to form a 2-amino-2-deoxy-glucose (Heyns rearrangement), in contrast with glucose, in which case Amadori rearrangement occurs (Danehy, 1987). However, there has been no
report on the formation of 3DG from a Heyns rearrangement
compound. Kato et al. (1969) reported that 3DG is formed
from fructose itself at pH 5.5 at 100°C in the absence of
amino compound.

Table 3 shows the results of the reaction between succinylated lysozyme and glucose or fructose. Succinylated
lysozyme incubated with glucose did not polymerize and no
arginine residue was impaired, but in the case of fructose,
succinylated lysozyme polymerized to a small extent and one
residue of arginine was impaired. These results indicate
that 3DG was generated also from the fructose without participation of amino groups, and that it polymerized the
succinylated lysozyme. In the case of glucose, the generation of 3DG, which is considered to be formed from Amadori
compounds, has been suppressed by the modification of lysine
residues. However, the degree of polymerization of succinylated lysozyme was much lower than that of intact lysozyme incubated with fructose. It is considered that intramolecular crosslinks were formed instead of intermolecular
ones, because of anionic intermolecular repulsion by abundant carboxyl anions in succinylated lysozyme.

TABLE 3. Polymerization and loss in amino acid residues of
lysozyme and succinylated lysozyme incubated with glucose
or fructose at 37°C for 28 days (Shin et al., 1988).

	Lysozyme			Succinylated lysozyme		
	None	Glc	Fru	None	Glc	Fru
Polymerization(%)	0	6	40	0	0	3
Lys*	5.9	4.4	4.9	6.0	6.1	6.0
Arg*	10.6	10.2	9.0	10.8	10.6	9.6
Trp*	5.5	4.5	4.9	5.4	5.4	5.3

* Amino acid residues are expressed as a molar ratio
taking the value for leucine to be 8.0.

The results described above postulate that 3DG is the
crosslinker responsible for the glucose- and fructose induced polymerization of proteins under physiological conditions. Then, we examined the reaction of proteins with 3DG.

5) Reaction of Various Protiens with 3DG

Highly purified 3DG was prepared according to the method of the previous papers (Kato, 1962; Kato et al., 1987a). One hundred mM 3DG or glucose were incubated with 10mg/ml each of lysozyme, RNase A, human immunoglobulin G (Ig G) or human serum albumin (HSA) in 0.2M sodium phosphate buffer (pH 7.4) at 37°C for 28 days. Table 4 shows polymerization and loss in lysine and arginine residues of each incubated protein. When incubated with 3DG, lysozyme, RNase A and Ig G were severely polymerized, whereas HSA was not polymerized so much, but the loss of lysine and arginine residues was almost the same for each protein. Glucose impaired mainly lysine residues, whereas 3DG impaired much arginine residues than lysine ones.

TABLE 4. Polymerization and remaining amounts of lysine and arginine residues of proteins after incubation with glucose or 3DG at 37°C for 28 days (Kato et al., 1987b).

	Lysozyme		RNase A		Ig G		HSA	
	Glc	3DG	Glc	3DG	Glc	3DG	Glc	3DG
Polymerization(%)	5	53	6	45	11	64	0	9
Lys(%)*	89	80	92	69	90	80	81	79
Arg(%)*	96	28	94	49	94	50	96	58

* The amino acid residues in the proteins incubated without glucose or 3DG remained unchanged (100%).

The time-course of the impairment of lysine and arginine residues and sodium dodecyl sulfate-polyacrylamide gel electrophoresis (SDS-PAGE) of lysozyme incubated with 3DG are shown in Fig. 3. After only 3 days incubation, a much amount of arginine residues was attacked by 3DG and the formation of some oligomers was observed.

These results confirm that, under physiological conditions, 3DG is able to cause crosslinking of proteins with impairment of arginine and lysine residues.

6) A Fluorescent Advanced-Stage Product "Peak L₁" in the Maillard Reaction in Vitro and in Vivo

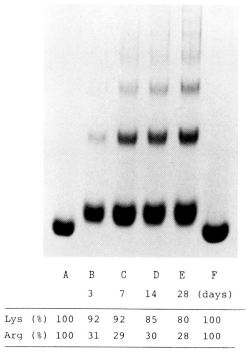

	A	B	C	D	E	F
		3	7	14	28	(days)
Lys (%)	100	92	92	85	80	100
Arg (%)	100	31	29	30	28	100

Figure 3. SDS-PAGE and loss(%) in lysine and arginine resi-
sues of lysozyme after incubation with 3DG for 3(B), 7(C),
14(D) and 28(E) days at 37°C in 0.2M phosphate buffer (pH
7.4); A, intact lysozyme; F, lysozyme incubated without
3DG (Kato et al., 1987b).

In the advanced-stage of the Maillard reaction, proteins polymerize with development of fluorescence and browning. In order to obtain a good indicator for the advanced-
stage reaction, BSA (0.3mM) was incubated with glucose (56
and 112mM) under the same condition for 7, 14 and 28 days,
and the reaction mixtures were hydrolyzed with 6N HCl at
95°C for 30 hours, and then fluorescent products in the hydrolysates were analyzed by high performance liquid chroma-
togrph (HPLC). Waters HPLC (Tokyo) and ODS-120T column
(Toyo Soda Co. Ltd., Japan), 4.6mm×25cm, were used, and 7mM
H_3PO_4 was used as a solvent and flow rate was 1ml/min. As
the experimental result, one peak named peak late number 1

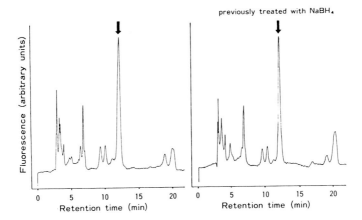

previously treated with NaBH₄

Figure 4. HPLC of Peak L₁ (arrows) in hydrolysates from BSA (0.3mM) incubated with glucose (112mM) at 37°C for 28 days with or without NaBH₄ pretreatment (Oimomi et al., 1988a). An excitation wavelength of 370nm and an emission one of 440nm were used according to Monnier et al. (1984).

Figure 5. HPLC of hydrolysates from rat aortas of 90 (A) and 50 (B) weeks of age; each arrow indicates Peak L₁ (Oimomi et al., 1988b).

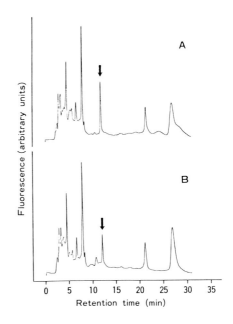

(Peak L_1) was selected; the height of this peak increased with glucose concentration and incubation time. Peak L_1 was eluted at a retention time of ca. 12 min and was not affected by treatment with sodium borohydride before acid hydrolysis, as shown in Fig. 4.

On the other hand, the Peak L_1 from in vivo samples was investigated. Abdominal aortas were resected from 5 rats each (Wistar ST strain, male) of ages 4, 14, 20, 33, 50, 70, 90 and 120 weeks. After adipose and connective tissues surrounding the aortas were stripped off, the aorta (50mg) was hydrolyzed. Figure 5 shows the examples of HPLC patterns of acid hydrolysates from rat aortas. Peak L_1 from rat aortas of 90 weeks of age was significantly higher than that from rats of 50 weeks of age.

Figure 6 shows the effect of age on the levels of Peak L_1 and furosine in the hydrolysates from the aortas of rats and on the level of glycated hemoglobin in the blood of the same rats. The level of furosine, which is an early-stage product, increased with aging to reach a maximum value in rats of 50 to 70 weeks of age and thereafter decreased. By contrast, the level of Peak L_1, which is a fluorescent advanced-stage product, reached a maximum value in rats of 90 weeks of age and remained at the maximum level in 120 weeks of age. On the other hand, the level of glycated hemoglobin showed no significant change with aging (Fig. 6). These results propose that Peak L_1 is useful as an indicator for evaluating the progress of the advanced-stage reaction. Peak L_1 was clearly detected also in human cataractous lens from diabetic patients and non-diabetic senile subjects (Oimomi et al., 1988a).

7) Formation of "Peak L_1" on the Reaction of Proteins with 3DG

In order to examine the role of 3DG in the formation of Peak L_1, lysozyme and BSA were incubated with 3DG of high purity in the concentration of 16.5 and 8.25mM under the same condition for 14 and 28 days. Figure 7 shows an example of HPLC pattern of the hydrolysate of a reaction mixture; lysozyme incubated with 3DG indicated the formation of Peak L_1, and the control incubated without 3DG also showed a small Peak L_1, suggesting that the lysozyme preparation had been partly glucosylated. Peak L_1 increased with incubation

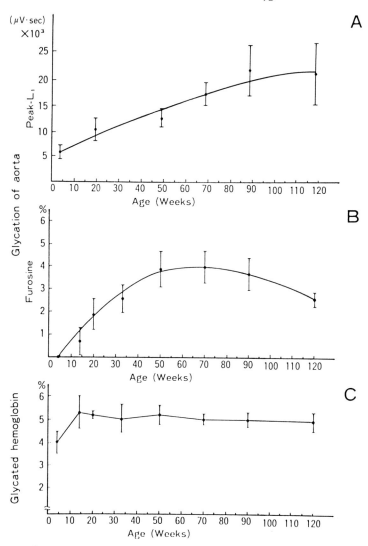

Figure 6. Effect of age of rats on the height of Peak L_1 and on the levels of furosine and glycated hemoglobin (Oimomi et al., 1988b). Height of Peak L_1 (A) was evaluated according to the method of Oimomi et al. (1988a); furosine content (B) was determined by using tyrosine as an standard according to the method of Schleicher and Wieland (1981); glycated hemoglobin (C) was determined by affinity column chromatography on a Glyc-Affin System (Isolab, Akron, Ohio).

time similarly as in the case of BSA-glucose reaction.

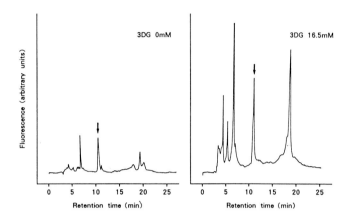

Figure 7. HPLC of Peak L_1 (arrows) in the hydrolysates of lysozyme (10mg/ml) incubated with 3DG (0 and 16.5mM) in 0.2M phosphate buffer (pH 7.4) at 37°C for 28 days.

The experimental results described above disclose that Peak L_1 is one of the major fluorescent products in the advanced-stage reaction and that 3DG is involved in the formation of Peak L_1 in vitro and in vivo. Chemical characterization of the fluorescent substance responsible for Peak L_1 is under way.

REFERENCES

Anet EFLJ (1960). Degradation of carbohydrates. I. Isolation of 3-deoxyhexosones. Australian J Chem 13:396-403.
Bunn HF, Higgins PJ (1981). Reaction of monosaccharides with proteins: possible evolutionary significance. Science 213:222-244.
Cho RK, Okitani A, Kato H (1985). Polymerization of proteins and impairment of their arginine residues due to intermediate compounds in the Maillard reaction. In Fujimaki M, Namiki M, Kato H (eds): "Amino-Carbonyl Reactions in Food and Biological Systems", Tokyo-Amsterdam: Kodansha-Elsevier, pp439-448.
Danehy JP (1986). Maillard reaction: Nonenzymatic browning in food systems with special reference to the development of flavor. Adv Food Res 30:77-138.

Kato H (1960). Studies on browning reactions between sugars and amino compounds. V. Isolation and characterization of new carbonyl compounds, 3-deoxyosones formed from N-glycosides and their significance for browning reaction. Bull Agric Chem Soc Japan 24:1-12.

Kato H (1962). Chemical studies on amino-carbonyl reaction. I. Isolation of 3-deoxypentosone and 3-deoxyhexosones formed by browning degradation of N-glycosides. Agric Biol Chem 26:187-192.

Kato H, Shin DB, Hayase F (1987b). 3-Deoxyglucosone crosslinks proteins under physiological conditions. Agric Biol Chem 51:2009-2011.

Kato H, Tsusaka N, Fujimaki M (1970). Isolation and identification of α-ketoaldehydes in calf and rabbit livers. Agric Biol Chem 34:1541-1548.

Kato H, Yamamoto M, Fujimaki M (1969). Mechanisms of browning degradation of D-fructose in special comparison with D-glucose-glycine reaction. Agric Biol Chem 33:939-948.

Kato H, Cho RK, Okitani A, Hayase F (1987a). Responsibility of 3-deoxyglucosone for the glucose-induced polymerization of proteins. Agric Biol Chem 51:683-689.

Kato H, Yamada Y, Izaka K, Sakurai Y (1961). Studies on browning mechanisms of soybean products. I. Separation and identification of 3-deoxyglucosone occurring in soysauce and miso. J Agric Chem Soc Japan 35:412-415.

Monnier VM, Cerami A (1983). Nonenzymatic glycosylation and browning of proteins in vivo. In Waller GR, Feather MS (eds): "Maillard Reaction in Foods and Nutrition", Washington, DC: American Chemical Society, pp431-449.

Monnier VM, Kohn RR, Cerami A (1984). Accelerated age-related browning to human collagen in diabetes mellitus. Proc Nat Acad Sci USA 81:583-587.

Oimomi M, Maeda Y, Hata F, Kitamura Y, Matsumoto S, Baba S, Iga T, Yamamoto M (1988a). Glycation of cataractous lens in non-diabetic senile subjects and in diabetic patients. Exp Eye Res 46:415-420.

Oimomi M, Maeda Y, Hata F, Kitamura Y, Matsumoto S, Hatanaka H, Baba S (1988b). A study of the age-related acceleration of glycation of tissue proteins in rats. J Gerontology 26: in press.

Okitani A, Cho RK, Kato H (1984). Polymerization of lysozyme and impairment of its amino acid residues caused by reaction with glucose. Agric Biol Chem 48:1801-1808.

Reynolds TM (1963). Chemistry of nonenzymic browning. I. The reaction between aldoses and amines. Adv Food Res 12:1-52.

Schleicher E, Wieland OH (1981). Specific quantitation by HPLC of protein (lysine) bound glucose in human serum albumin and other glycosylated proteins. J Clin Chem Clin Biochem 19:81-87.

Shin DB, Hayase F, Kato H (1988). Polymerization of proteins caused by reaction with sugars and the formation of 3-deoxyglucosone under physiological conditions. Agric Biol Chem 52:1451-1458.

Weber K, Osborn M (1969). The reliability of molecular weight determinations by dodecyl sulfate-polyacrylamide gel electrophoresis. J Biol Chem 244:4406-4412.

Wolfrom ML, Schuetz RD, Cavalieri LF (1948). Chemical interactions of amino compounds and sugars. III. The conversion of D-glucose to 5-(hydroxymethyl)-2-furaldehdye. J Amer Chem Soc 70:514-517.

The Maillard Reaction in Aging,
Diabetes, and Nutrition, pages 85–107
© 1989 Alan R. Liss, Inc.

THE CHEMISTRY OF THE MAILLARD REACTION UNDER PHYSIOLOGICAL CONDITIONS: A REVIEW

F. George Njoroge and Vincent M. Monnier
Institute of Pathology, School of Medicine, Case Western Reserve University Cleveland, Ohio 44106

ABSTRACT: The chemistry of the Maillard reaction is one of the most challenging to study due to its extreme complexity. When it comes to elucidating the structure of Maillard products bound to macromolecules, whether in foodstuffs or biological proteins, the difficulty becomes enormous. Although the structure of a variety of Maillard compounds has been elucidated in model systems at higher temperature, it is presently unknown to what extent they occur in vivo. Past and current approaches to obtain clues on the chemical nature of Maillard products formed under physiological conditions are reviewed.

INTRODUCTION

The discovery that nonenzymatic reactions between carbonyl groups of carbohydrates and free amino group on proteins, peptides, amino acids and organic amines can occur at physiological conditions of temperature, pH and concentration has aroused considerable interest in biomedical researchers working in the field of diabetes and aging. This reaction, commonly referred to as Maillard or nonenzymatic browning reaction, has been the subject of extensive review in the past (Hodge, 1953; Ellis, 1959; Paulsen, 1980). Several more recent reviews have focused on modification of proteins with greater emphasis on biological significance of this reaction (Harding, 1985; Brownlee, 1988; Kennedy and Baynes, 1984). However, although substantial amount of work has been undertaken in order to understand the biology of this reaction, relatively little progress has been achieved towards understanding the chemistry of the Maillard reaction under physiological conditions. For this reason, we have decided to review current knowledge in this area, hoping that it will serve as a frame for future research on the Maillard reaction in vivo.

BACKGROUND CHEMISTRY

The Maillard reaction can be divided into four steps namely: (1) The reversible formation of glycosylamine, (2) the Amadori rearrangement of the glycosylamine to the ketose-amine, 1-amino-1-deoxyketose, (3) degradation and dehydration of the amino sugar, and (4) reaction of amino groups with intermediates formed in step 4 and subsequent rearrangements to form advanced Maillard products. The sequence of these steps is outlined in figure 1. Steps 1 and 2 are commonly referred to as initial stages while 3 is an intermediate and 4 the final or late stage of Maillard reaction.

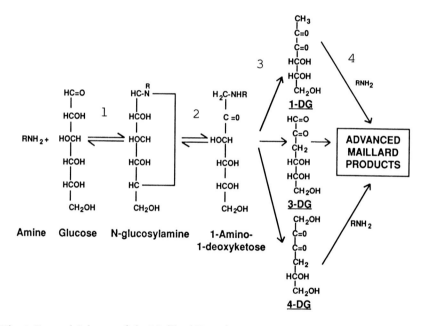

Fig. 1 General Scheme of the Maillard Reaction

FORMATION OF GLYCOSYLAMINES

Reducing sugars react with primary and secondary amines in non-polar or polar solvents (Hodge, 1953) and in absence of acid catalyst to give rise to N-substituted glycosylamines derivatives in which the glycosidic hydroxyl group is replaced by an amino group (Ellis, 1959), The reaction can be effected with alkyl- and arylamines, ammonia, esters of amino acids, and urea derivatives. Under acidic conditions, glycosylamines either undergo Amadori rearrangement to 1-amino-1-deoxy-2-ketoses or they are hydrolysed back to their starting materials i.e. glucose and amine (Paulsen, 1980). Glycosylamines have been of interest to pharmaceutical chemists in the field of nucleoside chemistry since nucleoside analogues can be formed via a reaction between the e.g. amino group of a pharmaceutical product and glucose (Paulsen, 1980).

FORMATION OF AMADORI PRODUCTS

One of the most extensively studied product resulting from non-enzymatic glycosylation is the ketoamine which is formed via Amadori rearrangement of glycosylamines (Hodge, 1953, 1955). The interest in the study of this product stems from the fact that its presence has been confirmed and well characterized in proteins such as hemoglobin, whereby the level of glycated hemoglobin was found to be a useful measure of average glycemia over several weeks (Koenig et al. 1976). Other proteins which are also known to be modified by formation of this ketoamine are plasma membranes, lipoproteins, lens crystallins, extracellular matrix and nerve protein to mention just a few. The biomedical aspects of nonenzymatic glycosylation have been recently reviewed (Brownlee et al. 1988) and a discussion of the Amadori product in proteins is provided by Baynes in this volume.

DEGRADATION OF AMADORI PRODUCTS

Although the Amadori product is a rather stable compound, with time, it undergoes a number of transformations as shown in Figure 1. At higher pH, the 1-amino-deoxy-ketose enolizes in position 2-3 and eliminates the amine from C-1 to form 1-deoxyglucosone (1-DG) (Anet, 1964). At lower pH, the ketoamine undergoes a 1-2 enolization leading to the formation of 3-deoxyglucosone (3-DG). Another diketone formed through this pathway is 4-deoxyglucosone (4-DG) (Fig. 1).

Of the three dicarbonyl compounds mentioned above, 3-deoxyglucosone has so far received the greatest attention. Although it was first suggested by Nef (1910) as an intermediate in the formation of metasaccharinic acids, direct experimental evidence was obtained by Machell and Richards (1960) who isolated this compound as an amorphous powder from treatment of 3-O-benzyl sugar with sodium hydroxide. It has also been prepared from the action of acid on fructose (Anet, 1962; 1962b). Kato (1960; 1962) reported isolation of the 2,4-dinitrophenylhydrazone of 3-DG and its free form by heating N-butyl-D-glucosamine in acetic acid. Other workers who recently reported improved synthesis of 3-DG are Madson and Feather (1981), and Khadem et. al.(1972). In biological systems, 3-DG has been isolated from beef liver by Eguyd (1972). Of interest is that the liver contains enzymes that can metabolize 3-DG (Hata et al. 1988). This points out to the presence of a biological defense mechanism against the advanced Maillard reaction.

1-deoxyglucosone (1-DG) is a lesser studied diketone. It has been identified as an intermediate in the formation of D-glucosaccharinic acid by Ishizu et. al. (1967) In a recent paper, Beck et. al. (1988) described the isolation of this diketone as a quinoxaline derivative from the degradation of 1-deoxy-1-piperidino-D-fructose and the subsequent reaction with O-phenylenediamine. This latter procedure might be a useful tool for quantitation of deoxyglucosones in biological specimens.

Of the three dicarbonyls described, 4-deoxyglucosone is the least known. So far it has not been isolated from Maillard degradation products but a preparation method has been described by Machell and Richards (1960).

The three deoxy compounds described above, either degrade to form compounds such as furfuraldehyde (Taufel and Iwainsky, 1952), reductones (Hodge and Rist, 1952), pyranones (Mills et al. 1970) or react further with amino groups to form compounds such as pyrroles (Kato and Fujimaki (1968), pyridines (Pachmayr et al., 1986) and pyrrolinone reductones (Ledl and Fritsch, 1984). These late products of Maillard reactions are UV active but are generally not colored. On standing, they may react further with amines or other carbonyls to form brown, fluorescent compounds, the structure of which is poorly understood. Some of these colored compounds are melanoidins, i.e. highly polymerized nitrogenous substances which are unlikely to be found in vivo.

One of the major problems biological chemists are facing when searching for the presence of advanced Maillard products in vivo is that the model compounds described in food science have been obtained using reaction conditions that were non-physiological. In addition, the relative abundance of each of these compounds is generally low, thus making the task of selecting a particular model for in vivo investigation very difficult. Below, we describe our approach towards elucidation of the structure of glucose-derived advanced Maillard compounds formed under physiological conditions.

REACTION BETWEEN SUGARS AND AMINES AT PHYSIOLOGICAL CONDITIONS

In order to alleviate the difficulties associated with isolation and purification of Maillard compounds of ε-amine lysine, neopentylamine was used as a substitute (Njoroge et al., 1987a). Neopentylamine was chosen because it allowed unequivocal structural assignments by proton and ^{13}C-NMR. Neopentylamine was incubated with glucose in sodium phosphate buffer at 37°C and the reaction mixture was monitored for formation of UV absorbing chromophores at 254 nm. Figure 2 shows an HPLC chromatogram of samples analyzed at various times using a Vydac C-18 reverse phase column and acetonitrile/water as eluting solvent. From these chromatograms, it was evident that a wide range of compounds with varying degree of polarity were formed.

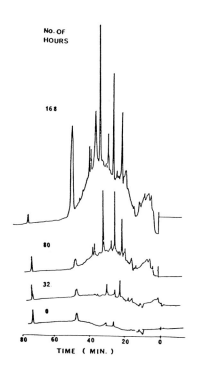

Fig. 2. HPLC profile of the reaction mixture of glucose and neopentylamine at 37°C and pH 7.2. (unpublished).

However, some compounds were predominant and their isolation and characterizization was pursued. Upon removal of the high molecular weight polymerized compounds by filtration, the less polar compounds were portioned between petroleum ether and dimethyl ether. The two fractions were then subjected to flash chromatography using hexane/ethyl-acetate in combinations as shown below:

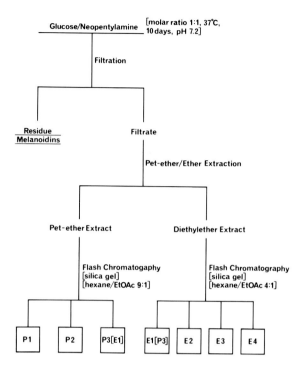

Fig. 3. Isolation of advanced Maillard products from the reaction of glucose with neopentylamine under physiological conditions.

Using this procedure we were able to isolate 3 major pyrrole compounds i.e. compounds 1, 2, and 3, and a gamma-pyranone E 2 (Njoroge et al., 1987b).

Although these four compounds had previously been detected in reaction mixtures at higher temperatures (Arnodi et al. 1987; Lewis et al., 1947, Cerrutti et al., 1985) this was the first report of their formation at physiological conditions.

From the same reaction mixture, an additional compound, 5, was obtained and fully characterized using ^{13}C-NMR, MS, IR, and UV spectroscopy (Njoroge et al., 1987b):

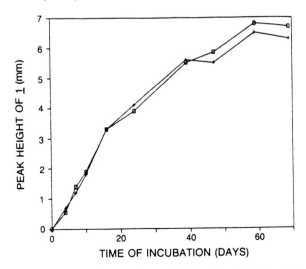

Compound 5, 3-(D-erythro-trihydroxypropyl)-1-neopentyl pyrrole-2-carboxaldehyde was found to form at the same rate either in oxygen or nitrogen thus excluding a fragmentation mechanism dependent oxygen radicals (figure 4). Its mechanism of formation was postulated to proceed via condensation of 3-deoxyglucosone with glycolaldehyde, followed by reaction with amino group of neopentylamine and subsequent dehydration. However, it is also possible that it may have formed from fragmentation of the glucosyl pyrrole 6 recently described by Farmar et. al.(1988).

Fig. 4. Kinetics of formation of glucosyl pyrrole 5 under air (□) and nitrogen with EDTA (+). From Njoroge et al. (1987). J. Carbohydr. Chem. 6:553:568.

The pyrrole compounds described above (i.e., 1, 2, 3, 5) represent advanced glycosylated end products of Maillard reaction. They all contain a functional group that is capable of reacting further to give rise to crosslinking compounds as shown below (Fig. 5). To investigate whether such molecules can form in biological systems, Hayase et al. (1989) have used an immunological approach to detect the pyrrole carboxaldehyde 5. This approach was necessary since acid hydrolysis destroyed the compound thus precluding its quantitation in proteins. Enzyme-linked immunosorbent assay of this molecule, now given the trivial name "pyrraline", indicates that it is found in increased amounts in albumin from diabetic subjects.

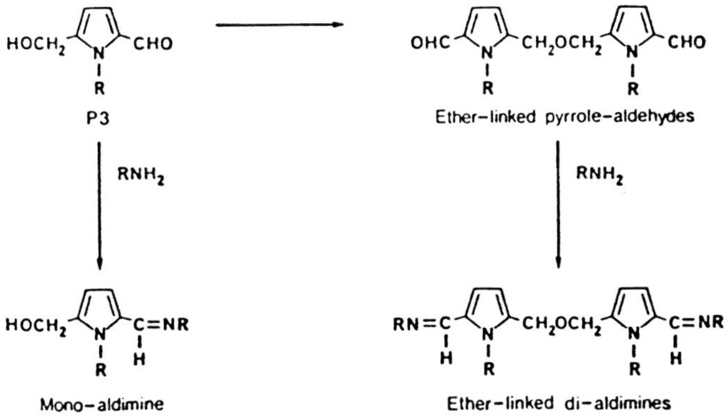

Fig. 5. Possible crosslinks of pyrraline.

The potential biological significance of glucose-derived pyrroles is apparent from comparison with toxicity resulting from chronic exposure to hexane. In this condition, 2,5-hexanedione is formed which reacts with amines of axonal proteins (DeCaprio, 1982 & 1986), thus leading to neurotoxic disease (Allen et al. 1985) (Figure 6). Hexane-induced neuropathy may serve as a model for diabetic neuropathy whereby glucose-derived instead of hexane-derived pyrrole would modify neurofilaments in diabetic neuropathy.

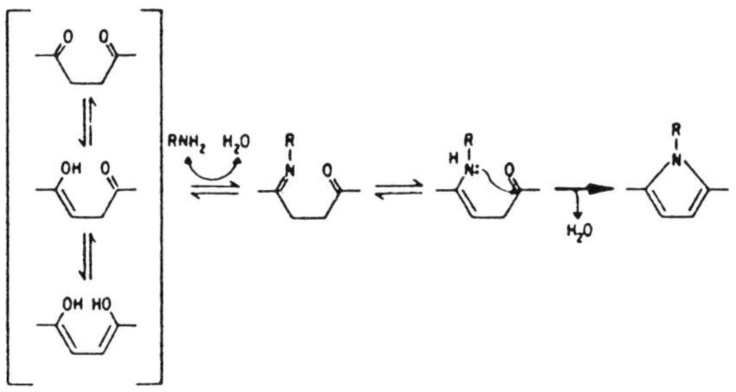

Fig. 6. Formation of pyrrole in the reaction of 2,5-hexanedione with primary amines (from Graham et al. (1982) Toxicol. Appl. Pharmacol. 64:415)

It has further been documented that hexane-derived pyrroles can undergo autoxidation (DeCaprio, 1986) and induce formation of inter or intramolecular protein crosslinks (Graham et al., 1982). The nature of the crosslinked chromophores is still poorly understood. However, in a study of reaction between ethanolamine and 2,5-hexanedione Graham et.al (1982) detected formation of 1-(2-hydroxyethyl)-2, 5-dimethylpyrrole. The latter pyrrole was found to autooxidize forming an orange, sodium borohydride reducible chromophore that showed maxima at 320 and 445 nm.

Pyrrolic chromphores were also observed when BSA or ovalbumin were reacted with various diketones; polyacrylamide gel electrophoresis revealed that these proteins had polymerized to form dimers, trimers, tetramers and higher-order polymers. The presence of pyrrole compounds in biological system has triggered considerable of interest because of the ease with which these five-membered heterocycles are formed from diketones.In a recent study, Lynn et.al.(1987) isolated and characterized pyrrole compound 7 from the roots of pisum sativum. It is possible that pyrrole compound 7 is derived from the reaction of glucose and homoserine, and these investigators propose that it may have cell cycle regulatory properties.

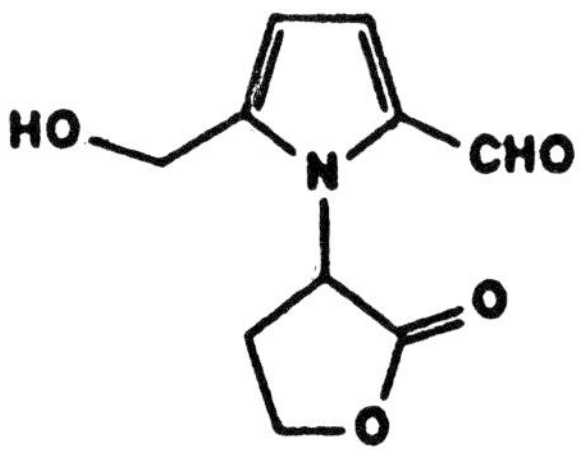

7

Other interests in pyrrole compounds stem up from the fact that lysyl pyrraline (carboxaldehyde pyrrole 3) has been found to be a competitive inhibitor of both aminopeptidase N and carboxypeptidase A (Oeste, 1987). This antiproteolytic property may influence the utilization of dietary proteins if this pyrrole is present in sufficient amount of the diet.

Finally it has been shown by Yen and Lee (1986) that nitroso derivatives of 2-acetylpyrrole, pyrrole 2-carboxaldehyde, and pyrrole 2-carboxylic acid are mutagenic. Omura and coworkers (1984) have also shown lysyl pyrraline to be mutagenic. The formation of such mutagen in food may have important implications for food safety since chronic ingestion of such foods might contribute to carcinogenesis in the gastrointestinal tract.

REACTION BETWEEN SUGARS AND AMINO ACIDS AT PHYSIOLOGICAL CONDITIONS

Reaction of amino acids with sugars differ from those of amines or peptides in two ways: (a) their acidity facilitates formation of Amadori product without the need of adjusting the pH to lower values (Finot, 1969) (b) the α-amino group reacts easily with α-dicarbonyl compounds rendering the amino acid prone to oxidative decarboxylation through a Strecker degradation (Nyhammar, 1983). Through this degradation, the amino group is transferred to the carbonyl compound which is thereby reduced and the remaining part of the α-amino acid is converted into an aldehyde.

Two of the most widely used model systems for study of the Maillard reaction between amino acids and sugars at 37°C are the reaction between either glycine or lysine with sugars. Borsook and Wasteneys (1925) investigated the reaction between glycine and glucose, glucose 6-phosphate, fructose, fructose 6-phosphate and found it to be highly accelerated by the presence of phosphate buffer. Glucose 6-phosphate was the most reactive in terms of brown color formed. Fructose was less reactive than glucose except in the case of unbuffered solutions where fructose was found to give more brown color than glucose. The implication of fructose in the Maillard reaction is of particular importance to diabetes since fructose levels are increased as a consequence of activated aldose reductase pathway. Recent studies on modification of proteins by fructose are discussed by G. Suarez and D. Walton in this volume (See also: Suarez et al., 1988,

McPherson et al. 1988). Burton and coworkers (1963) examined closely the development of chromophores in glucose-glycine and sucrose-glycine systems. Through organic solvent extraction, using ether, trichloroethylene and cyclohexanone, this group quantitated extractable material at successive stages of the reaction and examined, among other things, the development of the larger darker compounds from the smaller, less colored compounds. They found that during these reactions a number of conjugated, unsaturated compounds that were reactive towards phenylhydrazine were formed. They also found that while sulfites slowed down the rate of formation of these conjugated unsaturated carbonylic and fluorescent compounds, presence of sodium pyrophosphate seemed to increase their rate of production. Presence of iron also accelerated the rate of formation of these chromophores, apparently by a mechanism different from that observed with phosphates.

In the sucrose-glycine system, Burton et al (1963) also found a reaction pathway analogous to that of glucose-glycine with the difference that in the early stages of browning there were indications of a rapid utilization of the fructose formed.

In a more recent study, Hashiba (1986) reported formation of 2-hydroxy-2, 5-dihydroxy-1(4-pyridone) acetic acid 8 from the reaction of fructose-glycine under atmospheric oxygen and in presence of Fe(II). Compound 8 had a max at 298 which changed according to pH.

Benzing-Purdie and Nikiforuk (1985) have isolated the enaminol compound <u>9</u> shown above from the reaction of xylose and glycine in high yields using Sephadex G-10 gel chromatography.

Reaction between the ε-amino group of lysine with various sugars has always been of interest to researchers in food sciences since the modification of this group renders lysine chemically and nutritionally unavailable (Bujard & Finot, 1978). In biological systems, amino groups of lysine have been found to progressively decline as proteins such as serum albumin are incubated with glucose (Mohammad et al., 1949).

In 1951, Patton and Chism studied the reaction between α-N-acetyllysine with glucose at 37°C using paper chromatography. They identified four compounds, one of which gave a bright purple fluorescence under a ultra-violet light and, on elution, showed a pronounced peak at 288 nm. The precise chemical nature of these compounds remained undetermined. Subsequently, Hannan and Lea (1952) studied in more details the reaction between the free terminal amino groups of polypeptide-bound lysine and glucose without the side effects introduced by the presence of other reactive groups. Reaction conditions included (a) initial pH at 6.3 (b) 37°C (c) only a small excess of glucose and (d) controlled low water content obtained by freeze-drying and equilibrating with known relative humidities. Although the precise mechanism of the reaction between glucose and lysine, was not elucidated these researchers found many similarities with the reaction of casein and polylysine. A primary colorless reaction product formed which upon isolation and storage produced browning and insolubility. Retrospectively, it is likely that this product might have been the Amadori product of glucose.

More recently, Candiano and coworkers (1985) have studied the reactivities of amino acids with trioses and hexoses under physiological conditions. The most reactive species were found to be lysine, glyceraldehyde, and 2-amino-2-deoxyglucosone. Yellow, oligomeric compounds having molecular weights in the range 500-1000 daltons and pI values from 4 to 6 were obtained. In the lysine-glyceraldehyde adduct, the ε-amino group was found to be incorporated into pyrrole-type structure as evidenced by a positive Pauly reagent test.

REACTION OF GLUCOSE WITH PEPTIDES AND PROTEINS AT PHYSIOLOGICAL CONDITIONS

Because of its relevance to diabetic complications, the reaction between glucose, peptides and proteins was studied in great detail and several reviews on the subject have already been published (Kennedy & Baynes, 1984, Brownlee 1988). Therefore, we shall focus below mainly on a few studies which stress the chemical nature of the modified residue.

Conclusive evidence for the formation of Amadori products in hemoglobin was obtained by Koenig et. al. (1975) who demonstrated using ^{1}H-NMR spectroscopy the structural identity between 1-deoxyfructosyl valyl histidine isolated from the B-chain of HbA_{Ic} and the synthetic Amadori product of valylhistidine. Amadori products, however, were also found to form in the reaction between glyceraldehyde and hemoglobin S in which glyceralehyde was being evaluated as potential anti-sickling agent (Acharya & Manning, 1980 a,b).

Formation of di-hexosyl adducts was noted to occur between the ϵ-amino group of the tripeptide Ac-Tyr-Lys-Gly-NHz acetate and sodium glucuronate under physiological conditions. The major product was the sodium salt of Actyr-N-(D-arabino-5-carboxy-5-carboxy-2,3,4,5,-tetratrydro-1-pentenyl)-N-(D-arabino-5-carboxy-3,4,5-trihydroxy-2-oxopentylidene) Lys-Gly-NHz <u>10</u> (Takeda, 1977). The structure was elucidated on the basis of ^{1}H and ^{13}C NMR, UV spectra, and pH titration. The structure of compound <u>10</u> shown here reveals two sugars bound to an amino group via a conjugated enol-ketolimmonium structure. It is unknown whether the compound is fluorescent.

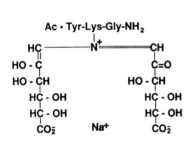

<u>10</u>

Although numerous studies have been devoted to the chemistry and biology of protein-bound Amadori products, few studies have been carried out to elucidate the precise structure of protein-bound Maillard products. This may be attributable to the extraordinary difficulty associated with structure elucidation of adducts and crosslinks of nonenzymatically browned proteins.

The possibility that nonenzymatic browning of proteins might occur in vivo was catalyzed by the observation that lens crystallins incubated at 37°C with hexoses underwent browning and crosslinking as observed in aging human and cataractous lenses (Monnier and Cerami, 1981). The presence, in the human lens, of a borohydride reducible molecule that co-cochromatographed with a similar molecule isolated from the brown reaction mixture of glucose and ϵ-amino lysine was detected but its structure remains unknown (Monnier and Cerami, 1983).

Two groups have used poly-L-lysine to investigate the structure of advanced products of the Maillard reaction. Pongor and coworkers (1984)incubated polylysine or bovine serum albumin with glucose for 28 days and observed gradual increase in absorbance as well as in fluorescence at 440nm upon excitation at 370nm. The polypeptide was acid hydrolyzed and the dry residue was basified with ammonium hydroxide. A deep yellow compound was extracted into chloroform and structure elucidation revealed presence of a furoyl imidazole (FFI). Further investigation on the mechanism of formation of the compound, however, revealed that it is formed from acid hydrolyzed Amadori products via condensation between free ammonia and furyl glyoxal that are released from the glycated protein (Njoroge et al. 1988).

Boissel and coworkers (1986) have also used poly-L-lysine as a model protein to study the relationship between fluorescence and polymerization. On incubating polylysine with glucose at 37°C in sodium phosphate buffer (pH 7.4), they observed a gradual increase in both fluorescence and polymerization of polylysine. When glycated polymer was incubated in the presence of [^{3}H]-L-Lysine, lysine was found to be rapidly incorporated into the glycated polylysine with subsequent release of a fluorescent low molecular weight component and depolymerization. The structure of the fluorescent molecule remains unknown.

The ability of glucose to form crosslinks and to impair protein function was studied in detail by Eble and coworkers (1983) using RNase as a model. Analysis of the modified protein by sodium dodecyl sulfate polyacrylamide gel electrophoresis revealed a time dependent formation of dimer and trimer. Polymerization rate was first order with respect to glucose, but was approximately first order with respect to protein concentration. Overall, their results supported the following type of reaction scheme for glucose - dependent crosslinking of proteins under physiological conditions:

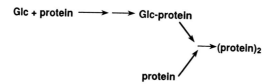

The structure of the crosslink was not elucidated in this study. Additional studies were carried out by the same group to characterize the conformation of the Amadori product, and the target amino acids as a in function of reaction conditions. Based on the intensity of the various ^{13}C-NMR resonances, demonstration was made that the pyranose conformation was predominant (Neglia et al. 1983 & 1985). In further experiments, it was noted that phosphate led to an enhanced rate of inactivation of the enzyme relative to the rate of modification of lysine residues, suggesting preferential modification of active site residues (Watkins et al., 1985, Ahmed, 1984). The ϵ-amino group of lys-1 was identified as the primary site (80-90%) of initial Schiff base formation of RNase. In contrast, lys-41 and lys-7 in the active site accounted for about 38% and 29%, respectively, of ketoamine adducts formed via the Amadori rearrangement. Other sites reactive in ketoamine formation included N-α-lys-1 (15%), N-ϵ-lys-1 (9%) and lys-37 (9%) which are adjacent to acidic amino acids. The remaining six lysine residues, which are located on the surface of the molecule, were found to be relatively inactive in forming either Schiff base or Amadori adduct. The kinetics of glycation and inactivation of RNase were substantially faster in phosphate buffer than in TAPSO, an organic, cationic buffer. This was explained by a phosphate catalyzed preferential modification of lysyl residues in the active site.

In studies on events occurring during the later stages of the Maillard reaction, Ahmed and coworkers (1984) have identified N-carboxymethyllysine (CML) as an oxidative degradation product of Amadori compounds. CML accounted for about 35% of total glycated of lysine residues in lysozyme after a 4 week incubation. The formation of CML requires oxygen, and the reaction proceeds by a metal catalyzed, free radical mechanism (Figure 7).

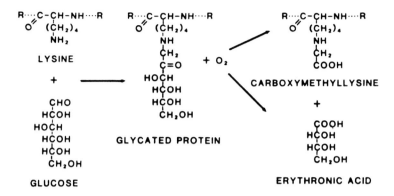

Fig. 7. Formation of N ε-carboxymethyl - lysine from glycated protein. (From Ahmed et al. J. Biol. Chem. 261:4889-4894, 1986).

Only trace amounts of CML were detectable in incubations carried out under nitrogen or in the presence of strong chelators. CML has been identified in human urine (Wadman et al. 1975) and in hydrolysates of human lens proteins (Ahmed et al., 1986), suggesting that degradation of glycated proteins to CML takes place in vivo. In another study, Liardon and coworkers (1987) have identified CML in urine samples from various groups of rats on the basis of mass spectral and capillary GC retention data. Urinary concentration of CML varied in relation to composition of the diet. Thus, additional studies will be needed to assess dietary versus endogenous production of CML, if CML is to be used as a marker for oxidative mechanisms in vivo.

In most of the studies on the reaction of sugars with proteins at physiological conditions, there has been no single report that identifies the specific compounds formed during the advanced stage of the Maillard reaction. However, in studies with Ehrlich's reagent, Scott and coworkers (1983) could detect the presence of an Ehrlich's chromogen in collagen cross-links which seems to be of pyrrolic nature. Using Pauly's reagent Ghiggeri and associates (1985) were also able to detect pyrrole formation in human serum albumin that had been reacted with aldoses (C_3-C_6) at 37°C. Although a positive Ehrlich's test supports the existence of protein-bound pyrrole in glucose incubated protein, the origin of collagen-bound pyrroles remains to be determined. Nevertheless, these results are in agreement with the recent immunological detection of pyrraline in albumin from diabetic subjects (Hayase et al., 1989).

Finally, Oimomi et al. (1988a) recently reported the presence of a fluorescent peak (peak L_1) with excitation/emission maxima at 370/440 nm in the reverse phase chromatogram of acid hydrolysate of bovine serum albumin incubated with glucose at 37°C. The peak increased with incubation time and with glucose concentration. Due to the inability of sodium borohydride reduction to prevent the formation of peak L_1, the authors concluded that the fluorescent molecule is an advanced product of the Maillard reaction. A similar peak was detected in senile and cataractous human lenses and in aortic collagen from senescent rats (Oimomi et al. (1988b).

CONCLUSION

Substantial amount of research has been done since Maillard first reported his finding in 1912. Most of the work has been centered on characterizing the early products of the browning reaction, particularly with proteins. Yet, relatively little information on structures of advanced Maillard products with physiological sugars is available. For use as probes of the Maillard reaction in vivo, many of the compounds described in model systems will need to be synthesized from the target amino acids, chemically stabilized if necessary or used as hapten such that antibodies can be raised for their detection in vivo. With exception of preliminary data on protein-bound pyrroles in diabetes, the structure of browned proteins is yet unknown. The slow progress in structure elucidation of advanced products of the Maillard reaction is attributable to various factors that include the complexity of the reaction products, often their lability to acid hydrolysis, their presence in low yields and the generation of multitude of artefacts during the hydrolytic steps that are necessary for their isolation.

ACKNOWLEDGEMENTS

This work was supported by grants AG 05601 and AG 06927 from the National Institute on Aging and grant EY07099 from the National Eye Institute.

REFERENCES

Acharya AS, Manning JM (1980). Amadori rearrangement of glyceraldehyde-hemoglobin schiff base adducts. J Biol Chem 255:7218-7224.

Acharya AS, Manning JM (1980). Reactivity of the amino groups of carbomonoxyhemoglobin S with glyceraldehyde. J Biol Chem 255:1406-1412.

Ahmed MU, Thorpe SR, Baynes JW (1986). Identification of N^{ϵ}-carboxymethyllysine a degradation product of fructose lysine in glycated protein. J Biol Chem 261:4889-4894.

Allen N, Mendell JR, Billmaier DJ, Fontaine, RE O'Neil (1975). Toxic polyneuropathy due to methyl n-butyl ketone. Arch Neurol 32: 209-218.

Anet EFLJ (1962). Formation of furan compounds from sugars. Chem Ind (London) 262.

Anet EFLJ (1962b). Thin layer chromatography of 2,4-dinitrophenylhydrazine derivatives of hydroxycarbonyl compounds. J Chromatog 9:291.

Anet EGLJ (1964). 3-Deoxyglycosuloses (3-deoxy-glucosones) and the degradation of carbohydrates. Adv Carbohydr Chem 19:181-218.

Arnodi A, Arnodi C, Baldi O, Griffin A (1987). Strecker degradation of leucine and valine in a lipidic model system. J Agric Food Chem 35:1035-1038.

Beck J, Ledl F, Severin T (1988). Formation of 1-deoxy-D-erythro-2,3-hexodiulose from Amadori compounds. Carbohydr Res 178:240-243.

Benzing-Purdie L, Nikiforuk JH (1985). Reaction of xylose and glycines: Identification of the major water soluble component. J Carbohydr Chem 4:15-27.

Boissel JP, Kasper T, Bunn HF (1986). Protein crosslinking during in vitro non-enzymatic glycation In: Amino-Carbonyl Reactions in Food and Biological Systems Fujimaki M Namiki M Kato H (Eds) 1986 Kodansha Ltd. pp 433-438.

Borsook H, Wasteneys H (1925). The interaction of free amino-nitrogen and glucose. Biochem J 19:1128-1137.

Brownlee M, Cerami A, Vlassara H (1988). Advanced glycosylation end products in tissue and the biochemical basis of diabetic complications. N Engl J Med 318:1315-1321.

Bujard E, Finot PA (1978). Mesure de la disponibilite et du blocage de la lysine dans les laits industriels. Ann Nutr Alim 32:291-305.

Burton HS, McWeeny DJ, Biltcliffe DO (1963). Non-enzymic browning; Development of chromophores in the glucose-glycine and sucrose-glycine systems. J Fd Sci 28:631

Cerrutti P, Resnik SL, Seldes A, Fontan CF (1985). Kinectics of deteriorative reactions in model food systems of high water activity. Glucose loss, 5-HMF accumlation and fluorescence development due to nonenzymatic browning. J Fd Sci 50:627-630.

Candiano G, Ghiggeri GM, Delfino G, Quierolo C, Cuniberti C, Gianazza E, Righetti PG (1985). Reaction of lysine with aldoses. Carbohydr Res 145:99-112.

DeCaprio AP (1986). Mechanism of in vitro pyrrole adduct autoxidation in 2,5 hexanedione treated protein. Mol Pharmacol 30:452-458.

DeCaprio AP, Olajos EJ, Weber P (1982). Covalent binding of a neurotoxic n-hexane metabolite Conversion of primary amines to substituted pyrrole adducts by 2,5-hexane-dione. Toxicol Appl Pharmacol 65:440-450.

Eguyd LG (1972). The isolation of 3-deoxy-D-erythro-hexos-2-ulose from beef livers. Carbohydr Res 23:307-310.

Eble AS, Thorpe SR, Baynes JW (1983). Nonenzymatic glucosylation and glucose-dependent crosslinking of protein. J Biol Chem 258:9406-9412.

Ellis GP (1959). The Maillard reaction. Adv Carbohydr Chem 14:63-133.

Farmar JG, Ulrich PC, Cerami A (1988). Novel pyrroles from sulfite-inhibited Maillard reactions Insight into the mechanism of inhibition. J Org Chem 53:2346-2349.

Finot PA, Mauron J (1969). Le blocage de la lysine par la reaction de Maillard I Synthese de N-(desoxy-1-D-fructosyl-1)-et N-(Desoxy-1-D-lactulosyl-1)-L-lysines. Helv Chim Acta 52:1488-1494.

Ghiggeri GM, Candiano G, Delfino G, Queirolo C, Vecchio G, Gianazza E, Righetti PG (1985). Reaction of human serum albumin with aldoses. Carbohydr Res 145:113-122.

Graham DG, Anthony DC, Boekelheide K, Maschmann NA, Richards RG, Wolfram JW, Shaw BR (1982). Studies of the molecular pathogenesis of hexane neuropathy II Evidence that pyrrole derivatization of lysyl residues leads to protein crosslinking. Toxicol Appl Pharmacol 64:415-422.

Hannan RS, Lea CH (1952). Studies of the reaction between proteins and reducing sugars in the 'dry' state. VI The reactivity of the terminal amino groups of lysine in model systems. Biochem Biophys Acta 9:293-305.

Harding JJ (1985). Nonenzymatic covalent posttranslational modification of proteins in vivo. Adv Protein Chem 37:247-334.

Hashiba H (1986). Oxidative browning of Amadori compounds-color formation by iron with Maillard reaction products In: Amino-Carbonyl Reactions in Food and Biological Systems Fujimaki H Namiki M Kato H Eds Kodansha Ltd p 155.

Hata F, Igaki N, Nakamichi T, Masuda S, Nishimoto S, Oimomi M, Baba S, Kato H (1988). Suppressive effect of α-ketoaldehyde dehydrogenase on the advanced process of the Maillard reaction. Diab Res Clin Pract 5:5413

Hayase F, Nagaraj RH, Miyata S, Njoroge FG, Monnier VM (1989). Aging of proteins: immunological detection of a glucose-derived pyrrole formed during Maillard reaction in vivo. J Biol Chem (In press).

Hodge JE (1955). The Amadori rearrangement. Adv Carbohydr Chem 10:169-205.

Hodge JE, Rist CE (1953). The Amadori rearrangement under new conditions and its significance for non-enzymatic browning reactions. J Amer Chem Soc 1953 75:316-322.

Hodge JE (1953). Chemistry of browning reactions in model systems. J Agric Food Chem 1:928-943.

Hodge JE, Rist CE (1952). N-Glycosyl derivatives of secondary amines. J Am Chem Soc 74:1494-1499.

Ishuzu A, Linderberg B, Theander O (1967). 1-Deoxy-D-erythro-2, 3-hexodiulose an intermediate in the formation of D-glucosaccharinic acid. Carbohydr Res 1967 5:329-334.

Kato H (1962). Chemical studies on amino-carbonyl reaction: Part I Isolation of 3-deoxypentosone and 3-deoxyhexosones formed by browning degradation of N-glycosides. Agr Biol Chem (Tokyo) 26:187-191.

Kato H (1960). Studies on browning reactions between sugars and amino compounds. Isolation and characterization of new carbonyl compounds, 3-deoxyosones formed from N-glycosides and their significance for browning reaction. Agric Biol Chem (Tokyo) 24:1-12.

Kato H, Fujimaki M (1968). Formation of N-substituted pyrrole-2-aldehydes in the browning reaction between D-xylose and amino compounds. J Fd Sci 33:445-449.

Kennedy L, Baynes JW (1984). Nonenzymatic glycosylation and the chronic complications of diabetes: an overview. Diabetologia 26:93-98.

Khadem H, EL Horton D, Meshreki MH, Nashed MA (1971). New route for the synthesis of 3-deoxyaldos-2-uloses. Carbohydr Res 17:183-192.

Koenig RJ, Peterson CM, Jones RL, Lehrman M, Cerami A (1976). Correlation of glucose regulation and hemoglobin A_{Ic} in diabetes mellitus. New Engl J Med 295:417-420.

Koenig RJ, Cerami A (1975). Synthesis of hemoglobin A_{Ic} in normal and diabetic mice: potential model of basement membrane thickening. Proc Natl Acad Sci USA 72:3687-3691

Ledl F, Fritsch G (1984). Formation of pyrrolinone reductones by heating hexose with amino acids. Z. Lebensm Unters Forsch 178:41-44.

Ledl F, Fritsch G, Severin T (1982). Melthylene reductinic acid: a new reductone from glucose. Z Lebensm Unters Forsch 175:208-210.

Lewis NR, Doty DM (1947). Partial characterization of a compound involved in blackening of white potatoes. J Am Chem Soc 27:521-523.

Liardon R, Weck-Gaudard D, Philippossian G, Finot PA (1987). Identification of N^{ϵ}- carboxymethylysine: A new Maillard reaction product in rat urine. J Agric Food Chem 35:427-431.

Lynn DG, Jaffe K, Cornwall M, Tramontano W (1987). Characterization of an endogenous factor controlling the cell cycle of complex tissues. J Am Chem Soc 109:5858-5859.

Machell G, Richards GN (1960). Mechanism of saccharinic acid formation Part II The αß-dicarbonyl intermediate in formation of D-glucometasaccharinic acid. J Chem Soc 1932-1944.

Machell G, Richards GN (1960). Mechanism of saccharinic acid formation Part III The α-keto-aldehyde intermediate in formation of D-glucometasacharinic acid. J Chem Soc 1945-1950.

Madson MA, Feather MS (1981). An improved preparation of 3-deoxy-D-erythro-hexos- 2-ulose via the bis (benzoylhydrazone) and some related constitutional studies. Carbohydr Res 94:183-191.

McPherson JD, Shilton B, Walton DJ (1988). Role of fructose in glycation and crosslinking of proteins. Biochemistry 27:1901-1907.

Mills FD, Wersleder D, Hodge JE (1970). 2,3-Dihydro-3,5-dihydroxy-6-methyl-4H-pyran-4-one, a novel nonenzymatic browning product. Tet Lett 15:1243-1246.

Mohammad A, Fraenkel-Conrat H, Olcott HS (1949). The "browning" reaction of proteins with glucose. Arch Biochem Biophys 24:157-163.

Monnier VM, Cerami A (1981). Nonenzymatic browning in vivo: possible aging process for long-lived proteins. Science 211:491-493.

Monnier VM, Cerami A Detection of nonenzymatic browning products in the human lens. Biochem Biophys Acta 760:97-103.

Nef JU (1910). Dissoziationsvorgaenge in der Zuckergruppe, Ueber das Verhalten der Zuckerarten gegen Aetzalkalien. Ann 376:1-118.

Neglia CI, Cohen HJ, Garber AR, Thorpe SR, Baynes JW (1985). Characterization of glycated proteins by ^{13}C NMR spectroscopy. J Biol Chem 260:5406-5410.

Neglia CI, Cohen HJ, Garber AR, Ellis PD, Thorpe SR, Baynes JW (1983). ^{13}C NMR investigation on nonenzymatic glucosylation of protein: Model studies using RNaseA. J Biol Chem 258:14279-14283.

Njoroge FG, Fernandes AA, Monnier VM (1987b). 3-(D-Erythro-trihydroxypropyl)-1-neopentyl pyrrole-2-carboxaldehyde, a novel nonenzymatic browning product of glucose. J Carbohydr Chem 6:553-568.

Njoroge FG, Fernades AA, Monnier VM (1988). Mechanism of formation of the putative advanced glycosylation and protein cross-link 2-(2-furoyl)-4 (5)-(2-furanyl)-1H-imidazole. J Biol Chem 263:10646-10652.

Njoroge FG, Sayre LM, Monnier VM (1987a). Detection of D-glucose-derived pyrrole compounds during Maillard reaction under physiological conditions. Carbohydr Res 167:211-220.

Nyhammar T, Olsson K, Pernemalm P-A (1983). In: Maillard Reactions in Food and Nutrition Waller G Feather MS (Eds) ACS Sympos 215:71-90.

Oimomi M, Maeda Y, Hata F, Kitamura Y, Matsumoto S, Baba S, Iga T, Yamamoto M (1988a). Glycation of cataractous lenses in non-diabetic senile subjects and diabetic subjects. Exp Eye Res 46:415-420.

Oimomi M, Maeda Y, Hata F, Kitamura Y, Matsumoto S, Hatanaka H, Baba S (1988b). A study of the age-related acceleration of tissue proteins in rats. J Gerontol 43:B98-101.

Omura H, Johan N, Shinohara K, Mukarami H (1984). Formation of mutagens by the Maillard reaction. In: the Maillard reaction in Foods and Nutrition, Waller GR and Feather MS, Eds. ACS Symp Ser 215:537-564.

Öste RE, Miller R, Sjostorm H, Noren O (1987). Effect of Maillard reaction products on protein digestion Studies on pure compounds. J Agric Food Chem 35:938-942.

Pachmayr O, Ledl F, Severin T (1986). Formation of 1-alkyl-3-oxypyridinium betaines from sugars. Z Lebensm Unters Forsch 182:1-4.

Paulsen H, Pflughaupt K-W (1980). In: The Carbohydrates: Chemistry and Biochemistry Pigman W, Horton D (Eds) Academic Press (New York) p 881-926.

Patton AR, Chism P (1951). Paper chromatography of browning reaction fluorogens. Nature 167:406.

Pongor S, Ulrich PC, Bencsath FA, Cerami A (1984). Aging of proteins: Isolation and identification of a fluorescent chromphore from the reaction of polypeptides with glucose Proc Natl Acad Sci USA 81:2684.

Scott JE, Qian RG, Henkel W, Glainville RW (1983). An Ehrlich chromagen in collagen crosslinks Biochem J 209:263-264.

Suarez G, Rajaram R, Bheyan KC, Oronsky AL and Goidl JA (1988). Administration of aldose reductase inhibitor induces a decrease of collagen fluorescence in diabetic rats. J Clin Inv 82:624-627.

Takeda Y, Kyogoku Y, Ishidate M (1977). The reaction of sodium D-glucuronate with an L-lysine containing peptide. Carbohydr Res 59:363-377.

Taufel T-L, Iwainsky H (1952). J Food Sci 50:627-631.

Wadman SK, DeBree PK, Van Sprang FJ, Kamerling JP, Haverkamp J, Vliegenthart JFG, (1975). N^ϵ-carboxymethylysine, a constituent of human urine. Clin Chim Acta 59:313-320.

Watkins NG, Thorpe SR, Baynes JW (1985). Glycation of amino groups in protein. J Biol Chem 260:10629-10636.

Watkins NG, Neglia-Fisher CI, Dyer DG, Thorpe SR, Baynes JW (1987). Effect of phosphate on the kinectics and specificity of glycation of protein. J Biol Chem 262:7207-7212.

Yen G-C, Lee T-C (1986). Mutagen formation in the reaction of Maillard browning products, 2-acetylpyrrole and its analogues, with nitrite. Chem Toxic 24:1303-1308.

The Maillard Reaction in Aging,
Diabetes, and Nutrition, pages 109–122
© 1989 Alan R. Liss, Inc.

NON-ENZYMATIC GLYCOSYLATION OF FIBROUS AND BASEMENT MEMBRANE
COLLAGENS

Allen J. Bailey and M.J. Christine Kent

AFRC Institute of Food Research - Bristol,
Langford, Bristol BS18 7DY, U.K.

ABSTRACT.   Physical and biochemical techniques
have clearly demonstrated that a second stage of
reaction of the hexosyl-lysines initially formed
on   non-enzymatic   glycosylation   of   collagen
involves   the   formation   of   intermolecular
crosslinking of the collagen molecules. We have
identified an early product of this crosslinking
reaction   as   a   putative   crosslink   and   its
structure is currently being elucidated. Similar
changes occurred with both the tightly packed
fibrous collagen and the open network of the
basement membrane collagen. The effect of these
crosslinks on the optimal functioning of basement
membrane is likely to be more dramatic than on
fibrous   collagen,   particularly   in   regard   to
flexibility and permeability of capillaries.

INTRODUCTION

Considerable interest has been generated in the nonenzymatic glycosylation of collagen in view of its extracellular nature, its long biological half-life permitting
long-term exposure to interstitial glucose, its importance in
the optimal functioning of many body organs and consequently
its   potential   relevance   to   complications   of   long-term
diabetes.

The mechanism of the initial stage of non-enzymatic
glycosylation has now been established: the condensation of

D-glucose with an amino group, either an α-amino group of a terminal amino acid, or the ε-amino group of a peptide bound lysine. The Schiff base or aldimine intermediate thus formed is unstable and reversible, but can be stabilised by slowly undergoing an Amadori rearrangement to form a keto-amine. The reaction is directly related to the glucose concentration, pH, time and temperature (Gottschalk 1972; Bunn & Higgins 1981; Brownlee et al. 1980).

The initial studies on collagen demonstrated the formation of N-ε-hexosyl-lysine and hydroxylysine (Robins & Bailey 1972; Tanzer et al. 1972) following stabilisation by sodium borohydride prior to hydrolysis. The detection of mannosyl-lysine confirmed that the initial aldimine had undergone the Amadori rearrangement. The extent of glycosylation increased with the age of the tissue (Bailey & Shimokomaki 1971; Robins et al. 1973). Detailed studies on the collagen from streptozotocin-induced diabetic rats confirmed that glucose was preferentially bound, particularly to hydroxylysine, and that the complex underwent an Amadori rearrangement. Further incubation of the diabetic collagen with glucose revealed a decreased reaction suggesting that some sites were already blocked and therefore more reactive (Le Pape et al. 1981).

The increase in glucose binding observed with most proteins amounts to about 1-2 residues of hexose. Collagen is similar but increases with age of the tissue, and is approximately doubled in diabetic subjects. Consequently, several workers have suggested that such a small effect is unlikely to be a primary cause of the late complications observed in diabetic patients (Trueb et al. 1984). However, it is possible that the residues could attach to sensitive points of the molecule, for example, the collagenase site, the cell or glycoprotein interacting sites. In the case of basement membrane collagen the latter could affect the selective filtration properties of the membrane. Indeed, Tarsio et al. (1987) reported a three-fold reduction in the affinity of type IV basement membrane collagen for fibronectin and heparan sulphate following glycosylation of these proteins. The interactions of these proteins are crucial to the optimum effect of basement membrane in filtration. In the same way a single additional crosslink between two linear polymers could significantly affect the mechanical properties of such a protein. It would appear therefore that there is a _prima facie_ case that limited glycosylation of proteins, particularly collagen, may have a significant effect on their properties and hence the overall biological efficiency of this tissue and therefore be worthy of investigation.

At the same time several workers had reported the increased stability of collagen obtained from diabetic patients, for example, reduced solubility, increased resistance to collagenase, and increased shrinkage temperature compared to age-matched controls. These changes were interpreted as 'accelerated ageing' of the collagen in diabetics (Hamlin et al. 1975; Schnider & Kohn 1981). Several mechanisms were proposed, from an increase in the normal enzymic crosslinking mechanism, stabilisation by non-covalent bonds, altered disulphide bonding, to decreased synthesis leading to a higher proportion of mature crosslinks in the collagen. Studies on other proteins have revealed evidence of crosslinking, for example, ribonuclease (Eble et al. 1983), and albumin (Day et al. 1980), although Rucklidge et al. (1980) were unable to repeat the results of the latter studies.

Our own studies on streptozotocin treated rats clearly demonstrated an increase in tensile strength of the intact fibre, and an increase in the tension generated during thermal denaturation compared to controls and to insulin treated rats (Andreassen et al. 1981; Kent et al. 1985). We proposed that the introduction of stable intermolecular crosslinks between the collagen molecules could account for these changes in properties. Further studies revealed that the stabilisation was not an enhancement of the normal enzymic ageing process.

Clearly the changes in physical properties of collagen causing 'accelerated ageing', i.e. an enhancement of the ongoing maturation of collagen through the formation of stable mature crosslinks, must involve additional cross-linking mediated by the hexosyl-lysines initially formed.

To confirm the hypothesis of the formation of new covalent crosslinks a system in which tissue or purified protein could be glycosylated in a controlled manner and be chemically and mechanically analysed is required. In this paper we review the evidence for increased stability using a simple in vitro system for the glycosylation of tendons as examples of fibrous collagen and lens capsules as examples of non-fibrous basement membrane collagens and present evidence of a common crosslink.

GLYCOSYLATION OF FIBROUS COLLAGEN IN VITRO

Following non-enzymic glycosylation by incubation in vitro the mechanical strength of the fibres increases and the fibres become more brittle. Such additional contraints imposed on the structure strongly suggested increased crosslinking within the fibre.

A more definitive technique to demonstrate crosslinking is to determine the thermal properties of the fibre. Increased covalent crosslinking occurring between collagen molecules within a fibre is known to increase the temperature at which the fibre shrinks to approximately one-quarter of its original length. The average shrinkage temperature of mature collagen is 65–67° depending on the age of the tissue, but increases up to 90° can be observed following incubation of fibres with glucose in vitro.

The formation of heat-stable intermolecular crosslinks was further supported by isometric tension on heating at constant length (Fig. 1). In the case of rat-tail tendon the fibre readily ruptures on further heating, but following glycosylation the tension generated is increased and the fibre does not rupture. Similarly, other collagenous tissues show elevated hydrothermal contraction forces under isometric conditions and also a higher residual tension even after heating to 90°C. At these temperatures the residual strength of the denatured collagen (gelatinised) fibre must be due to the presence of heat-stable covalent crosslinks.

It was interesting to note that the compressor tendon in the rabbit foot (which contains predominantly heat-labile crosslinks) showed a dramatic increase in isometric tension, in contrast to the extensor tendon (which contains predominantly heat-stable crosslinks) where the effect of glycosylation was minimal (Fig. 1).

Supporting evidence for covalent crosslinking was provided by the CNBr peptide maps of glycosylated tendon which showed a significant accumulation of high molecular weight material as would be expected if crosslinking occurred. Similar findings were observed with highly

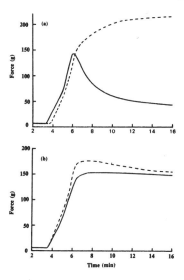

Fig. 1. Isometric tension curves of control and glycosylated rabbit tendon: (a) compressor tendon; ——— control, - - - glycosylated; (b) extensor tendon; ——— control, - - - glycosylated.

purified reprecipitated collagen, demonstrating that the reaction did not involve a minor impurity in the native tendon.

In all these studies the control incubation in the absence of glucose showed a similar but much less marked change in physical properties. These changes in the normal crosslinking observed in vitro follow the age-related changes occurring with increasing age in vivo (Robins & Bailey 1977). The mechanism of this process is fairly well established as an enzymic reaction initially occurring through lysine-derived aldehydes to form aldimines and keto-imines, and subsequently progressing to multivalent crosslinking thus stabilising the molecules within the fibres in a three-dimensional network (Bailey et al. 1974; Bailey & Light 1985).

These studies demonstrating enhanced stabilisation following non-enzymatic glycosylation clearly indicate that the hexosyl-lysine or hexosyl-hydroxylysine undergo further reaction to produce covalent intermolecular crosslinks. The mechanism of formation of these crosslinks has not been elucidated although several proposals have been made. A possible candidate is the fluorescent compound isolated from acid hydrolysates of glycosylated bovine serum albumin or poly-L-lysine. This advanced reaction product was identified as 2-(2-furoyl)4(5)-(2-furanyl)-IH-imidazole (or FFI) and despite its absence of reactive side groups would appear to have the right properties for a crosslink (Pongor et al. 1984). Using immunoassays Chang et al. (1985) detected the presence of FFI in proteolytic digests of glycosylated protein indicating it was not a degradation product of the acid hydrolysis. Although not isolated from collagen, some recent studies by Kennedy (1987) have detected FFI in diabetic patients using immunoassays with an antibody to FFI. However, further evidence is required to confirm that the compound is a crosslink between two molecules and not a side reaction. In addition, the reactions leading up to the formation of this compound and the possibility of other complex compounds need to be established. For example, further reaction with glucose rather than lysine could lead to dicarbonyl sugars which would then act as crosslinking agents (Anet 1964).

Isolation of glucose mediated crosslinks clearly presents considerable difficulty in view of the highly complex series of reactions of glucose and amino acids subsequent to the initial Maillard reaction. These reactions are particularly sensitive to pH concentration and temperature. Unless the compound is stable attempted isolation following acid hydrolysis could lead to further reactions or degradation of the putative crosslink. The imidazole FFI isolated by Pongor et al. (1984) clearly comes into this category although the antibody studies discussed earlier suggest that at least the main structure is not modified.

In an attempt to stabilise the potential crosslink components to acid hydrolysis, we reduced the glycosylated collagen with sodium borohydride. This technique has the added advantage of tritium labelling the potential crosslink for ease of detection.

A potential lysine–glucose crosslink must satisfy several requirements. The crosslink should be labelled by ^{14}C-glucose and ^{3}H-lysine, it may be reducible and, if so, carry an additional ^{3}H-label. The component should increase in quantity with time of incubation and possess a molecular weight in excess of hexosyl-lysine. The final test of the role of any compound as a crosslink must be the isolation of a peptide fragment of two or more chains crosslinked by the compound.

From an analysis of the acid hydrolysate fragments separated on ion-exchange columns it was possible to identify a limited number of compounds that satisfied these various criteria (Fig. 2).

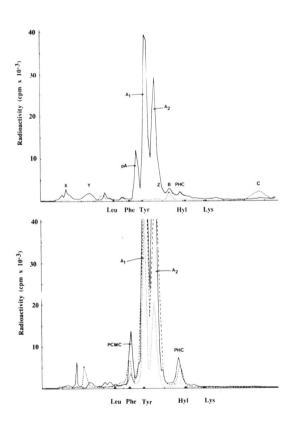

Fig. 2. Ion-exchange column elution profiles of acid hydrolysate of borohydride reduced normal (.....) and glycosylated collagen (top) and polylysine (bottom) 2 days (.....); 2 weeks (- - -); 8 weeks (————).

Additional evidence was also obtained in a simplified system in which glucose was incubated with poly-lysine. The major new component in this system was found to correspond with one of the major components in the collagen-glucose system (Fig. 2b).

Isolation and purification of this pre-hydroxylysine peak (PHC) revealed that it contained primary amine groups and had an apparent molecular weight of 470-530. The isolation of sufficient quantities of the material to carry out a chemical determination of the structure is continuing. It is therefore only possible to speculate on the possible mechanism at this time. For example, the Amadori rearrangement hexosyl-lysine could react through the keto-group with a further lysine of an adjacent molecule resulting in a divalent crosslink. Further reaction could occur through a third lysine group by reaction with the keto-group thus formed to provide a trivalent crosslink (Fig. 3).

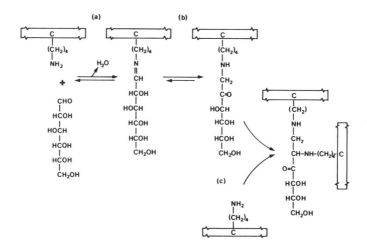

Fig. 3. Theoretical schemes for the formation of an inter-molecular crosslink from glucitol-lysine.

The lysines and hydroxylysines involved in these reactions would occur along the backbone of the tropocollagen molecules thus producing inter-triple-helical crosslinks, in addition to the head-to-tail crosslinking of collagen through the normal enzymic polymerisation (Fig. 4).

NORMAL CROSS-LINKING

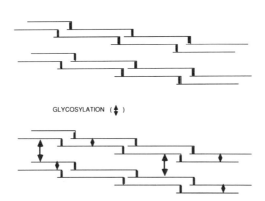

Fig. 4. Diagrammatic representation of the probable cross-link locations of glucose-mediated crosslinks and the normal enzymically formed crosslinks.

GLYCOSYLATION OF NON-FIBROUS COLLAGEN - BASEMENT MEMBRANE IN VITRO

One of the characteristic manifestations of long-term diabetes mellitus is the thickening of the basement membrane (Vrako 1978) resulting in diabetic microangiopathy, which is believed to lead to renal failure, blindness and arterio-sclerosis (Spiro 1976). Non-enzymatic glycosylation of the type IV collagen of basement membrane has been reported by Cohen et al. (1980).

The type IV collagen of thin basement membrane ($\sim$20 nm) would certainly be expected to be more sensitive to glycosylation than the thick fibres of the type I collagen. Consequently crosslinking, as shown to occur with the fibrous collagens, could have a more dramatic effect on the mechanical properties of membranes. Lens capsule was used as a model membrane as it does not possess the underlying fibrous network typical of most membranes.

As in the case of the fibrous collagen, we found that non-enzymatic glycosylation rendered lens capsules increasingly brittle, together with a dramatic reduction in breaking strength (Fig. 5). Such changes clearly indicate the formation of additional intermolecular crosslinks.

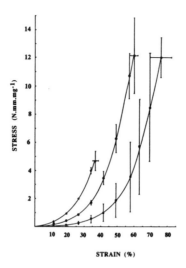

Fig. 5. Stress-strain curves of bovine lens capsule. Fresh control ——■—— ; incubated 12 weeks without glucose ——●—— ; incubated 12 weeks with glucose ——✕—— .

We also examined the change in thermal stability of the type IV collagen of lens capsule. The thermograph of lens capsule obtained by differential scanning calorimetry reveals two peaks, the first at 53-55°C (Tm^1) which is believed to be due to the collapse of the triple helix on thermal denaturation, and a second peak at 88-90°C (Tm^2) believed to be due to the denaturation of the highly stable 7S region. Marked increases in the denaturation temperature of both Tm^1 and Tm^2 occurred following incubation with glucose although the increase in Tm^2 was relatively small (Fig. 6).

The location of glucose-mediated crosslinks between the helices of the laterally packed molecules of the fibrous collagens is readily conceptualised, but the intermolecular crosslinking of the open structure of type IV molecules in basement membrane presents more of a problem. The current model is based on an open chicken wire type of network, the component arms being single triple-helical type IV molecules (Timpl et al. 1981). We have suggested that this would be a

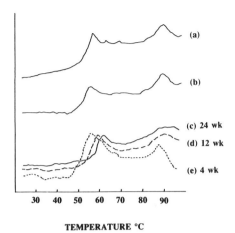

TEMPERATURE °C

Fig. 6. DSC thermograms of bovine lens capsule: (a) fresh lens capsule; (b) after incubation without glucose; (c), (d) and (e) after incubation with glucose for 4, 12 and 24 weeks.

fragile framework and, based on X-ray diffraction analysis of stretched lens capsules, that some lateral aggregation of the molecules probably occurs (Barnard et al. 1987). The proposal is also supported by the increase in Tm of the single type IV molecule at 43–45 and the type IV structure in lens capsules at 53–55°. If some lateral aggregation occurs it would be possible for intermolecular crosslinking of the collagen molecules to take place in basement membrane and account for the resultant change in its mechanical properties. The effect of crosslinking could increase pore size and reduce the flexibility of the network due to the tighter packing of the molecules. In this modified model the glucose-mediated crosslinks would involve interaction of lysine and hydroxylysine residues along the arms of the network. As in the case of the fibrous collagen, the normal crosslinking of the type IV network only involves the terminal regions of the molecules, particularly the 7S region. The location of the crosslinks are basically different, and may account for the rapid change in breaking strength.

Chemical analysis for the crosslink following

borohydride reduction of lens capsule after glycosylation revealed several active peaks and once again we observed the PHC peak previously recorded in both fibrous collagen and polylysine after glucose incubation. Thus stabilisation of the basement membrane of lens capsules appears to occur by the same mechanism as for the fibrous collagen.

In conclusion, physical and biochemical techniques have been employed to demonstrate an increase in crosslinking of both fibrous and basement membrane collagen by non-enzymatic glycosylation. The nature of the crosslink has not been elucidated but the same putative crosslinking occurs in both systems.

This mechanism of increased stabilisation via glucose-mediated crosslinks as shown here for an in vitro system also occurs in tissues of diabetic patients. In these subjects this mechanism is in addition to the normal age-related stabilisation of collagen, the mechanism of which is now fairly well established. The tissues of diabetic patients are therefore referred to as undergoing 'acccelerated ageing'. Such effects are likely to be more dramatic in terms of malfunctioning of tissue with basement membrane than thick collagenous fibres. The changes in the capillaries and the glomerular basement membrane are already well known and it is likely that non-enzymatic glycosylation is a significant factor in determining the extent of these effects.

REFERENCES

Andreassen TT, Seyer-Hansen K, Bailey AJ (1981). Changes in thermal isometric tension, reducible cross-links and mechanical properties of rat tail tendon induced by experimental diabetes. Biochim Biophys Acta 677:313-317.
Anet EFLJ (1964). 3-deoxyglycosuloses (3-deoxyglycosones) and the degradation of carbohydrates. Adv Carbohydr Chem 19:181-218.
Bailey AJ, Light ND (1985). Intermolecular crosslinking in fibrotic collagen. In "Fibrosis", Ciba Foundation Symposium 114, London: Pitman, pp 80-96.
Bailey AJ, Shimokomaki M (1971). Age related changes in the reducible cross-links of collgen. FEBS Lett 16:86-88.
Bailey AJ, Robins SP, Balian G (1974). Biological signi-ficance of the intermolecular crosslinks of collgen.

Nature 251:105-109.

Barnard K, Gathercole LJ, Bailey AJ (1987). Basement membrane collagen - evidence for a novel molecular packing. FEBS Lett 212:49-52.

Brownlee M, Vlassara H, Cerami A (1980). Measurement of glycosylated amino acids and peptides from urine of diabetic patients using affinity chromatography. Diabetes 29:1044-1047.

Bunn HF, Higgins PJ (1981). Reaction of monosaccharides with proteins: possible evolutionary significance. Science 213: 222-224.

Chang JCF, Ulrich PC, Bucala R, Cerami A (1985). Detection of an advanced glycosylation product bound to proteins in situ. J Biol Chem 260:7970-7974.

Cohen MP, Urdanivia E, Surma M, Wu VY (1980). Increased glycosylation of glomerular basement membrane collagen in diabetes. Biochem Biophys Res Commun 95: 765-769.

Day JF, Thorpe SR, Baynes JW (1980). Glucose dependent chemical cross-linking of proteins in diabetes. Fed Proc 39:2179.

Eble AS, Thorpe SR, Baynes JW (1983). Non-enzymatic glucosylation and glucose-dependent cross-linking of protein. J Biol Chem 258(15):9406-9412.

Gottschalk A (ed) (1972). "The Glycoproteins." New York: Elsevier.

Hamlin CR, Kohn RR, Luschin JH (1975). Apparent accelerated aging of human collagen in diabetes mellitus. Diabetes 24: 902-904.

Kennedy L - personal communication.

Kent MJC, Light ND, Bailey AJ (1985). Evidence for glucose-mediated covalent crosslinking of collagen after glycosylation in vitro. Biochem J 225:745-752.

Le Pape A, Muh J-P, Bailey AJ (1981). Characterisation of N-glycosylated Type I collagen in streptozotocin induced diabetes. Biochem J 197:405-412.

Pongor S, Ulrich PC, Bencsath FA, Cerami A (1984). Aging of proteins: isolation and identification of a fluorescent chromophore from the reaction of polypeptides with glucose. Proc Natl Acad Sci USA 81:2684-2688.

Robins SP, Bailey AJ (1972). Age-related changes in collagen: the identification of reducible lysine-carbohydrate condensationi products. Biochem Biophys Res Commun 48:76-84.

Robins SP, Shimokomaki M, Bailey AJ (1973). The chemistry of the collagen cross-links. Age-related changes in the reducible components of intact bovine collagen fibres.

Biochem J 131:771-780.

Rucklidge GJ, Bates GP, Robins SP (1983). Preparation and analysis of the products of non-enzymatic protein glycosylation and their relationship to cross-linking of proteins. Biochim Biophys Acta 747:165-170

Schnider GL, Kohn RR (1981). Effects of age and diabetes mellitus on the solubility and non-enzymatic glucosylation of human skin collagen. J Clin Invest 67:1630-1635.

Spiro RG (1976). Search for a chemical basis of diabetic microangiopathy. Diabetologia 12:1-14.

Tanzer ML, Fairweather R, Gallop PM (1972). Collagen cross-links. Isolation of reduced N^9-hexosylhydroxylysine from borohydride-reduced calf skin insoluble collagen. Arch Biochem Biophys 151:137-141.

Tarsio JF, Reger LA, Furcht LT (1987). Decreased interaction of fibronectin, type IV collagen and heparin due to non-enzymatic glycosylation. Implications for diabetes mellitus. Biochemistry 26:1014-1020.

Timpl R, Weidemann H, van Delden V, Furthmayr H, Kuhn K (1981). A network model for the organization of type IV collagen molecules in basement membrane. Eur J Biochem 120:203-211.

Trueb B, Fluckiger R, Winterhalter KH (1984). Non-enzymatic glycosylation of basement membrane in diabetes mellitus. Coll Rel Res 4:239-251.

Vrako R (1978). In Kefalides NA (ed): "Biology and Chemistry of Basement Membrane", New York: Academic Press, pp 483-493.

The Maillard Reaction in Aging,
Diabetes, and Nutrition, pages 123–139
© 1989 Alan R. Liss, Inc.

NONENZYMATIC GLYCOSYLATION (GLYCATION) OF LENS CRYSTALLINS
IN DIABETES AND AGING

Edathara C. Abraham, Mruthinti S. Swamy and
Ronald E. Perry.

Department of Cell and Molecular Biology,
Medical College of Georgia, Augusta, Georgia
30912-2100.

ABSTRACT.   Lens crystallin glycation, thiol oxidation
and aggregation showed parallel changes in streptozotocin-diabetic and aging rats. The levels of the
disulfide-linked HMW aggregates were essentially the
same in the diabetic and senile cataracts, but glycation was significantly lower in the latter. Inhibition of glycation by acetylating potential glycation
sites by aspirin during in vitro glycation and in diabetic rats has led to inhibition of protein thiol
oxidation and aggregation. A predominance of glycated
crystallins, γ crystallin in particular, was noticed
in the HMW aggregates. Likewise, the glycated portion
of the whole crystallin preparation showed an enrich-
ment of the HMW aggregates. These observations
strongly suggest a significant contribution by
crystallin glycation in the formation of disulfide-
linked aggregates.

INTRODUCTION

The lens crystallins are extremely long-lived proteins,
and turn over very slowly or not at all. This provides a
great opportunity for post-translational modifications such
as nonenzymatic glycosylation or glycation to occur. In
glycation glucose reacts with free amino groups (α-NH$_2$ and
and ϵ-NH$_2$ groups) first forming a reversible Schiff-base
(aldimine) intermediate which undergoes an Amadori rearrangement to form a stable practically irreversible ketoamine structure (Bunn et al., 1978; Cerami and Koenig, 1978;

Mayer and Freedman 1983; Abraham, 1985). Beyond these "early glycation" steps, the glycated residues can undergo a sequence of dehydration and rearrangement reactions to form advanced glycation end products which are fluorescent and have cross-linking properties (Cerami et al., 1978). Since the levels of glycated proteins are influenced by the time averaged glucose concentration and the half-life of the protein, in diabetes increased level of glycated lens crystallins are expected to be found. In fact, studies done in various laboratories have shown that this indeed is true (Stevens et al., 1978; Ansari et al., 1980; Monnier et al., 1979; Perry et al., 1987; Garlick et al., 1984). Glycated crystallins were also shown to be increased with aging (Chiou et al., 1981; Garlick et al., 1984; Swamy and Abraham, 1987), although a comparison of their levels in diabetes vs aging does not exist.

The role of glycation in cataractogenesis is not clearly understood. It is believed to initiate or enhance protein aggregation leading to the formation of high molecular weight (HMW) aggregates (Stevens et al., 1978; Ansari et al., 1980; Perry et al., 1987; Swamy and Abraham, 1987) that are responsible for light scattering. Different types of HMW aggregates that are noncovalently-linked, covalently-linked through disulfide bonds, and covalently-linked trough nondisulfide bonds exist in cataract lens (Harding and Crabbe, 1984; Spector, 1984; Perry et al., 1987; Swamy and Abraham, 1987). Although the recent focus is on advanced glycation mediated protein cross-linking (Cerami et al., 1987) considerable attention needs to be given to disulfide-linked aggregates which seem to constitute the major portion of the water insoluble lens proteins (Perry et al., 1987; Swamy and Abraham, 1987). It has been postulated that glycation leads to protein conformational changes or protein unfolding (Liang and Chakrabarti, 1981) and aggregation. Although this is an attractive hypothesis no direct evidence still exists to strengthen this. Moreover it remains to be seen whether glycation and thiol-oxidized protein aggregation will be a common mechanism for diabetic and senile cataracts.

MATERIALS AND METHODS

Studies in Streptozotocin-Diabetic Rats

We had performed two sets of in vivo studies utilizing
control and streptozotocin-diabetic rats over a period two
years. The first set was designed to study the progressive
changes in lens crystallin glycation and aggregation leading
to cataract development, and to determine the extent of
glycation of HMW aggregates, different crystallins and their
subunits. Fifty Sprague-Dawley (Harlan Sprague-Dawley,
Inc., Madison, WI) rats (100-150 g weight and 1 month old)
were divided into control and diabetic groups (20 controls
and 30 diabetics). The diabetic group was injected with
65 mg Kg^{-1} streptozotocin through tail vein as detailed in
an earlier report (Perry et al., 1987). Four to five
animals in each group were sacrificed every 30 days after
streptozotocin injection. In the second study diabetic
animals were used as an in vivo model to study the effect of
aspirin feeding (to block NH$_2$-groups that are potential
glycation sites by acetylation) on lens protein glycation
and aggregation. Four groups of rats were used: diabetics,
diabetics fed daily powdered rat chow mixed with aspirin
(acetylsalicylic acid or ASA) (200 mg/Kg/body weight/day),
controls, and controls receiving ASA.

In Vitro Glycation Studies

The purpose of these studies was to demonstrate that in
vitro glycation also can lead to protein aggregation and
that in vitro acetylation by ASA inhibits lens crystallin
glycation thereby inhibiting aggregation. Water-soluble
lens crystallin solution (2.5 mg protein/ml of 50 mM sodium
phosphate, pH 7.0) was sterile-filtered through a series of
5, 0.8 and 0.45 micron filters (Gelman Services, Ann Arbor,
MI). Incubations were done with 50 mM glucose, 50 mM
glucose and 20 mM ASA, and with no additives. Each
incubation also contained 50 µl of streptomycin-penicillin.

Crystallin preparation. The water-soluble (WS) and the
urea-soluble (US) fractions were prepared according to the
modified procedure of Herbrink and Bloemendal (1974) as
described in detail before (Perry et al., 1987; Swamy and
Abraham, 1987).

Reduction with NaBH4. For reduction with NaBH4 a 100 molar excess of NaBH4 (1 M solution of NaBH4 or [^{3}H]NaBH4 prepared in 100 mM potasium phosphate, pH 6.0) was added to the protein and reacted at room temperature for 10 min followed by an additional reaction for 50 min at 4°C and dialyzed extensively against water.

Quantification of glycated crystallins. The glycated proteins (GP) in the WS and US fractions were determined by affinity chromatography with phenylboronate agarose resin using Glyc-Affin microcolumns from Isolab Inc. (Akron, OH) as described in previous communications (Perry et al., 1987; Swamy and Abraham, 1987).

Sulfhydryl titration. Free protein thiols were deter-mined by titration with parachloromercuribenzoate according to the method of Boyer (1954).

Molecular sieve high pressure liquid chromatography (HPLC) of proteins in WS and US preparations. Previously described methodologies were used for the separation of the HMW aggregates and other proteins in the WS and US fractions (Perry and Abraham, 1986; Perry et al., 1987; Swamy and Abraham, 1987).

Reverse-phase HPLC separation of crystallin subunits. Reverse-phase HPLC on Vydac C4 column was used for the separation of crystallin subunits of the WS and US fractions (Perry and Abraham, 1986).

Other Methods. The plasma glucose levels were deter-mined by the glucose oxidase assay (Raabo and Terkildsen, 1960) provided in kit from Sigma Chemical Company. Glycated hemoglobin (GHb) was determined with the Isolab Glyc-Affin microcolumns (Isolab Inc. Akron, OH) (Abraham et al., 1983). Protein concentrations were determined by the Bio-Rad protein assay.

RESULTS AND DISCUSSION

As shown by markedly increased levels of plasma glucose and GHb, rats responded well to streptozotocin administra-tion and developed diabetes (Fig. 1A). Glycated proteins of the WS and US fractions were determined by affinity chroma-tography. In the control rats the levels of GP showed a small age-related increase whereas the diabetic animals showed substantial increases at all ages; the US fractions consistently contained higher level of GP than the WS (Fig.1B). Utilizing sensitive molecular sieve HPLC techniques HMW aggregates and the various crystallins were separated from both WS and US fractions. In the control rats there was an age-dependent increase in HMW aggregates, in both the soluble and insoluble fractions (Fig. 1C). In

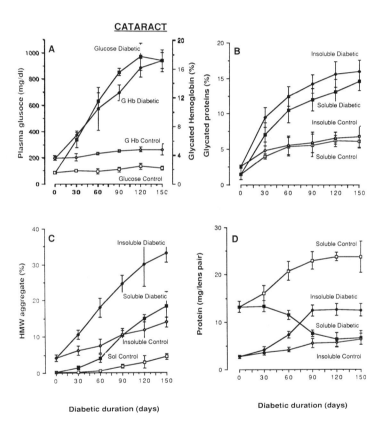

Fig. 1. Progressive changes in streptozotocin-diabetic rats of A. plasma glucose and glycated hemoglobin; B. soluble and insoluble glycated proteins; C. soluble and insoluble HMW aggregates; D. soluble and insoluble protein content.

creases in these aggregates were much higher in the diabetic animals. Again the US fractions contained higher levels of aggregates than the WS fractions. Similar changes in GP and HMW aggregates were reported in an earlier study (Perry et al., 1987; Swamy and Abraham, 1987). As shown in Fig. 1D the insoluble protein fraction increased and the soluble fraction decreased as diabetes advanced. In the control animals at the same time both the soluble and insoluble proteins increased due to the normal growth of the lens occurring during the early months.

Aged or senile rats and diabetic young rats develop cataract. The mechanism of these cataracts are considered different. We wanted to show whether the levels of the HMW aggregates and the glycation status are the same or not at the precataract and cataract stages in these two types of cataracts. It was possible to compare the levels of GP and HMW aggregates in the WS and US fractions of senile rats (20 to 32 month-old, 32 month-old rats having cataract) and dia-betic rats (60-150 day diabetic rats, 90-150 day diabetics having cataract) (Fig. 2). Interestingly, the proportions of the HMW aggregates in the WS and US fractions were nearly the same in both groups of animals. The GP values, on the contrary, were markedly lower in the senile rats (about half of the level in the diabetics). Thus, it appears that glycation is not a predominant factor in senile cataract.

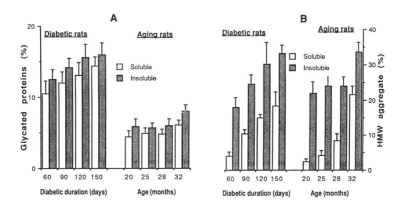

Fig.2. Comparative profile of the levels of (A)glycated proteins and (B) HMW aggregates in WS and US proteins of diabetic and aging rats.

It is generally believed that the HMW aggregates of the WS fraction are formed by noncovalently-linked aggregation and those of the US fraction by covalent bonds. To determine the nature of these linkages in the various aggregates in our system, the WS fraction was dialyzed against 7 M urea and the US fraction against 7 M urea containing 0.1 M β-mercaptoethanol. HPLC separations after these treatments showed complete absence of any aggregates in the soluble fraction confirming the absence of any covalent linkage and the disappearance of about 95% of the aggregates in the insoluble fraction substantiating the presence of disulfide as the predominant form of linkage in the insoluble aggregates (Fig. 3). The type of covalent linkage in the remaining of the aggregates (seen after mercaptoethanol reduction) is not known. Thus, in diabetes and aging protein aggregation appears to involve protein unfolding and thiol oxidation.

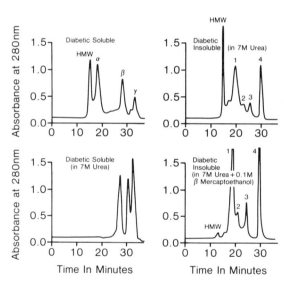

Fig. 3. Molecular sieve HPLC separation of the water soluble fraction in the presence and absence of 7 M urea and of the water-insoluble (urea-soluble) fraction in the presence and absence of 0.1 M β-mercaptoethanol

The first approach to show that glycation contributes to lens protein aggregation was to utilize [^{3}H]NaBH$_4$ reduction followed by molecular sieve HPLC to demonstrate that HMW aggregates have increased content of GP compared to other protein components of the insoluble fraction. Fig. 4 shows the separations of the proteins in the insoluble fraction isolated from a 5 month-old control rats and diabetic rats having cataract. As expected, the diabetic cataract

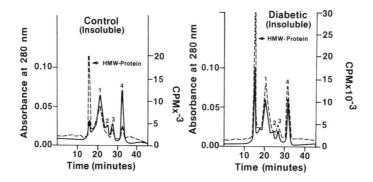

Fig. 4. Molecular sieve HPLC separation of [3H]NaBH4-reduced insoluble fraction from age matched controls and 120 day diabetic rats having cataract (age 5 months).

showed increased radioactivity i.e. increased GP, in all the protein components. The specific activity of the HMW aggregate peaks was significantly higher than all other peaks in both the chromatograms confirming increased presence of GP in the aggregates. The next step was to identify the major source of the label, i.e. to identify the glycated crystallins, in the insoluble fraction. The β-mercaptoethanol-reduced US fraction was chromatographed on reverse-phase HPLC column with developers containing TFA, acetonitrile and water and effluent fractions counted for radioactivity. Under these conditions all the crystallin subunits could be readily separated. Fig. 5, shows the separation of the crystallin subunits in the US fraction from a diabetic cataract after reduction with [3H]NaBH4 and Table I shows the specific activities of the crystallin subunits. The identities of the protein components were based on comparison of the amino acid analysis data and the retention times on reverse-phase column with those already established for crystallin subunits (Perry and Abraham, 1986). It appeared that all the crystallin subunits were glycated in vivo, the γ crystallin being glycated the most. The specific activities of the crystallin subunits were higher in the diabetic cataract than in the control. The protein composition of the insoluble HMW aggregates and the extent of glycation of each

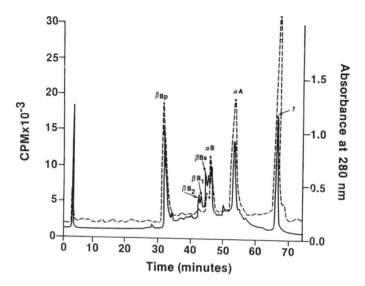

Fig. 5. Reverse phase HPLC separation of [3H]NaBH4-reduced insoluble fraction from 120 day diabetic rats (age 5 months).

Table 1.

Lens Protein Fraction	Crystallin Subunit						
	βBP	βB1	βB2	βBs	αB	αA	γ
	Specific Activity (cpm/mg protein)						
Control Insoluble	1,830	140	110	260	1,965	2,350	4,895
Cataract Insoluble	5,250	405	310	461	4,830	6,923	19,480

component could be determined by reverse-phase HPLC of the HMW aggregates isolated from [³H]NaBH₄-reduced US proteins (Fig. 6).

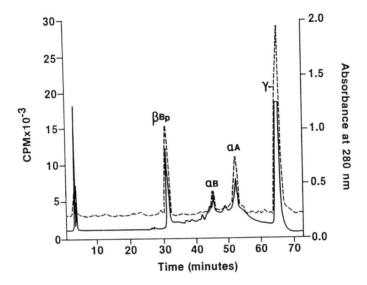

Fig.6. Reverse phase HPLC separation of insoluble HMW aggregate. Insoluble fraction from 120 day diabetic rat lens was reduced with [3H]NaBH₄, dialysed and the insoluble HMW aggregate was separated on molecular sieve HPLC, pooled and rechromatographed on Vydac C4 reverse phase HPLC after reduction with β-mercapto-ethanol.

The insoluble HMW aggregate contained all crystallins, however, the proportion of γ crystallins seems to be higher than other crystallins and the radioactivity of this peak was also higher, which underscores that the γ crystallins are predominant constituents of this aggregate. It is an interesting finding in relation to our previous observation that the proportion of γ crystallin in the soluble fraction decreases with diabetes and aging (Perry et al., 1987; Swamy and Abraham, 1987). It is possible that this fate of γ crystallin is governed by the fact it is excessively glycat-ed. Since we have shown that the HMW aggregates contain a substantial level of glycated proteins, we could rationalize that the glycated portion of the total crystallins, if separated, should contain more HMW aggregates than the nonglycated portion. In fact, molecular sieve HPLC analysis of the affinity chromatography-purified glycated and nonglycated proteins of the US fraction clearly showed a predominance (three-fold) of HMW aggregates in the glycated fraction (Fig. 7).

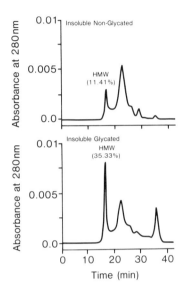

Fig. 7. Molecular sieve HPLC of phenyl boronate affinity chromatography separated non-glycated and glycated proteins.

All the studies described thus far have strongly indicated that glycation is an important factor in protein aggregation. But the most direct and convincing evidence came from the studies where glycation could be inhibited by blocking potential glycation sites by acetylation with ASA while keeping the glucose level high. Acetylation of lysine residues (Day et al., 1979) by ASA was previously shown to inhibit glycation of hemoglobin (Rendell et al., 1986), plasma proteins (Rendell et al., 1986) and lens proteins (Swamy and Abraham, 1988; Huby and Harding, 1988). Whole lens crystallin preparations were incubated with 50 mM glucose for up to 15 days in the presence and absence of 20 mM ASA. At the end of each incubation period an aliquot of the incubation mixture was mixed with 14 M urea to ensure complete dissociation. Protein thiols and HMW aggregates were determined immediately whereas GP was separated after reduction with NaBH₄. Just as we have shown in diabetic animals (Fig. 1), during cell-free glycation with 50 mM glu-

cose there was a time-dependent increase in GP, oxidation of
protein thiols, and protein aggregation; all these were inhibited by ASA (Fig. 8). Interestingly, a parallel increase
in glycation and thiol oxidation were seen whereas HMW aggregation lagged behind for about 5 days, indicating that
protein unfolding and thiol oxidation are the immediate
effects of glycation. The formation of disulfide-linked

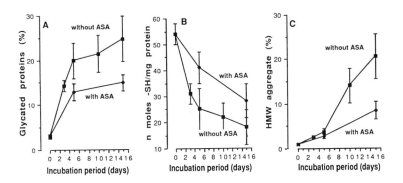

Fig. 8. Effect of aspirin on in vitro glycation and
glycation-induced lens protein changes. A. Glycated
proteins; B. Protein thiols and C. HMW aggregates.

low molecular weight aggregates during the early period of
incubation cannot be ruled out. Incubation of protein alone
did not generate any aggregates whereas incubation of
protein with ASA alone showed an increase in protein aggregation, but this increase was relatively small compared to a
17-fold increase in aggregation observed with 50 mM glucose.
Most interestingly, as reported before (Francois et al.,
1965; Harding, 1972; Perry et al., 1987; Swamy and Abraham,
1987) in diabetic and aging rats, there was a significant
decrease in γ crystallin during in vitro glycation, which
presumably was appearing in the HMW aggregates (Fig. 9).

In vivo studies where streptozotocin-diabetic rats were
fed ASA containing diet complemented the observations made
by the in vitro studies. Significant inhibition of glycation could be achieved by ASA feeding, as evident by markedly reduced level of GHb and glycated proteins (Fig. 10).

Inhibition of glycation resulted in a corresponding level of inhibition of the formation of both disulfide-linked (insoluble) and noncovalently-linked (soluble) aggregates. In fact, inhibition of glycation has led to a delay of cataractogenesis for about 30 days. As seen in in vitro studies, ASA treatment in the control animals did show a slight increase in HMW aggregates (data not given) sug-

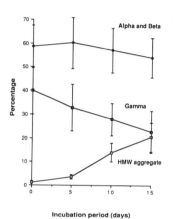

Fig. 9. Changes in lens crystallins and HMW aggregate during in vitro glycation. After incubation with 50 mM glucose, lens protein aliquots were removed, solubilized with an equal volume of 14 M urea, and separated on molecular sieve HPLC columns with mobile phase containing 7 M urea.

gestive that acetylation has a destabilizing effect on lens protein structure, but this effect was only minimal compared to the marked effect glycation had on protein stability and aggregation. In essence acetylation is less harmful than glycation and in a hyperglycating system blocking glycation sites by acetylation certainly has a beneficial effect. These findings may explain the various reports, based on clinical experience, on the effect of ASA therapy on cataractogenesis in human (Rao et al., 1985; Cotlier, 1981; Van Heyningen and Harding, 1986; Seigel et al., 1982; Kewitz et al., 1986).

In this work we have focussed on the effect of the ketoamine formation or early glycation on protein aggregation. A large portion of urea-soluble proteins is in fact cross-linked by disulfide and early glycation seems to influence the formation of these aggregates. Almost 95% of the proteins in these aggregates could be fully dissociated by β-mercaptoethanol and the remaining aggregates may represent the proteins cross-linked by other means. Glycation also influences the formation of non-covalently linked aggregates. As mentioned earlier, the level of glycated crystallins in the senile cataract was only about half of

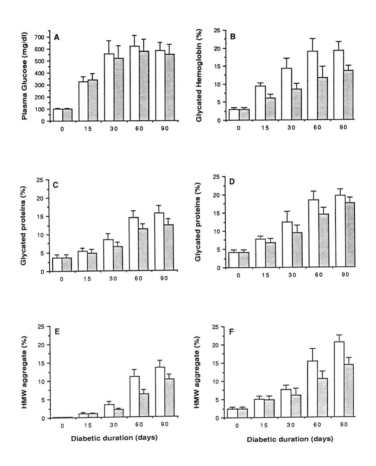

Fig.10. Inhibition of glycation and glycation-induced changes by aspirin in diabetic rat lens. A. Plasma glucose; B. Glycated hemoglobin;C. Glycated lens soluble proteins;D. Glycated lens insoluble proteins; E. Soluble HMW aggregates and F. Insoluble HMW aggregates.
□ Diabetics □ASA fed diabetic

that seen in the diabetic cataract, but the levels of HMW aggregates were equally high in both, which might indicate that glycation is not the only factor in senile cataractogenesis. It is difficult to determine the minimum level of glycation needed to initiate protein unfolding. Our in vitro and in vivo studies showed significant protein aggregation only after a level of about 10% glycation has achieved. However, we measured only the super aggregates and protein unfolding and aggregation might have started at an earlier stage. Moreover, other posttranslational modifications such as deamidation, oxidation, C-terminal degradation and carbamylation are also expected to play a significant role in cataractogenesis. An argument against the glycation theory and for the sorbitol theory came from the finding that inhibition of aldose reductase with sorbinil in galactosemic rats prevented or markedly delayed cataract without affecting galactosylation (Chiou et al., 1988). This rationale is weakened by the fact that inhibition of aldose reductase builds up NADPH and the reduction potential in the lens which is expected to prevent excessive thiol oxidation. Interestingly in a recent study by feeding butylated hydroxytoluene, a chain breaker in free radical reactions, prevented galactosemic cataract in rats without decreasing galactitol levels (Das et al., 1988).

ACKNOWLEDGEMENT

This work was supported by a grant from National Institutes of Health (EY-07394).

REFERENCES

Abraham EC (1985). Glycosylated hemoglobins: Methods of analysis and clinical applications. Mercel and Decker, New York and Basel, pp 33-58.

Ansari NH, Awasthi YL, Srivastava SK (1988). Role of glycosylation in disulfide formation and cataractogenesis. Exp Eye Res 31: 9-19.

Boyer PD (1954). Spectrophotometric study of the reaction of protein sulfhydryl groups with organic mercurials. J Am Chem Soc 76: 4331-4337.

Bunn HF, Gabbay KH, Gallop PM (1978). The glycosylation of hemoglobin: Relevance to diabetes mellitus. Science 200: 21-27.

Cerami A, Koenig RJ (1978). Hemoglobin AI$_C$ as a model for the development of the sequelae of diabetes mellitus. TIBS 3: 73-75.

Cerami A, Vlassara H, Brownlee M (1987). Glucose and aging. Scientific American 256: 90-96.

Chiou S-H, Chylack LT, Bunn HF and Kinoshita JH (1980). Role of nonezymatic glycosylation in experimental cataract formation. Biochem Biophys Res Commun 95: 844-901.

Chiou S-H, Chylack LT, Tung WH, Bunn HF (1981). Nonenzymatic glycosylation of bovine lens crystallins: Effect of aging. J Biol Chem 256: 5176-5180.

Cotlier E (1981). Senile cataracts: Evidence for acceleration by diabetes and deceleration by salicylate. Can J Ophthalmol 16: 113-118.

Das B, Ansari NH, Hair GA, Srivastava SK (1988). Decreased defense against oxidants:A possible cause of sugar cataractogenesis. Proceedings of the International Society for Eye Research, Volum V, San Francisco, CA. Abs #136, pp 128.

Day JF, Thornbug RW, Thorpe SR, Baynes JW (1979). Nonenzymatic glucosylation of rat albumin. Studies in vitro and in vivo. J Biol Chem 254: 9394-9340.

Francois J, Rabaey M, Stockman L (1965). Gel filtration of the soluble proteins from normal and cataractous human lenses. Exp Eye Res 4: 312-318.

Garlick RL, Mazer JS, Chylack LT, Jr., Tung WH, Bunn HF (1984). Nonenzymatic glycosylation of human lens crystallin: Effect of aging and diabetes mellitus. J Clin Invest 74: 1742-1749.

Harding JJ (1972). The origin of urea-insoluble protein isolated from the rat lens. Exp Eye Res 14: 289-290.

Harding JJ, Crabbe MJC (1984). The lens: Development, proteins, metabolism and cataract. In Davson H (ed): "The Eye," 3rd Edition, New York: Academic Press, pp 294-308.

Herbrink P, Bloemendal H (1984). Studies on β-crystallin. I. Isolation and partial characterization of the principle polypeptide chain. Biochim Biophys Acta 336: 370-382.

Huby R, Harding JJ (1988). Nonenzymatic glycosylation (glycation) of lens proteins by galactose and protection by aspirin and reduced glutathione. Exp Eye Res 47:53-59.

Kewitz H, Nitz M, Gaus V (1986). Aspirin and cataract. Lancet ii, 689.

Monnier VM, Stevens VJ, Cerami A (1979). Nonenzymatic glycosylation, sulfhydryl oxidation and aggregation of lens proteins in experimental sugar cataracts. J Exp Med 50: 1098-1107.

Perry RE and Abraham EC (1986). High performance liquid chromatographic separation of lens crystallins and their subunits. J Chromatog 351: 103-110.

Rao GN, Lardis MP, Cotlier E (1985). Acetylation of lens crystallins: A possible mechanism by which aspirin could prevent cataract. Exp Eye Res 40: 297-311.

Rendell M, Nierenberg J, Brannan C, Valentine JL, Stephen PM , Dodds S, Mercer PO, Smith PK, Walder J (1986). Inhibition of glycation of albumin and hemoglobin by acetylation in vitro and in vivo. J Lab Clin Med 108: 286-293.

Seigel D, Speraduto RD, Ferris FL (1982). Is aspirin therapy for cataracts justified? Can J Ophthalmol 17: 135-136.

Spector A (1984). The search for a solution to senile cataract: Proctor lecture. Invest Ophthalmol Vis Sci 25: 130-146.

Stevens VJ, Rouzer CA, Monnier VM, Cerami A (1978). Diabetic cataract formation: Potential role of glycosylation of lens crystallins. Proc Natl Acad Sci USA 75: 2918-2922.

Swamy MS, Abraham EC (1987). Lens protein composition, glycation and high molecular weight aggregation in aging rats. Invest Ophthalmol Vis Sci 28: 1693-1701.

Swamy MS and Abraham EC (1988). Influence of glycation inhibitors on thiol oxidation and aggregation of lens crystallins in vitro. Invest Ophthalmol Vis Sci (Suppl) 29: 30.

van Heyningen R and Harding JJ (1986). Do aspirin-like analgesics protect against cataract? A case-control study. Lancet i: 1111-1113.

The Maillard Reaction in Aging,
Diabetes, and Nutrition, pages 141–162
© 1989 Alan R. Liss, Inc.

NONENZYMATIC BROWNING OF PROTEINS AND THE SORBITOL PATHWAY.

Gerardo Suarez

Department of Biochemistry, New York Medical
College, Valhalla, New York 10595

ABSTRACT. As a result of the operation of the
sorbitol pathway fructose levels increase in
various tissues in diabetes. In vitro glycation
of protein by fructose (fructation) leads to
protein bound fluorescence generation at a rate
ten times that resulting from glycation by
glucose (glucation), possibly by a faster
conversion of Amadori groups to fluorophores.
Therefore, tissue protein fluorescence might, in
part, result from fructation. Evidence is
presented for the occurrence of in vivo
fructation of skin collagen and soluble lens
proteins in diabetic rats. Fructation-induced
protein functional alterations might underlie
complications of diabetes in tissues where the
sorbitol pathway is active.

INTRODUCTION

Nonenzymatic glycation of proteins has been primarily
thought of as the result of the covalent attachment of
glucose to protein amino groups. Increased levels of this
posttranslational modification in diabetes has been
correlated with hyperglycemia (Thorpe and Baynes, 1982).
Search for in vivo glycation of proteins by sugars other
than glucose has been restricted almost exclusively to gal-
actation, i.e., glycation by galactose, in view of its
relevance to galactosemia, an inherited metabolic disorder
(Urbanowski et al., 1982a). We have suggested in recent

TABLE 1

METABOLITES OF SORBITOL PATHWAY IN VARIOUS TISSUES

Organ or tissue	Glucose concentration		Fructose concentration		Sorbitol concentration		References
	Control	Diabetic	Control	Diabetic	Control	Diabetic	
Eye lenses (Rats)	0.5	8.1	0.7	16.3	1.5	31.3	Kinoshita et al., 1979
Eye lenses (Rats)	0.222	5.55	0.55	8.66	n/d	n/d	Kuck, 1979
Eye lenses (Rats)	0.8	4.23	0.55	3.2	0.33	12.2	Gonzalez et al.,1983
Eye lenses (Rats)	n/d	n/d	0.689	3.8	0.137	1.291	Stribling et al., 1985
Eye lenses (human)	0.7–2.2	3.0–4.5	0.4–1.4+	1.2–12+	0.3–2.4+	1.7–9.5+	Jedziniak et al.,1981
Sciatic nerve (Rats)	0.84	6.11	0.49	5.95	0.17	6.11	Tomlinson et al., 1985
Sciatic nerve (Rats)	3.81	11.33	0.58	2.68	0.237	0.780	Finegold et al., 1983
Sciatic nerve (Rats)	1.94	11.47	0.942	5.73	0.108	1.83	Poulsom et al., 1983a
Sciatic nerve (Rats)	1.65	9.45	0.790	6.51	0.150	1.30	Poulsom et al., 1983b
Sciatic nerve (Rats)	2.65	3.97	1.04	2.67	0.11	0.26	Hotta et al., 1985
Sciatic nerve (human)	0.46	1.61	0.08	1.24	0.09	0.39	Mayhew et al., 1983
Retina (Rats)	5.38	3.8-29.23	0.805*	2.44*	0.66*	2.38*	Heath and Hamlett., 1976
Retina (Rats)	0.81	5.78	0.054	0.68	0.061	0.660	Poulsom et al., 1983a
Kidney (Rats)	4.33	30.1	0.370	1.92	0.300	0.570	Poulsom et al., 1983b
Seminal vesicles(Rats)	1.05	20.6	2.43	6.50	0.200	0.640	ibid

+: (mM) ; * : Sucrose fed. umoles/lens; n/d: not determined
Unless otherwise indicated values are expresed as umole/g wet tissue

years (Suarez et al., 1984; Suarez et al., 1986) that
glycation of proteins by fructose (fructation) should also
be considered as relevant to the development of the
abnormalities in diabetes. In this article, we will outline briefly the metabolic, clinical and chemical evidence
for increased protein fructation in diabetes and the
possible significance of this reaction in the development
of complications in this disease. Furthermore, animal experimentation has indicated that fructose might induce
lesions similar to those found in diabetes.

Metabolic Basis for Nonenzymatic Protein Fructation in
vivo.

    In various organs and tissues where complications
arise in long-standing diabetes, the sorbitol pathway
operates at rates that are commensurate with the supply of
glucose to the intracellular space. The sorbitol pathway
is a metabolic shunt that mediates the conversion of
glucose into fructose with only one intermediate, i.e.,
sorbitol (Gabbay, 1975). The overall process proceeds by
means of the activities of two enzymes that catalyze two
consecutive reactions: 1. aldose reductase, which cata-
lyzes the NADPH-dependent reduction of glucose (and other
aldohexoses) to sorbitol (or the polyol corresponding to
the original sugar) and 2. sorbitol dehydrogenase, by which
sorbitol is oxidized to fructose with NAD+ as a cofactor.
The activity of the sorbitol pathway has been demonstrated
in the eye lens (Jedziniak et al., 1981), erythrocytes
(Morrison et al., 1970), peripheral nerve (Tomlinson et
al., 1985), arteries (Ludvigson and Sorenson, 1980) and
retina (Heath and Hamlett, 1976), among other organs.
Glucose diffuses freely into these organs and tissues in an
insulin-independent fashion and, as a result of the activity of the sorbitol pathway, the concentrations of both
sorbitol and fructose rise significantly in diabetes. So
far, attention has been focused on fluctuations in sorbitol
concentrations in efforts to explain the generation of diabetic complications. However, fructose levels
rise in parallel with those of sorbitol and glucose. Table
1 summarizes documented increases of fructose concentration
and compares them with the rise of glucose or sorbitol in
organs with an active sorbitol pathway. It can be seen
that the increase in fructose concentration is in several
cases comparable to that of sorbitol and glucose. Further-

more, in one of the cases shown, corresponding to a 23-fold
rise in the lens fructose level, the concentration of this
sugar surpassed that of glucose (Kinoshita et al., 1979).
Based on these findings, the role of fructose as a pathogenetic metabolite should be considered at least as
legitimate as that of glucose or sorbitol. Also, although
fructose concentrations are in most cases lower than those
of glucose, the higher reactivity of the former (see below)
may overcome concentration discrepancies and so, significant fructation should be expected.

Clinical Observations Suggesting In Vivo Protein Fructation.

Monitoring of glycated proteins has become a standard
procedure for the diagnosis and management of diabetes
mellitus and the assessment of glycemic control. Since it
is considered an indicator of the glucose levels that
prevailed during the life span of the particular protein,
the levels of glycated protein, especially hemoglobin Alc,
afford information on the blood glucose values integrated
over that time (Bunn et al., 1978). However, an increasing
number of clinical findings do not appear to conform to the
parallelism between the glycemia and the extent of protein
glycation. In most of these cases, a high level of
circulating fructose would be expected. For example, a
group of children with juvenile diabetes who were receiving
large amounts of fructose in their diet showed increased
levels of glycated hemoglobin despite a rigorous control of
the glycemia (Burden, 1984). Glycated hemoglobin returned
to normal values following a restriction of fructose
ingestion. Patients with hereditary fructose intolerance,
who have increased levels of circulating fructose, also
exhibited higher than normal levels of HbAlab, a glycated
minor component of hemoglobin (Bohles et al., 1987). Other
studies documented increased fluorescence, with the
characteristics of advanced glycation products, in plasma
proteins of relatively high turnover (Jones et al., 1986).
These observations are difficult to explain solely on the
basis of the Maillard reaction initiated by glucose, a very
slow condensation process between a sugar and protein amino
groups. However, protein fructation, a much faster
posttranslational modification (see below), is more likely
to generate the fluorescence in these proteins. This view
becomes more plausible on consideration of the higher serum

fructose concentrations in diabetic patients, compared with normal subjects, following the administration of sucrose (Sekimoto et al., 1988).

Results from Animal Experimentation.

Although the specific role of protein glycation has not been expressly addressed in these studies, investigators have found that long term administration of fructose in the diet has led to lesions similar to diabetic microangiopathy in rats (Cohen et al., 1977). Similar results have been induced with sucrose, where the authors determined that fructose was the retinopathic agent (Boot-Handford and Heath, 1980). Although the mechanism of the generation of these lesions may be multiple, the particular role of protein fructation should be investigated.

RESULTS

In Vitro Protein Fructation.

In vitro studies on protein glycation have dealt with galactose (Urbanowski et al., 1982b), mannose, fucose (Zaman and Vergilhen, 1981), sialic acid (McKinney et al., 1982), glucose 6-phosphate (Haney and Bunn, 1970) and xylose (Monnier et al., 1980), in addition to glucose. Glycation by fructose (fructation) has not received sufficient specific attention and has been only peripherally mentioned in comparative studies involving various sugars (Monnier et al., 1980; Bunn and Higgins, 1981). We have been attempting to characterize the reactivity of fructose toward protein amino groups in order to provide a basis for the possible occurrence of this modification in vivo. The reactivities of glucose and fructose with protein were compared by incubating these sugars with bovine serum albumin (BSA) for extended periods of time (Suarez et al., 1989). Whereas formaldehyde release upon periodate oxidation, an indicator of the generation of Amadori groups (Gallop et al., 1981), increased with time in the glucated protein at a rate that was about double that of the fructated protein, protein-bound fluorescence of the latter rose at a rate ten times greater (Fig. 1). In addition, the figure shows that, in contrast to short-term incubations (Bunn and Higgins, 1981), the rate of blocking

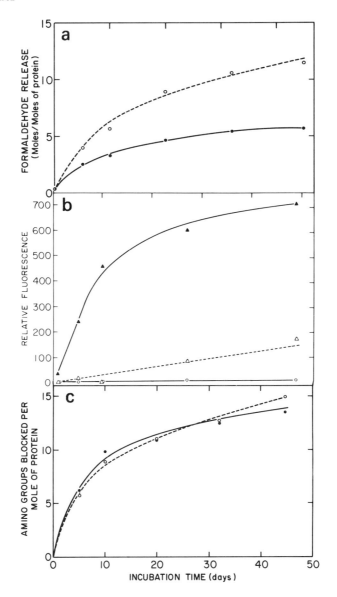

Figure 1. <u>Time course of the Maillard reaction</u>. BSA, 6 mg/ml, was incubated with 0.5 M glucose (---) or 0.5 M fructose (——). a) Formaldehyde release; b) fluorescence generation (exc.:340nm;em:410 nm); c) blocking of primary amino groups.

of amino groups by glucose and fructose are very similar.
So the former results cannot be accounted for by differences in the rate of adduct formation, but rather by
differences in the rate of intramolecular rearrangements in
the more advanced stages of the Maillard reaction or
structural differences between the products of glycation by
each of the two sugars. Formaldehyde release upon periodate
oxidation was introduced by Gallop et al. (1981) as an
assay for glycated hemoglobin. We have exploited this

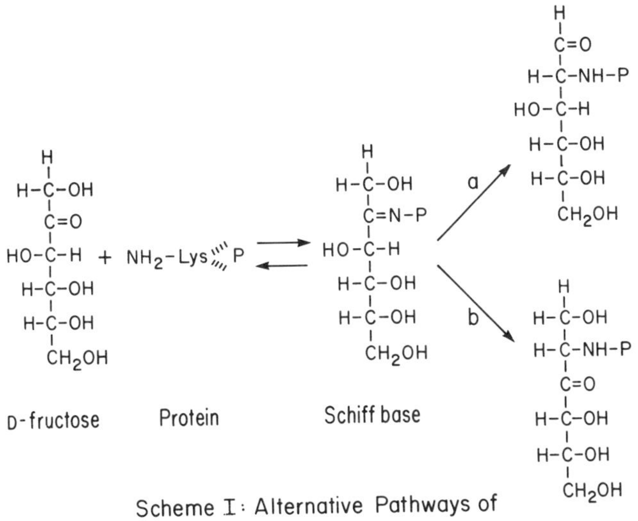

Scheme I: Alternative Pathways of
Amadori Rearrangement from fructose

reaction with the aim of gaining insight into the possible
structures of the moieties that result from the Amadori
rearrangement of nonenzymatically fructated (NEF) BSA.
This reaction has been studied for some time and has been
termed the Heyns rearrangement. The description of this
rearrangement was based on reactions carried out with
nonprotein models under nonphysiological conditions (Heyns
and Meinecke, 1953). Examination of Scheme I reveals that,
in principle, the Amadori rearrangement following the
addition of fructose to a protein may proceed by two
alternative routes, one involving C-1 and the other with
participation of C-3. Since cleavage of -C-C- bonds by
periodate oxidation proceeds according to well established
patterns known as Malaprade's rules (Bobbitt, 1956),
information on the structure of the Amadori products can be
extracted by examining the molar yield of formaldehyde.
For that purpose, NEF BSA and glucated (NEG) BSA were

generated by incubating the protein with 0.5 M sugar for 17
days. After exhaustive dialysis, removal of the Amadori
structures was accomplished by oxidation with sodium
periodate (20 mM). Both the control and oxidized protein
were reduced with sodium borohydride (Suarez, et al.,
1989) and the reduced proteins reisolated by tetrahydro-
furan precipitation. The ratio between the loss of
formaldehyde releasing ability and the number of regenerated amino groups upon oxidation was determined. From
these values, the stoichiometry of formaldehyde release was
computed after correcting for the effect of borohydride
reduction on the formaldehyde release. It was determined
that the Amadori group derived from glucose (GA) yields 0.8
mol formaldehyde and the fructose initiated Amadori group
(FA) yields 0.47 mol formaldehyde. The first value
conforms fairly well with the values of 1 reported by
Gallop et al. (1981). The formaldehyde yield of FA is
consistent with the participation of both C-1 and C-3 in
the Amadori rearrangement. As illustrated in Fig. 2A,
exclusive participation of C-1 would result in the absence

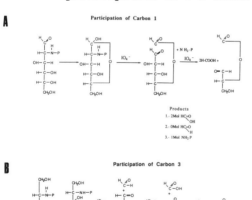

Figure 2. Amadori re-
arrangement of **NEF**
BSA. Products of
periodate oxidation of
Amadori groups as
predicted by Mala-
prade's rules A)Parti-
cipation of carbon 1.
B)Participation of
carbon 3 (Adapted from
Suarez et al., 1989).

of formaldehyde release, which would be in conflict with
our experimental results (Fig. 1). On the other hand,

exclusive participation of C-3 (Fig. 2B) would lead to a stoichiometry of 1 for formaldehyde release, which is higher than our experimentally determined value. So, we conclude, that both pathways might be involved in the Amadori rearrangement from fructose.

To explain the rate of the generation of formaldehyde-yielding capacity during glucation and fructation as depicted in Fig. 1, the Maillard reaction was treated as a sequence of two consecutive irreversible reactions. The first reaction is pseudo-first order with respect to protein amino group concentration and leads to the formation of the Amadori products. The second reaction is first order with respect to Amadori groups and defines the further transformations of these groups to fluorophores and other structures:

$$\text{Sugars + P-NH2} \xrightarrow{k_1} \text{Amadori groups} \xrightarrow{k_2} \text{Fluorophores and other structures}$$

It can be shown (manuscript in preparation) that the rate of generation of Amadori groups according to this simplified kinetic model can be expressed as:

$$Am(t) = \frac{(NH_2)o \, k_1}{k_2 - k_1} (e^{-k_1 t} e^{-k_2 t})$$

Am: Amadori groups; $(NH2)o$:initial concentration of protein amino groups; t:incubation time; k_1 and k_2:first order rate constants.

To assess the validity of this model, formaldehyde release values were expressed as Amadori group concentrations on the basis of the stoichiometries mentioned above. From the rate of Amadori group generation, k_1 values were computed for arbitrarily chosen values of k_2 by means of a program (SAS Institute, Cary, N.C. 27511) which processes the partial derivative of the model expression with respect to k_1. Best fits were obtained for k_2 values of 0.044 days^{-1} and 0.075 days^{-1} for glucation and fructation, respectively, from which the corresponding k_1 values of 0.017 days^{-1} and 0.02 days^{-1} were computed. Theoretical curves were constructed from these constants and the initial amino group concentration, $(NH2)o$, and compared with the observed time course of Amadori group generation during glucation and fructation. As is shown in

Fig. 3, there was a good agreement between the theoretical and the experimental values, except for the last days of incubation. Higher k_2 value for fructation would explain the greater rate of fluorescence generation and earlier attainment of maximum formaldehyde releasing ability in NEF BSA (Fig. 1).

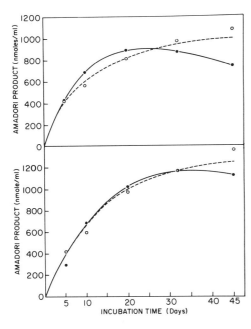

Figure 3. Rate of Amadori group generation of BSA. Rate constants were computed according to the kinetic model as described in the text. Top:nonenzymatic fructation. Bottom:nonenzymatic glucation. (———): theoretical curve, drawn from the initial amino group concentration and the computed constants. (---): experimental curve.

Binding of Model Fructose-derived Fluorophores to Proteins.

The lysine derivative, N-α-acetyl-lysine-N'-methylamide (NALMA) was chosen as a model for lysine residues in proteins because it has both the α-amino and the carboxyl group blocked. When this compound, at a concentration of 2.5 mM, was incubated for 32 days at 37°C with 0.5 M sugar, fluorescence was generated. The fluorophores that developed had excitation spectra with a maximum at 340 nm, when emission was monitored at 410 nm. These spectra were almost identical to those of NEF BSA. Also, since the excitation spectrum of fructated NALMA (fNALMA) overlaps to a large extent with the emission spectrum of tryptophan residues in proteins (Fig. 4), it was conjectured that the effect of the NALMA fluorophore on the tryptophan

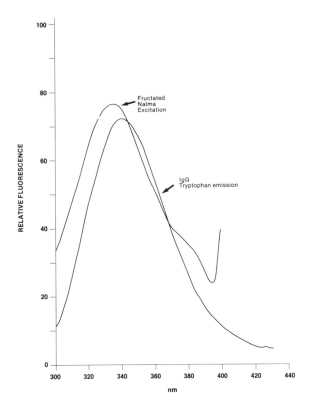

Figure 4. <u>Superposition of fluorescence spectra</u>. Emission spectrum of IgG (Exc.:278 nm) and excitation spectrum of fNALMA (em.:410 nm). IgG and fNALMA were prepared as described in text.

fluorescence intensity might give information as to the binding of advanced Maillard products to proteins. To test the validity of this approach, bovine serum albumin and immunoglobin G (IgG) were chosen as acceptor proteins.

IgG was obtained from sera of mice immunized with BSA. Balb/c mice were immunized by injecting intraperitoneally 20 µg of BSA (Sigma, crystallin, fatty acid-free) with complete Freund's adjuvant. Intraperitoneal injections were repeated after 2 and 4 weeks with incomplete Freund's adjuvant. A final intravenous injection was done at day 51 without Freund's adjuvant. Anti-BSA antibody was purified by affinity chromatography on columns of immobilized BSA as

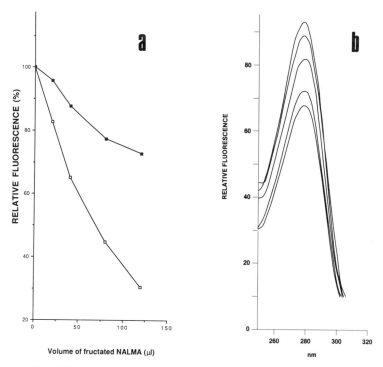

Figure 5. Titration of BSA with fNALMA. BSA (37 µg/ml,
1 ml) was mixed with increasing volumes of fNALMA. a)
Relative fluorescence (exc.:278 nm;em.:340 nm).
□—□:before dialysis; ■—■:after dialysis (protein conc.:15
µg/ml). b)Excitation spectra (em.:340 nm) of dialyzed
mixtures of BSA with fNALMA; from top to bottom, 0, 20, 40,
80, 120 µl fNALMA.

described (Fuchs and Sela, 1978). Immobilization was
accomplished by coupling 20.5 mg of BSA with Affi-Gel 15,
an activated affinity support, following the procedure of
the manufacturers (Bio-Rad, Bulletin 1085). The affinity-
purified antibody was characterized as an immunoglobulin G
by SDS gel electrophoresis (Phastsystem, Pharmacia).

Interaction of these proteins with the fNALMA
fluorophore was investigated by measuring the fluorescence
at 340 nm, using an excitation wavelength of 278 nm, in the
presence of increasing concentrations of the NALMA
derivative. Fig. 5 shows the results of titration of BSA.
Fluorescence decreased in a concentration dependent

fashion. At the highest concentration of fNALMA the
fluorescence was about 30% of that of the protein alone.
Similar quenching effects were observed with IgG (Fig. 6),
the fluorescence of which was reduced to less than 30%.

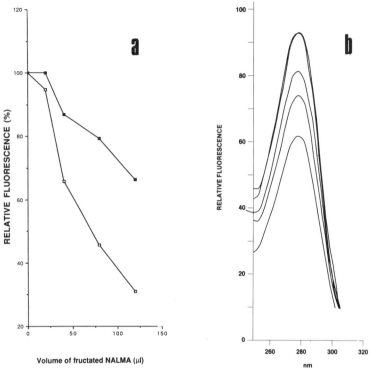

Figure 6. <u>Titration of IgG with fNALMA</u>. IgG (37 µg/ml, 1
ml) was mixed with increasing volumes of fNALMA. a)
Relative fluorescence (exc.:278 nm; em.:340 nm) □—□ :before
dialysis; ■—■ :after dialysis (protein concentration
15 µg/ml/ml). b)Excitation spectra (em.:340 nm) of
dialyzed mixtures of IgG with, from top to bottom, 0, 20,
40, 80, 120 µl fNALMA.

In order to exclude trivial filtering effects of the
dissolved fNALMA on the fluorescence, the mixtures
containing the protein and quencher were dialyzed overnight
against the dissolving buffer. As Figs. 5 and 6 show,
significant quenching was still observable. BSA fluorescence decreased to 72% and IgG to 66% at the highest
concentration of quencher. These results are consistent
with significant binding of the fNALMA fluorophore to the

proteins and can be interpreted as fluorescence energy transfer from tryptophan (donor) to the NALMA derivative (acceptor). Since the extent of this transfer is dictated by the distance between the donor and acceptor according to Forster theory (Lakowicz, 1985), this approach might give information on the binding of fructated proteins to specific domains in other proteins.

Evidence for <u>In Vivo</u> Nonenzymatic Protein Fructation.

Due to the lack of suitable probes or specific chemical assays for the products of nonezymatic fructation, their identification <u>in situ</u> is not possible at present. So, we have attempted to gather information on the occurrence of this modification in an indirect way. For this purpose, a study was undertaken that compared formaldehyde releasing ability and fluorescence in proteins obtained from diabetic rats treated with an aldose reductase inhibitor, with those found in proteins of untreated diabetic and control rats (Suarez et al., 1988). Diabetes was induced in male Sprague-Dawley rats (average weight:160 g) by means of the subcutaneous injection of a single dose of streptozotocin (80 mg/kg body weight). One group of these rats received in the diet sorbinil ([+]6-fluoro-spiro-[chroman-4,4^1-imidazolidine]-2^1,5^1-dione) in doses that have been shown to be effective at decreasing the fructose levels in tissues where the sorbitol pathway is active (Poulsom et al., 1983a; Poulsom et al., 1983b; Stribling et al., 1985). The rationale of this experiment was based on the assumption that sorbinil would affect the generation of Maillard products derived directly from protein fructation while leaving those originated from glucation unchanged, since the drug has no effect on the glycemia.

Figure 7 shows the fluorescence (exc. 350 nm; em.: 410 nm) associated with the skin collagen of the three groups of animals. Collagen was solubilized by digestion with purified Clostridium histolyticum collagenase as described (Suarez et al., 1988) and fluorescence was normalized with respect to the content of hydroxyproline, a marker of the parent collagenous material, in the digests. The fluorescence associated with collagen decreased from 117±7 in the collagen from the skin of untreated diabetic

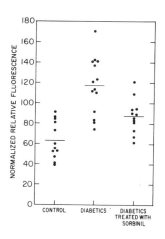

Fig. 7. Normalized relative fluorescence of collagenase digests from skin of normal and diabetic rats (Suarez et al., 1988).

rats to 87±4 in collagen from the sorbinil treated animals, which was highly significant (P<0.003). Control rat collagen had 63±5 relative fluorescence. Periodate induced formaldehyde release, an assay for the Amadori products as mentioned before, is difficult to interpret while dealing with collagen, due to interference by hydroxylysine. This amino acid, with a side chain having a vicinal aminol, releases formaldehyde as predicted by Malaprade's rules.

Since the lens is an organ with a very active sorbitol pathway, the effect of sorbinil administration was also investigated. Soluble protein was extracted from the lens by homogenization in a Dounce homogenizer in 0.01 M phosphate/0.1 M NaCl, pH 7.45, followed by centrifugation at 10,000 g for 20 min. The supernates were dialyzed vs 2 changes of a 200-fold volume of the same buffer. Formaldehyde release assays and fluorescence measurements were conducted in the dialyzed material. Fluorescence measurements were expressed in reference to the standard tetraphenyl butadiene to correct for small variations in instrument response.

Table 2 summarizes the results on formaldehyde release and fluorescence in these proteins. The formaldehyde release by lens proteins from diabetic rats was almost 2.5

greater than that of control lens proteins. Following administration of sorbinil, the formaldehyde releasing ability decreased from 3.7 nmol/mg protein to 2.57 nmol/mg protein. The difference between the values of the two diabetic groups was even more significant (P<0.0001) than the difference between the values of lenses from control and sorbinil-treated diabetic rats (P<0.001). Fluorescence values, normalized with respect to protein concentration, in both diabetic groups were significantly higher than those of the control group. However, there was no significant difference between the protein associated

Table 2
Soluble Lens Proteins

Animal group	Formaldehyde release*	Fluorescence**
Control n=12	1.50±0.23	8.77±0.68
Diabetic n=14	3.70±0.97	11.55±1.14
Sorbinil-treated diabetic n=12	2.57±0.39	10.88±0.79

*nmol/mg protein ± S.D.   **Normalized with respect to protein concentration. Lenses were from rats treated as described (Suarez et al., 1988).

fluorescence of the untreated and sorbinil treated diabetic rats (P=0.11).

DISCUSSION

The increase in fructose levels in several tissues with an active sorbitol pathway has been documented repeatedly in diabetes. In vitro studies have shown that fructose forms Schiff base adducts with hemoglobin at a rate that is about eight times faster than glucose, possibly a reflection of the higher proportion of the linear, reactive form in fructose solutions (Bunn and Higgins, 1981). We have shown that subsequent steps of the Maillard reaction that lead to the generation of fluorescence are also much faster during fructation. The increased rate of fluorescence generation might be due, possibly, to the higher reactivity of the aldehydic Amadori group resulting from fructation compared with the ketonic function originated during glucation, thus facilitating a faster conversion of these groups to fluorophores. The spectral properties of the fluorescence are, on the other hand, almost identical in both forms of glycated proteins and, therefore, the fluorescence observed in proteins obtained from tissues should not be attributed exclusively to glucation.

The significant overlap between the protein tryptophan emission and the excitation of Maillard reaction fluorophores provides a tool for the investigation of interactions between glycated proteins and other proteins. Our preliminary results indicate that fluorophores derived from a fructated lysine derivative bind strongly to BSA and IgG. The nature of this interaction has not been characterized thus far, but the relevance of these findings to the pathophysiology of diabetes warrants further exploration. An increased concentration of albumin at the site of the basement membranes of kidney from patients with diabetic nephropathy has been explained as the result of enhanced binding of this protein to the extracellular matrix (Michael and Brown, 1981). Also, albumin in association with IgG and IgM, was found at higher concentrations in the endoneurium of sural nerve biopsy samples from patients with diabetic polyneuropathy (Podulso et al., 1988). IgG has also been found increasingly bound to the glomerular membrane of diabetic kidney tissue (Westberg and Michael, 1972). These observations might be explained by a high affinity binding of extravasated serum proteins to glycated proteins of the extracellular matrix. Since the sorbitol pathway is operative in these organs, glycation by fructose is probable.

The decrease of collagen fluorescence induced by sorbinil supports the view that protein bound fluorescence might be originated from nonenzymatic fructation, a rather surprising process in a protein such as collagen, which in its mature form is found primarily in the extracellular space. However, sorbitol accumulation within the extracellular matrix has been recently invoked as a pathogenetic factor in the syndrome of limited joint mobility, a sequela of long-standing diabetes (Eaton, 1986). Furthermore, evidence has been adduced for significant diffusion of fructose to the extracellular space, on the basis of organ culture experiments with aortas (Morrison et al., 1972).

The lack of effect of sorbinil on lens protein fluorescence is in contrast with the significant effect found in skin collagen. Although both proteins have a low turnover, fluorescence in collagen was measured after solubilization of a predominantly insoluble protein, containing crosslinks originated from lysine derived aldehydes as well from Maillard reaction products. The results on lens proteins were obtained, on the other hand, on the soluble fraction. We conclude that Amadori groups in the soluble lens proteins, which apparently are significantly reduced by sorbinil administration, arise to a large extent from protein fructation and are not involved in protein, crosslinking, at least to a degree sufficient to induce insolubilization. In contrast, evidence has been presented for the involvement of fluorescent products in protein crosslinking and insolubilization as a result of glycation (Brownlee et al., 1986). Thus, it would be expected that fluorescence in the soluble proteins should not be so sensitive to fluctuations in glycation as collagen.

In this study, sorbinil had no effect on the blood sugar levels of the diabetic rats. This was in accordance with previous reports. Therefore, the decrease in collagen fluorescence or in formaldehyde release by soluble lens proteins cannot be the reflection of diminished direct glycation by glucose.

The Maillard reaction, as exemplified by fructation, and the operation of the sorbitol pathway might be linked in a unified pathogenetic mechanism.

REFERENCES

Bobbit JM (1956). Periodate oxidation of carbohydrates. Adv Carbohydr Res 11:1-14.
Bohles H, Schadle J, Endres W, Shin YS, Kollmann F, Bender SW, Kruse K (1987). Increased concentrations of HbAlab in

hereditary fructose intolerance and galactosemia. Padiatr Padol 22:25-31.

Boot-Handford R, Heath H (1980). Identification of fructose as the retinopathic agent associated with the ingestion of sucrose-rich diets in the rat. Metab. Clin Exp 29:1247-1252.

Brownlee M, Vlassara H, Kooney, A, Ulrich P, Cerami A (1986). Aminoguanidine prevents diabetes-induced arterial wall protein cross-linking. Science 232:1629-1632.

Bunn HF, Gabbay KH, Gallop, PM (1978). The glycosylation of hemoglobin: relevance to diabetes mellitus. Science 200:21-27.

Bunn HF, Higgins PJ (1981). Reaction of monosaccharides with proteins: possible evolutionary significance. Science 213:222-224.

Burden AC (1984). Fructose and misleading glycosylation data. Lancet 1984ii:986.

Cohen AM, Teitelbaum A, Rosenman E (1977). Diabetes induced by a high fructose diet. Metab Clin Exp 26:17-24.

Eaton RP (1986). Aldose reductase inhibition and the diabetic syndrome of limited joint mobility:implications for altered collagen hydration. Metab Clin Exp 35 (Suppl 1):119-121.

Finegold D, Lattimer SA, Nolle S, Bernstein M, Greene DA (1983). Polyol pathway activity and myo-inositol metabolism. A suggested relationship in the pathogenesis of diabetic neuropathy. Diabetes 32:988-992.

Fuchs S, Sela M (1978). Immunoadsorbents. In "Handbook of Experimental Immunology", Oxford:Blackwell, Vol 1, pp 10.1-10.6.

Gabbay KH (1975). Hyperglycemia, polyol metabolism, and complications of diabetes mellitus. Annu Rev Med 26: 521-536.

Gallop PM, Fluckiger R, Hanneken A, Mininsohn MM, Gabbay KH (1981). Chemical quantitation of hemoglobin glycosylation:Fluorometric detection of formaldehyde released upon periodate oxidation of glycoglobin. Anal Biochem 117:427-433.

Gonzalez AM, Sochor M, McLean P (1986). The effect of an aldose reductase inhibitor (sorbinil) on the level of metabolites in lenses of diabetic rats. Diabetes 32: 482-485.

Haney DN, Bunn HF (1976). Glycosylation of hemoglobin in vitro: Affinity labeling of hemoglobin by glucose-6-phosphate. Proc Natl Acad Sci USA 73:3534-3538.

Heath H, Hamlett YC (1976). The sorbitol pathway: Effect of streptozotocin induced diabetes and the feeding of a sucrose-rich diet on glucose, sorbitol and fructose in the retina, blood and liver of rats. Diabetologia 12: 43-46.

Heyns K, Meinecke K-H (1953). Uber Bildung und Darstellung von d- Glucosamin aus Fructose und Ammoniak. Chem Ber 86: 1453-1462.

Hotta N, Kakuta H, Fukasawa H, Kimura M, Koh N, Iida M, Terashima H, Morimura T, Sakamoto N (1985). Effects of fructose-rich diet and the aldose reductase inhibitor, ONO-2235, on the development of diabetic neuropathy in streptozotocin-treated rats. Diabetologia 28: 176-180.

Jedziniak JA, Chylack LT, Jr, Cheng H-M, Gillis MK, Kalustian AA, Tung WH (1981). The sorbitol pathway in the human lens: aldose reductase and polyol dehydrogenase. Invest Ophthalmol Vis Sc 20:314-326.

Jones AF, Jennings PE, Wakefield A, Winkles J, Lunec J, Barnett AH (1986). Collagen-linked fluorescence in diabetes mellitus. N Engl J Med 315:323-324.

Kinoshita JH, Fukushi S, Kador P, Merola LO (1979). Aldose reductase in diabetic complications of the eye. Metab Clin Exp 28 (Suppl 1):462-469.

Kuck JFR, Jr (1962). Glucose metabolism and fructose synthesis in the diabetic rat lens. Invest Ophthalmol 1:390-395.

Lakowicz JR (1983). "Principles of Fluorescence Spectroscopy." New York:Plenum, pp. 303-339.

Ludvigson MA, Sorenson RL (1980). Immunohistochemical localization of aldose reductase.1. Enzyme purification and antibody preparation-Localization in peripheral nerve, artery, and testis. Diabetes 29:438-449.

Mayhew JA, Gillon KRW, Hawthorne JN (1983). Free and lipid inositol, sorbitol and sugars in sciatic nerve obtained post-mortem from diabetic patients and control subjects. Diabetologia 24:13-15.

McKinney RA, Urbanowski JC, Dain JA (1982). Nonenzymatic glycosylation of albumin and fetuin by sialic acid. Biochem Int 4:127-133.

Michael AF, Brown DM (1981). Increased concentration of albumin in in kidney basement membranes in diabetes mellitus. Diabetes 30: 843-846

Monnier V, Stevens VJ, Cerami A (1980). Nonenzymatic glycosylation of hemoglobin and lens crystallins. In Srivastava SK (ed) "Red Blood Cell and Lens Metabolism,"

Amsterdam:Elsevier, pp 463-474.

Morrison AD, Clements RS, Jr, Winegrad AI (1972). Effects of elevated glucose concentrations on the metabolism of the aortic wall. J Clin Invest 51:3114-3123.

Morrison AD, Clements RS, Jr, Travis SB, Oski F, Winegrad AI (1970). Glucose utilization by the polyol pathway in human erythrocytes. Biochem Biophys Res Comm 40:199-205.

Podulso JF, Curran GL, Dyck PJ (1988). Increase in albumin, IgG and IgM blood-nerve barrier indices in human diabetic neuropathy. Proc Natl Acad Sci USA 85:4879-4883.

Poulsom R, Mirrlees DJ, Earl DCN, Heath H (1983a). The effects of an aldose reductase inhibitor upon the sorbitol pathway, fructose-1-phosphate and lactate in the retina and nerve of streptozotocin diabetic rats. Exp Eye Res 36:751-760.

Poulsom R, Boot-Handford RP, Heath H (1983b). The effects of long-term treatment of streptozotocin-diabetic rats with an aldose reductase inhibitor. Exp Eye Res 37:507-515.

Sekimoto H, Matsumoto M, Nakano T, Horibe N, Suzuki T, Morimoto E, Lin K, Ishikawa N, Tsuchiya H, Ikegaki H, Okuizumi M (1988). Clinical study on the metabolism of various sugars in diabetes mellitus. In Sakamoto N, Kinoshita JH, Kador PF, Hotta N (eds) "Polyol pathway and its role in diabetic complications", Amsterdam: Elsevier, pp 564-568.

Stribling D, Mirrlees DJ, Harrison HE, Earl DCN (1985). Properties of ICI 128,436, a novel aldose reductase inhibitor, and its effects on diabetic complications in the rat. Metab Clin Exp 34:336-344.

Suarez G, Novick J, Oronsky AL (1984). Non-enzymatic fructosylation of albumin:generation of a fluorophore. Fed Proc 43:2022 (Abstr).

Suarez G, Rajaram R, Bhuyan KC, Oronsky AL, Goidl JA (1986). Reduction of skin collagen fluorescence following treatment of diabetic rats with sorbinil: evidence for in vivo non-enzymatic fructosylation. In "International Symposium on the Polyol Pathway and its Role in Diabetic Complications." Kashikojima, Japan, p 38 (Abstr.)

Suarez G, Rajaram R, Bhuyan KC, Oronsky AL, Goidl JA (1988). Administration of an aldose reductase inhibitor induces a decrease of collagen fluorescence in diabetic rats. J Clin Invest 82:624-627.

Suarez G, Rajaram R, Oronsky, AL, Gawinowicz MA (1989).

Nonenzymatic glycation of bovine serum albumin by fructose (fructation). Comparison with the Maillard reaction initiated by glucose. J Biol Chem 264:3674.

Thorpe SR, Baynes JW (1982). Nonenzymatic glycosylation of proteins in vitro and in vivo. In Horowitz MI, Pigman W (eds.) "The Glycoconjugates", New York: Academic Press, Vol III, pp 113-131.

Tomlinson DR, Townsend J., Freeten P (1985). Prevention of defective axonal transport in streptozocin-diabetic rats by treatment with "Statil" (ICI 128436), an aldose reductase inhibitor. Diabetes 34:970-972.

Urbanowski JC, Cohenford MA, Levy HL, Crawford JD, Dain JA (1982a). Nonenzymatically galactosylated serum albumin in a galactosemic infant. N Engl J Med 306: 84-86.

Urbanowski JC, Cohenford MA, Dain JA (1982b). Nonenzymatic galactosylation of human serum albumin. In vitro preparation. J Biol Chem 257:111-115.

Westberg NG, Michael AF (1972). Immunohistopathology of diabetic glomerulosclerosis. Diabetes 21:163-174.

Zaman Z, Verwilghen RL, (1981). Non-enzymic glycosylation of horse spleen and rat liver ferritins. Biochim Biophys Acta 699:120-124.

ACKNOWLEDGEMENT

I gratefully acknowledge my colleagues R. Rajaram, A.L. Oronsky, K.C. Bhuyan, C. Raventos-Suarez, J. Maturana, J.A. Goidl and M.A. Gawinowicz for their participation in various stages of this research. Partially funded by the American Heart Association, the Milton Petrie Fund, and Lederle Laboratories. I thank Jeanne Appedu for her skillful typing of the manuscript.

The Maillard Reaction in Aging,
Diabetes, and Nutrition, pages 163–170
© 1989 Alan R. Liss, Inc.

FRUCTOSE MEDIATED CROSSLINKING OF PROTEINS

Donald J. Walton, John D. McPherson and Brian H. Shilton

Department of Biochemistry, Queen's University, Kingston, Ontario, Canada K7L 3N6

ABSTRACT.   10-20% of the hexose bound to human ocular lens proteins was found to be attached to ε-amino groups of lysyl residues via carbon 2. It was concluded that the proteins had undergone nonenzymatic reactions with endogenous fructose. This process may be important in some mammalian tissues, owing to the high crosslinking potential of fructose.

INTRODUCTION

In some mammalian organs, such as lens, peripheral nerve and kidney, fructose is synthesized by operation of the polyol pathway (Gabbay, 1973). Dr. Suarez, who is attending this symposium, noted that fructose reacts with proteins in neutral aqueous solutions, to give coloured, fluorescent products (Suarez et al., 1984 and 1986). We therefore proposed that this type of glycation reaction occurs in vivo, and that it might lead to protein crosslinking. This hypothesis was examined in three stages. (1) The chemistry of fructosylation of lysyl residues of human serum albumin (HSA) was studied, (2) fructosylated lysyl residues were identified in human lens proteins, and (3) the crosslinking potential of fructose was demonstrated, using a model protein.

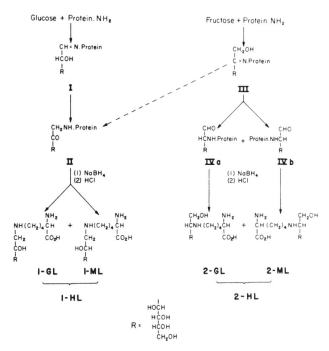

Figure 1. Reaction scheme showing glucosylation and fructosylation of a protein, and formation of deoxyhexitol derivatives of lysine. Reprinted with permission (McPherson et al., 1988). Copyright (1988) American Chemical Society.

CHEMISTRY OF FRUCTOSYLATION OF HSA

We had already established a method of analysis of glycated lysyl residues (Walton and McPherson, 1987). A glucosylated protein (II; Fig. 1) is treated with borohydride, and is then hydrolyzed to give 1-GL and 1-ML, the gluco and manno epimers of N^ϵ-(1-deoxyhexitol-1-yl)lysine (1-HL). 1-HL is isolated by phenylboronate affinity chromatography, and determined by HPLC of the phenylthiocarbamyl (PTC) derivative. This method was extended to the analysis of N^ϵ-(2-deoxyhexitol-2-yl)lysine (2-HL; a mixture of the epimers 2-GL and 2-ML).

Incubation of nonglyco-HSA with 0.5 M glucose in phosphate buffer (pH 7.4) at 37° for 1 week gave only

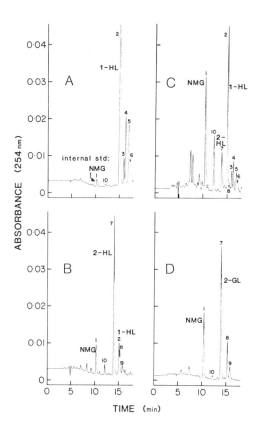

Figure 2. Separation of PTC hexitol amino acids by HPLC, using a C18 column (Walton and McPherson, 1987). NMG refers to N-methylglucamine, the internal standard. 3-6 and 8-9 are acid degradation products of 1-HL and 2-HL, respectively. Panels A-C represent hydrolysates of borohydride-reduced proteins: (A) nonglyco-HSA, incubated with glucose for 1 week; (B) nonglyco-HSA, incubated with fructose for 1 week; (C) water-soluble fraction of lens protein from 60-69 year old diabetic subjects. (D) Synthetic 2-GL, after being heated in 4 N HCl at 110°C for 24 h. Reprinted with permission (McPherson et al., 1988). Copyright (1988) American Chemical Society.

1-HL, i.e. all of the bound hexose was attached to lysines via C-1 (see Fig. 2A and Table 1). Incubation with fructose under similar conditions gave 1-HL and 2-HL in a ratio of 15:85 (see Fig. 2B and Table 1). It was assumed that 2-HL was derived from structures IVa and/or IVb (Fig. 1) which were formed by attachment of fructose to lysyl amino groups. Detection of 1-HL, which represents compound II, was not surprizing, since small quantities of 1-deoxyfructos-1-yl derivatives are formed when fructose reacts with amino acids (Heyns et al., 1957). However, the mechanism involved is not properly understood.

The interpretation of the results of analysis of hydrolysates of borohydride-treated proteins (below) was therefore based upon the following principles:
Detection of 1-HL Only. ϵ-Amino groups of lysyl residues were glucosylated. No fructosylation had occurred.
Detection of 2-HL. ϵ-Amino groups were fructosylated. In this case a relatively small quantity of 1-HL must be ascribed to fructosylation.

TABLE 1. Hexitol Lysine Content of HSA[a], Glycated in Vitro and Treated with Borohydride

Hexose used for incubation	mol/mol of HSA		
	Attached hexose (counting)[b]	1-HL	2-HL
glucose	12	14	0
fructose	1.5	0.2	1.3

[a]Nonglyco HSA incubated with hexose for 1 week.
[b]Hexose incorporated during incubation with [U-14C] hexose.

IN VIVO FRUCTOSYLATION OF HUMAN LENS PROTEINS

Borohydride-treated lens proteins gave a strong signal for PTC-1-HL (Fig. 2C), confirming previous reports

(Garlick et al., 1984; Liang et al., 1986) that they are glucosylated. All of the samples examined gave another, weaker, signal with the same retention time as that of synthetic 2-GL. It was concluded that lysine residues of these proteins had undergone nonenzymatic fructosylation in vivo. Presumably a small proportion of the 1-HL was attributable to fructosylation. 1-HL and 2-HL contents of proteins from several groups of lenses are given in Table 2. There were no significant differences between the 2-HL contents of proteins of clear and cataract-containing, or diabetic and nondiabetic categories.

TABLE 2. Hexitol-Lysine Content of Borohydride-Treated Proteins from Human Lenses[a]

Age (years)	With (+) or without (-) cataract	Diabetic (D) or non-diabetic (N)	Hexitol-lysine content[b] (mmol per mol protein) soluble 1-HL	2-HL	insoluble 1-HL	2-HL
41-55	-	N	16	2	16	6
41-55	-	N	14	1	14	1
41-55	-	N	5	1	6	1
41-55	+	N	16	3	11	2
41-55	+	N	9	1	10	2
41-55	+	N	10	2	c	c
56-70	-	N	15	4	14	4
56-70	-	N	5	1	5	1
56-70	-	N	6	5	c	c
60-69	+	D	32	5	61	6
60-69	+	D	34	8	61	6
60-69	+	D	c	c	56	7

[a]The data on each line were obtained from a pool of 4 lenses.
[b]Values are based upon crystallin monomer, molecular weight 20,000.
[c]Not determined.

CROSSLINKING POTENTIAL OF FRUCTOSE

Dr. Baynes has shown that bovine pancreatic ribonuclease A (RNase) is a useful model for studying hexose-induced protein crosslinking (Eble et al., 1983). In the work described here, RNase was incubated with 0.5 M glucose or fructose in phosphate buffer (pH 7.4) at 37°, and the fraction of crosslinked protein was then determined by scanning of Coomassie Blue-stained SDS-PAGE gels (run under reducing conditions).

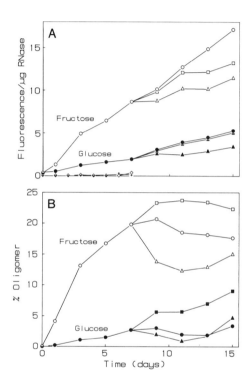

Figure 3. (A) Development of non-tryptophan fluorescence of RNase on incubation with hexoses. (B) Crosslinking of RNase.

Non-tryptophan fluorescence development (excitation and emission maxima 330 and 405 nm, respectively) (Fig. 3A; circles) and crosslinking (Fig. 3B; circles) were induced several times more rapidly by fructose than by glucose. After 10 days of incubation with either hexose crosslinking ceased while fluorescence continued to develop, suggesting that crosslinking preceded fluorophore formation. The removal of hexoses from incubation mixtures at 7 days did not prevent further fluorescence development or crosslinking (Figs. 3A and 3B; squares). It was therefore concluded that the order of events was (i) glycation, to afford a relatively stable protein derivative such as II or IV, (ii) reaction of the bound hexose with a nucleophile of another protein molecule to form a crosslink, and (iii) fluorophore formation.

After removal of hexose at 7 days, fluorescence and crosslinking were inhibited by 0.1 M D-penicillamine (Figs. 3A and 3B; triangles), which probably reacted with carbonyl groups of the bound hexose of II or IV.

CONCLUSIONS

We have demonstrated that at least one type of protein is nonenzymatically fructosylated in vivo, and that fructose induces protein crosslinking in vitro. Fructose mediated crosslinking merits further consideration, as it may cause some of the modifications of proteins that are associated with aging and diabetes.

ACKNOWLEDGMENT

The authors wish to thank the Canadian Diabetes Association for financial support of this work.

REFERENCES

Eble AS, Thorpe SR, Baynes JW (1983). Nonenzymatic glucosylation and glucose-dependent cross-linking of protein. J Biol Chem 258:9406-9412.

Gabbay KH (1973). The sorbitol pathway and the complications of diabetes. N Engl J Med 288:831-836.

Garlick RL, Mazer JS, Chylack LT, Tung WH, Bunn HF (1984). Nonenzymatic glycation of human lens crystallin. J Clin Invest 74:1742-1749.

Heyns K, Breuer H, Paulsen H (1957). Darstellung und Verhalten der 2-N-Aminosäure-2-desoxy-glucosen ("Glucose-Aminosäuren") aus Glycin, Alanin, Leucin und Fructose. Chem Ber 90:1374-1386.

Liang JN, Hershorin LL, Chylack LT (1986). Non-enzymatic glycosylation in human diabetic lens crystallins. Diabetologia 29:225-228.

McPherson JD, Shilton BH, Walton DJ (1988). Role of fructose in glycation and cross-linking of proteins. Biochemistry 27:1901-1907.

Suarez G, Novick J, Oronsky AL (1984). Non-enzymatic fructosylation of albumin: generation of a fluorophore. Fed Proc, Fed Am Soc Exp Biol 43:2022.

Suarez G, Rajaram R, Oronsky AL (1986). Selective removal of Amadori products from non-enzymatically fructosylated bovine serum albumin. Fed Proc, Fed Am Soc Exp Biol 45:1539.

Walton DJ, McPherson JD (1987). Analysis of glycated amino acids by high-performance liquid chromatography of phenylthiocarbamyl derivative. Anal Biochem 164:547-553.

The Maillard Reaction in Aging,
Diabetes, and Nutrition, pages 171–184
© 1989 Alan R. Liss, Inc.

ACTIVATION   OF   ALDOSE   REDUCTASE   BY   NONENZYMATIC
GLYCOSYLATION

Satish K. Srivastava, Naseem H. Ansari, Aruni
Bhatnagar, Greg Hair, Siqi Liu, and Ballabh Das
Department of Human Biological Chemistry & Genetics
University of Texas Medical Branch
Galveston, TX 77550

ABSTRACT

Incubation of human erythrocyte with 50 mM glucose
results in glycosylation of aldose reductase besides hemoglobin A and other proteins. The glycosylation of aldose
reductase is established by adsorption of the enzyme on
phenyl boronate (PBA-60) column. Furthermore, the enzyme
was purified to an apparent homogeneity from the erythrocytes incubated with 50 mM glucose and the glycosylation
was quantitated by reduction with tritiated sodium borohydride. The glycosylated aldose reductase exhibits lower Km
for glucose and NADPH as compared to unglycosylated enzyme
and is not inhibited by phosphorylated intermediates such
as ADP, 1,3-DPG, 2,3-DPG and 3-PGA, whereas physiological
concentrations of these intermediates almost completely
inhibit the unglycosylated enzyme. In addition, the glycosylated enzyme is less susceptible to aldose reductase
inhibitors such as sorbinil and alrestatin. In hyperglycemia, blood glucose higher than 11 mM, almost all the aldose
reductase is glycosylated.

INTRODUCTION

The mechanism of schiff-base formation between glucose
and α- or ϵ-amino group of lysine of proteins followed by
Amadori's rearrangement has already been discussed by
several speakers. A schematic diagram of the reaction of a
protein with glucose is presented in Fig. 1. I will
discuss the role of non-enzymatic glycosylation of
proteins, especially lens proteins, in the

pathophysiology of diabetic complications, mainly cataractogenesis.

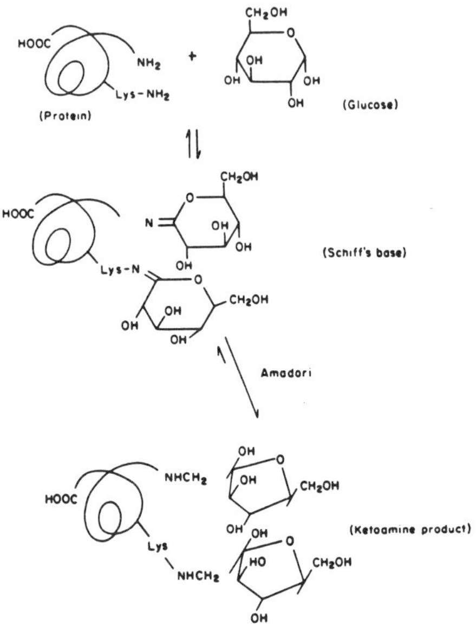

Figure 1. Reaction of a protein with glucose (From Ref. 1)

Although Maillard reaction has been known to and used by scientists to explain browning of food products for a long time, it's application in the pathophysiology of human diseases has been appreciated only during the past two decades. Nonenzymatic glycosylation of human hemoglobin A by glucose and its correlation with blood glucose levels over an extended period of time has proved to be a better indicator of diabetes as compared to one or two determinations of blood glucose. Increased glycosylation of lens crystallins in diabetic subjects and in animals with experimentally induced diabetes as well as in lenses incubated with high glucose or lens crystallins incubated for several days with glucose has been demonstrated by a number of investigators including us (1-8). Stevens et al. (8) in 1978 suggested that glycosylation of lens crystallins may make them more vulnerable to intra and inter-disulfide bond formation which may eventually result in high molecular weight protein aggregates leading to cataractogenesis. However, we (1,2) did not find a correlation between human lens crystallin glycosylation and disulfide bond formation in diabetic cataract. Pandey et al. (3) also did not find any correlation between increased glycosylation and opacification of the human lens. Liang et al. (5) have recently concluded that the extent of glycosylation depends on the accessibility of the surface areas of protein where lysine residues are located which in turn are correlated with protein conformation. Chiou et al. (4) studied the non-enzymatic glycosylation of bovine lens crystallins and concluded that it increases with aging and further demonstrated that treatment of galactosemic rats with aldose reductase inhibitor, sorbinil, prevented cataractogenesis but had no effect on the non-enzymatic glycosylation. Also, in db/db mice which have hereditary hyperglycemia, no cataract formation has been demonstrated. These studies indicate that modification of lens crystallins with nonenzymatic glycosylation may not be the primary cause of sugar induced cataractogenesis.

Thus the question arises, does glycosylation play a role in diabetic complications, especially cataractogenesis via a) modification of proteins such that the tertiary structure changes and sulfhydryl groups are exposed and become vulnerable to oxidation leading to formation of intra and inter-molecular disulfide bonds which may be responsible for protein aggregation and increased light scattering, b) glycosylation of enzyme proteins which may affect their catalytic properties.

Reports which indicate that modification of lens crystallins by glycosylation may not be the primary cause of sugar induced cataractogenesis have already been discussed (1-8). We will now discuss mainly the effect of glycosylation on aldose reductase which appears to be involved in sugar induced cataractogenesis because aldose reductase inhibitors such as sorbinil and alrestatin prevent diabetic and galactosemic cataractogenesis (9-13) and are of some help in other diabetic complications. The mechanism could be mainly via inhibition of aldose reductase or scavenging of free radicals.

$$\text{Glusoce} + \text{NADPH} + \text{H}^+ \xrightarrow{\text{aldose reductase}} \text{sorbitol} + \text{NADP}^+$$

$$\text{Sorbitol} + \text{NAD}^+ \xrightarrow{\text{sorbitol dehydrogenase}} \text{fructose} + \text{NADH} + \text{H}^+$$

Fig. 2   Enzymes of sorbitol pathway.

As shown in Fig. 2, aldose reductase is the first enzyme of the sorbitol pathway which reduces glucose to sorbitol in the presence of NADPH. The second enzyme, sorbitol dehydrogenase, oxidizes sorbitol to fructose in the presence of NAD. We have purified aldose reductase from a number of human tissues such as erythrocyte, lens, placenta, kidney, brain, and muscle and from bovine lens and kidney and have studied its kinetic, structural, and immunological properties (14-19).

Figure 3 shows the activity of erythrocyte aldose reductase from hyperglycemic subjects. As you can see there is an excellent correlation, correlation coeffecient >0.9, between blood glucose levels and aldose reductase activity (20).

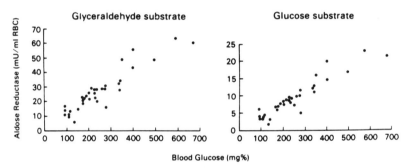

Fig. 3 Erythrocyte aldose reductase activity from hyperglycemic subjects. Aldose reductase activity was determined in the erythrocytes obtained from hyperglycemic subjects as described earlier (Taken from Ref. 20).

Increased levels of aldose reductase activity were observed in the lens also from diabetic subjects with hyperglycemia as compared to normal subjects (21).

One should therefore expect increased levels of aldose reductase activity in the erythrocytes incubated with higher concentrations of glucose. As shown in Table 1, we observed 2 to 4 fold increase in the enzyme activity in various experiments. As the glucose concentration in the medium increased, aldose reductase activity also increased. We also observed increased accumulation of sorbitol in the erythrocytes incubated with increasing levels of glucose for 6 hrs at 37°C (Fig. 4).

TABLE 1. Activation of human erythrocyte aldose reductase by glucose

Blood samples were incubated with varying concentrations of glucose for 6 h at 37°C and the enzyme was quantitated after partial purification by DE-52. Values are average ± SD: N = 4

Glucose (mM)	Aldose reductase (mu/ml RBC)	
	glyceraldehyde as substrate	glucose as substrate
-	10.5 + 3.9	3.1 + 0.8
5.5	11.9 + 4.8	3.1 + 0.6
15	18.1 + 1.4	5.2 + 0.8
30	38.4 + 8.2	9.8 + 1.4
50	46.4 + 8.0	12.5 + 0.9

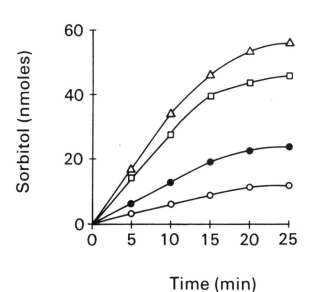

Fig. 4   Accumulation of sorbitol in erythrocytes incubated with glucose.   Human erythrocytes were incubated with glucose, 5.5 mM (0-0), 15 mM (●-●), 30 mM (□-□) and 50 mM (△-△) at 37°C for 6 h.   Sorbitol was determined fluorometrically as described earlier (20).

We subsequently studied the kinetic properties of aldose reductase purified from erythrocytes incubated with 5.5 mM and 30-50 mM glucose for 4 hrs at 37°C and from erythrocytes obtained from diabetic subjects with varying degrees of hyperglycemia (22). The enzyme obtained from 5.5 mM glucose incubated erythrocytes was designated normal or native or unactivated and the enzyme obtained from 30-50 mM glucose incubated erythrocytes or from hyperglycemic subjects with blood glucose levels higher than 200 mg% was designated activated enzyme.

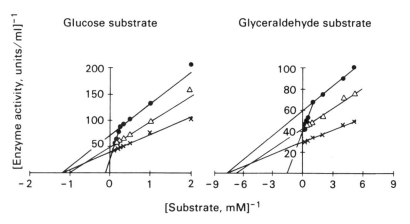

Fig. 5 Reciprocal plots of erythrocyte activity vs substrate concentration. Native enzyme (●-●), 30 mM glucose-incubated erythrocyte (x-x), and erythrocyte from hyperglycemic subjects, blood glucose 250 mg%(△-△) (Ref. 20).

As shown in Figure 5, the plots of the reciprocals of the enzyme velocity and substrate concentration were biphasic in the case of the native enzyme and were monophasic in the case of the activated enzyme obtained from 30 mM glucose incubated or hyperglycemic subjects when either glyceraldehyde or glucose was used as a substrate. The Km glucose of the activated enzyme was 0.8 mM while the Km glucose of the unactivated enzyme was 0.8 mM and 10 mM.

Native aldose reductase was almost completely inhibited by 15 uM ADP, 2,3-DPG, 3-PGA, and 1,3-DPG, whereas the activated enzyme was not inhibited (Table 2). The effect of phosphorylated intermediates on aldose reductase purified from erythrocytes subjects with varing degrees of

hyperglycemia was also studied.   As you can see, the inhibition by these four phosphorylated intermediates decreased
as the blood glucose levels increased. This would indicate
that under normoglycemic conditions aldose reductase could
be almost completely inhibited whereas in hyperglycemia the
enzyme becomes active and can efficiently reduce glucose.

TABLE 2. Effect of phosphorylated intermediates (PI) on
erythrocyte aldose reductase activity.

PI (15 uM)	Enzyme activity remaining (% of control)				
	normal	normal with 30 mM glc	diabetic (blood glc mg%)		
			<150	151-250	>250
− (control)	100	100	100	100	100
AMP	100	98	100	105	100
ADP	22	96	32	65	92
ATP	90	100	94	100	98
Glc-1-P	100	102	96	98	105
Glc-6-P	130	96	115	108	100
Fru-6-P	110	94	108	99	105
Fru-1,6-P_2	108	106	96	102	98
Gly-3-P	123	95	119	115	105
DHAP	84	99	106	95	97
1,3-DPG	0	94	24	68	85
2,3-DPG	0	89	12	56	79
PEP	88	90	96	89	100
3-PGA	3	92	21	69	88

The   activated enzyme was found to be less susceptible
to inhibition by aldose reductase inhibitors such as
sorbinil and alrestatin (20). The unactivated enzyme was
almost completely inhibited by 20 uM Sorbinil while the
activated enzyme was inhibited by only approximately 25%
when glyceraldehyde was used as the substrate (Fig. 6). As
the blood glucose concentration increased in diabetic
subjects, the enzyme became less susceptible to inhibition
by Sorbinil.

The obvious question, therefore, is what is the
mechanism of aldose reductase activation in erythrocyte and
lens? It is likely that under hyperglycemic conditions,
aldose reductase   gets glycosylated and the glycosylated
enzyme has different properties as compared to
unglycosylated enzyme.

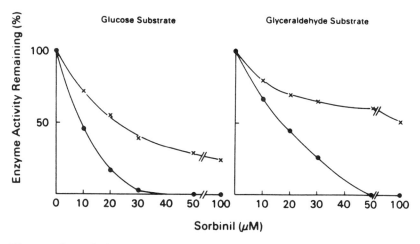

Figure 6. Inhibition of activated (x-x) and unactivated (•-•) erythrocyte aldose reductase by sorbinil (Ref. 20).

We therefore purified aldose reductase to an apparant homogeneity from human erythrocytes incubated with 5.5 and 50 mM glucose for 6 hr at 37°C. The enzyme obtained from 50 mM glucose incubated erythrocyte was glycosylated as determined by phenylboronate affinity chromotography and tritiated sodium borohydride reduction. Similarly, the enzyme obtained from erythrocytes of diabetic subjects with blood glucose levels higher than 200 mg% was more than 90% glycosylated.

Another interesting observation was that we were able to activate the native enzyme purified from erythrocytes of normoglycemic subjects, with a mixture of 10 uM each of glucose-6-P, NADPH and glucose. The activated enzyme had all the properties of the enzyme obtained from 50 mM glucose incubated erythrocytes and from erythrocytes of hyperglycemic subjects.

Two models have been proposed to explain the role of aldose reductase in sugar induced cataractogenesis. The first model (Fig. 7) is based upon osmotic changes due to increased accumulation of polyol as proposed by Kinoshita (23). In the second model (Fig. 8) it is shown that under normoglycemic conditions, aldose reductase is almost completely inhibited by phosphorylated intermediates, but

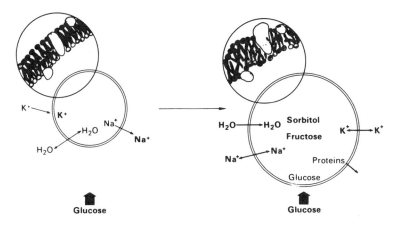

Fig. 7. Model for membrane dysfunction due to osmotic imbalance.

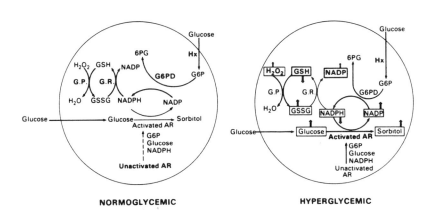

NORMOGLYCEMIC   HYPERGLYCEMIC

Figure 8 Model to show activation of aldose reductase in hyperglycemia and the effect of competition between aldose reductase and glutathione reductase for NADPH.

under hyperglycemic conditions, it gets glycosylated and activated and may compete for NADPH which is required for reducing the oxidants. Increased diversion of NADPH to reduce glucose may lead to decreased reduction of GSSG, increased efflux of GSSG, increased glutathione-protein mixed disulfide formation, increased H_2O_2 and lipid peroxides etc. The net result of prolonged hyperglycemia thus could be increased oxidative damage leading to cataractogenesis and other diabetic complications.

The results of two of our major experiments which favor the second hypothesis are summarized below: Human erythrocytes were incubated with 5.5 mM or 30 mM glucose at 37°C for 4 hrs. Subsequently the erythrocyte GSH was oxidized by t-butylhydroperoxide and the cells after washing were incubated with 5.5 mM glucose and the regeneration of GSH was followed. The 30 mM glucose-preincubated erythrocytes regenerated GSH much slower for the first 5 min as compared to the 5.5 mM glucose-preincubated (Fig. 9).

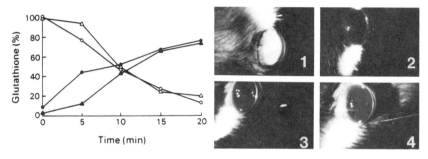

Figure 9.   Figure 10.

Figure 9 Regeneration of glutathione in the erythrocytes pre-incubated with 30 mM glucose. Whole blood was incubated with 5.5 mM (control) and 30 mM (experimental) glucose at 37°C for 6 h. The washed erythrocytes were treated with tertiary butyl hydroperoxide for 20 min at room temperature. The erythrocytes were washed with phosphate buffered-saline and suspended in two volumes of the medium. Final concentration of glucose was 5.5 mM. At different time intervals, aliquots were removed for GSH and GSSG determinations: Experimental - GSH = ▲-▲, and GSSG = △-△. Control - GSH = ●-●, and GSSG = O--O .

Figure 10 Prevention of cataract formation in galactosemic rats by butylated hydroxytoluene (BHT). Photographs of the lens were taken by slit lamp 23 days after feeding high-galactose diet to 6 wk old rats. 1) 50% galactose 2) 50% galactose + 0.4% BHT, 3) starch, 4) starch + 0.4% BHT. (From Ref. 24.)

TABLE 3.
Biochemical determinations in the lens of galactosemic rats

	Group 1		Group 2		Group 3		Group 4	
	Day 10	Day 23	Day 10	Day 23	Day 10	Day 23	Day 10	Day 23
Lens wt.	37.4±0.4	42.8±0.8	33.7±0.8	35.2±1.1	30.0±0.5	33.0±0.8	30.8±0.4	35.6±1.4
GSH	1.1±0.3	0	5.2±0.3	1.5±0.2	5.5±0.4	5.4±0.3	6.5±0.5	6.6±1.0
Prot-SH	58.0±3.9	41.6±5.4	55.8±3.3	53.8±3.3	53.7±4.5	54.2±5.7	58.3±3.9	57.8±5.3
Galactitol	102±9	83 ±16.7	96±12	186±31	ND	ND	ND	ND
AR	13.0±0.9	4.4±0.7	13.3±2.7	14.8±1.6	14.1±1.1	17.9±0.8	15.1±1.4	14.4±0.9

Group 1, Galactose; Group 2, galactose plus butylated hydroxytoluene (BHT); Group 3, starch; Group 4, starch plus BHT. Values are mean ± SD. ND, not detectable, AR = Aldose reductase.

Subsequently the rate increased and in approximately 15 min maximum regeneration of GSH was achieved in both the cases. This indicated lower reducing capacity of the erythrocytes, pre-incubated under hyperglycemic conditions.

In the second experiment (24), we had four groups of rats fed 50% galactose, galactose + butylated hydroxy-toluene (BHT), starch, and starch + BHT. We found that rats fed 50% galactose diet (Fig. 10, upper left) developed mature cataract in approximately 23 days whereas the rats which received 50% galactose plus butylated hydroxy toluene had no opacity on day 23 but they developed mature cataract in approximately 38 days. Important to note was that on day 10 the galactitol levels were comparable in the two groups, galactose and galactose + BHT and on day 23 the galactitol levels in the BHT treated group were more than twice as much as in the galactose treated group which had developed complete opacity (Table 3). The galactitol levels in the BHT plus galactose group on day 23 were 185 nmoles/mg pertein as opposed to galactose group which had 83 nmoles/mg protein. This should be enough to cause osmotic changes in galactose + BHT group but apparently it did not. This experiment would indicate that polyol accumulation leading to osmotic changes alone cannot explain sugar induced cataractogenesis. Oxidative damage may be the primary cause of sugar induced cataractogenesis and possibly other diabetic complications. This would be substantiated by increased activity of aldose reductase due to glycosylation in hyperglycemia, decreased activty of superoxide dismutase (25), a defense enzyme against oxidants, due to glycosylation, and decreased Na^+/K^+ ATPase acivity due to glycosylation (26).

ACKNOWLEDGEMENT

This work was supported in part by the PHS grants EY-01677 and DK-36118 awarded by the National Institutes of Health.

REFERENCES

1. Ansari, N.H., Awasthi, Y.C. and Srivastava, S.K. Role of glycosylation in protein disulfide formation and cataractogenesis. Exp. Eye Res., 31, 9-19, 1980.

2. Awasthi, Y.C., Ansari, N.H. and Srivastava, S.K. In: Red Blood Cell and Lens Metabolism, Elsevier North Holand, Inc. Ed. Srivastava, S.K., 1979.

3. Pande, A., Garner, W.H. and Spector, A. Glycosylation of human lens protein and cataractogenesis. Biochem. Biophys. Res. Comm., 89, 1260-1266, 1979.

4. Chiou, S.H., Chylack, L.T., Tung, W.H. and Bunn, F. Nonenzymatic glycosylation of bovine lens crystallins. J. Biol. Chem., 256, 5176-5180, 1981.

5. Liang, N., Hershorin, L.L. and Chylack, L.T. Nonenzymatic glycosylation in human diabetic lens crystallins. Diabetologia, 29, 225-228, 1986.

6. Lee, J.H., Shin, D.H., Lupovitch, A. and Shi, D.X. Glycosylation of lens proteins in senile cataract and diabetes mellitus. Biochem. Biophys. Res. Comm., 128, 888-893, 1984.

7. Chiou, S.H., Chylack, L.T., Bunn, F. and Kinoshita, J.H. Role of nonenzymatic glycosylation in experimental cataract formation. Biochem. Biophys. Res. Comm., 95, 895-901, 1980.

8. Stevens, V.J., Rouzer, C.A., Monnier, V.M. and Cerami, A. Diabetic cataract formation: Potential role of glycosylation of lens crystallins. Proc., Natl. Acad. Sci., 75, 2918-2922, 1978.

9. Foulds, G., O'Brien, M.M., Bianchine, J.R. and Gabbay, K.H. Kinetics of an orally absorbed aldose reductase inhibitor, sorbinil. ClinPharmTher 30, 693-700, 1981.

10. Dvornik, D., Sinard-Duquesne, N., Krami, M., Sestanj, K., Gabbay, K.H., Kinoshita, J.H., Varma, S.D. and Merola, L.O. Polyol accumulation in galactosemic and diabetic rats. Control by an aldose reductase inhibitor. Science, 182, 1146-1148, 1973.

11. Peterson, M.J., Sarges, R., Aldinger, C.E. and MacDonald, D.P. CP-45, 634: A novel Aldose Reductase inhibitor that inhibits polyol pathway activity in diabetic and galactosemic rats. Metabolism, 28 Suppl. 1, 456-612, 1979.

12. Judzewitsch, R., Jaspan, J.B., Pfeifer, M. A., Polonsky, K.S., Harlar, E., Vukadinovic, C. Richton, S., Gabbay, K. Inhibition of Aldose Reductase improves motor nerve conduction velocity in diabetics. Diabetes, 30 Suppl. 30A, 1981.

13. Gabbay, K.H., Spack, N., Loo, S., Hirsh, H.F. and Ackil, A.A. Aldose reductase inhibition: Studies with alrestatin. Metabolism 28, Suppl. 1, 471-476, 1979.

14. Petrash, J.M. and Srivastava, S.K. Purification and properties of human liver aldehyde reductases. Biochim. et Biophys. Acta 707, 105-14, 1982.

15. Das, B. and Srivastava, S.K. Purification and properties of aldehyde reductase from human placenta. Biochim. et Biophys. Acta 840, 324-333, 1985.

16. Das, B. and Srivastava, S.K. Purification and properties of aldose reductase and aldehyde reductase II from human erythrocytes. Arch. Biochem. Biophys. 238 670-679, 1985.

17. Das, B., Song, H.P., Ansari, N.H., Hair, G.A. and Srivastava, S.K. Purification and properties of aldose reductase and aldehyde reductase II from human lens. Lens Res. 4, 309-335, 1987.

18. Srivastava, S.K., Ansari, N.H., Hair, G.A., and Das, B. Aldose and aldehyde reductases in human tissues. Biochim. Biophys. Acta 800, 220-227, 1984.

19. Srivastava, S.K., Das, B. Hair, G.A., Gracy, R.W., Awasthi, S., Ansari, N.H. and Petrash, J.M. Biochemical and genetic interrelationship among human aldoketo reductases: Immunochemical, kinetic and structural properties. Biochim. Biophys. Acta 840 334-343, 1985.

20. Srivastava, S.K., Ansari, N.H., Hair, G.A., Jaspan, J., Rao, M.B. and Das., B.Hyperglycemia induced activation of human erythrocyte aldose reductase and alteration in kinetic properties. Biochim. Biophys. Acta 870 302-311, 1986.

21. Srivastava, S.K., Hair, G.A. and Das, B. Activated and unactivated forms of human erythrocytes aldose reductase. Proc. Natl. Acad. Sci. (USA) 82, 7222-7226, 1985.

22. Das, B., and Srivastava, S.K. Activation of aldose reductase from human tissues. Diabetes 34, 1145-1151, 1985.

23. Kinoshita, J.H.: Mechanism initiating cataract formation. Invest. Ophthalmol., 123, 713-724, 1974.

24. Srivastava, S.K. and Ansari, N.H. Prevention of sugar-induced cataractogenesis in rats by butylated hydroxytoluene. Diabetes 37, 1505-1508, 1988.

25. Arai, K., Magurchi, S., Fujii, S., Ishibashi, H., Oikawa, K. and Taniguchim N. Glycation and inactivation of human Cu-Zn-SOD: identification of the in vitro glycated sites. J. Biol. Chem, 262, 16969-16972, 1987.

26. Garner, M.H. and Spector, A. Direct stimulation of Na$^+$-k$^+$-ATPase and its glucosylated derivative by aldose reductase inhibitor. Diabetes, 36, 716-720, 1987.

The Maillard Reaction in Aging,
Diabetes, and Nutrition, pages 185–203
© 1989 Alan R. Liss, Inc.

NON-ENZYMATIC GLYCATION AND PROTEIN RECOGNITION

M.W. Bitensky↓†, A. Kowluru† and R. A. Kowluru†

Life Sciences † and Physics ↓ Divisions
Los Alamos National Laboratory, Los Alamos,
New Mexico 87545

Abstract:
Glycation of proteins increases their
negative charge and is a self-limiting
process. Glycation also changes the
recognition of proteins. The mammalian
nephron can discriminate between glycated
and unmodified albumin. Diabetes and ageing
both modify this discrimination. Abnormalities in protein recognition may contribute
to the pathological impact of glycation.
The increase in negative charge may explain
both the limit on glycation and its
capacity to change protein recognition.

I   Introduction:
     Non-enzymatic glycation (NEG) of most proteins occurs
slowly and continuously. The rate of this reaction is
accelerated in diabetes mellitus, reflecting increased
levels of glucose in plasma and cells (Brownlee and Cerami
1981; unn 1981; Bernstein 1987; and Gonen et al 1987).
There are numerous examples of altered protein function,
altered protein recognition and protein sequestration via
cross-linking, that follow NEG. E.g., glycated hemoglobin
exhibits reduced affinity for its modulator 2,3 DPG, (Ditzel
et al, 1975) and glycated calmodulin, reduced ability to
activate a variety of target enzymes (Kowluru et al, 1988a).
Glycated plasma albumin (in contrast to the unmodified form)
is avidly taken up by the micropinocytic vesicles of
endothelium (Williams et al, 1981). Glycated myelin basic
protein (and not the unmodified form) is readily ingested by
peritoneal macrophages (Vlassara et al, 1985). Glycated
lens crystalins are known to form higher molecular weight
aggregates (Monnier et al, 1979), while glycated tubulin

monomers form insoluble amorphous aggregates rather than ordered microtubules (Williams *et al*, 1982).

Here we summarize recent work on the processing of glycated albumin by the normal, diabetic and ageing nephron. Our data indicate that glycated albumin (in contrast with its unmodified antecedent) is less effectively reabsorbed by the proximal tubular epithelium. Moreover, reduced quantities of glycated albumin are filtered by the ageing glomerulus in contrast to the amount filtered by normal or diabetic glomeruli in younger animals. We also present recent data which illustrate that NEG is a self limiting process.

A simple model is presented which finds explanation for these observations in the fact that NEG reliably increases the global negative charge (I. e, decreases the pI) of the glycated protein (Williams and Siegal 1985; Kowluru *et al* 1987; 1988a; Krishnamoorthy *et al* 1986; Kondo *et al* 1987). This progressive increase in negative charge associated with glycation appears also to offer a plausible explanation for the apparent limit which is observed (for any particular protein) on the extent of its glycation.

II   Findings:

1)   Editing of NEG Albumin by the Mammalian Nephron:
The differential excretion of glycated and unmodified albumin by the mammalian nephron has been studied in some detail (Williams *et al* 1983; Williams and Pinter 1983; Ghiggeri *et al* 1984; 1985; Kowluru *et al* 1987). The phenomenon, which we term editing, manifests as a marked increase in the percent glycation of urinary albumin which can reach levels 16 times higher than that of plasma albumin in healthy young humans, and 35 times higher in urine vs. plasma in the young wistar rat (Table I, Fig. 1). We define the editing ratio as the percent glycation of urinary albumin divided by the percent glycation of plasma albumin. In calculating this ratio, no distinction was made between albumin molecules bearing 1, 2 or 3 ketoamines. This convention (glycated vs. unmodified) follows the separation characteristics of the phenyl boronate (Glycogel [R]) column used to separate the two classes of albumin (Kowluru *et al* 1987).

		GFR (ml/min/kg)	TOTAL URINARY GLUCO ALB (µg)	EDITING RATIO
SPRAGUE-DAWLEY RAT	NONDIABETIC	6.5	53.82	14.0
	OLD	5.1	26.64	7.2
	DIABETIC	13.30	227.85	3.1
WISTAR RAT	MANNITOL DIURESIS	5.23	159.60	20.5
	CONTROL	1.93	76.86	34.0

Table I)   Relationship between GFR, Urinary Glucoalbumin and Editing Ratios:
Creatinine clearance, urinary glucoalbumin and editing ratios were determined in young (2 mos), old (15 mos), and streptozotocin diabetic (3 mos) Sprague-Dawley males. These measurements were also done in Wistar rats (4 mos), before and at the peak of mannitol induced diuresis.

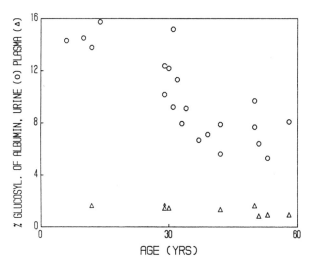

Fig. 1)   Age Dependent Attenuation of Editing in Humans:
Percent glucoalbumin in plasma and urine was measured in humans, (n = 21) between ages 5 and 58 (Kowluru et al 1987).

The total quantity of albumin in human plasma is in the range of 300 grams, while the normal daily excretion of albumin in the urine is less than 40 milligrams. Thus, the total daily excretion of glycated albumin is < 6 milligrams, which compares with a total mass of glycated albumin in the plasma of ≃ 3,000 milligrams. Clearly the urinary excretion of glycated albumin cannot serve as the principal mode by which it leaves the circulation. Moreover, the excretion of glycoalbumin in the urine does not explain the micro albuminuria of diabetes which primarily reflects an increase in glomerular filtration rate (GFR) (Mogensen 1976).

2.   Editing and the Proximal Tubular Reabsorbtion of Albumin:
The magnitude of editing is most striking in young mammals and gradually diminishes with age (Fig. 1 and see below). A key feature of editing, as observed in the absence of intrinsic renal pathology, is the absence of microscopical albuminuria. A most compelling explanation for this phenomenon is found in the proximal tubule, as contrasted with the glomerulus. The glomerulus cannot establish a filtration bias which would preferentially increase glycated albumin, (pI 4.5) which is more negatively charged than unmodified albumin (pI 4.7) (Kowluru *et al*, 1987). Thus a glomerular filtration bias would serve, if anything, to diminish the total amount of glycated albumin filtered.

However, it is in the proximal one third of the proximal tubule where unmodified albumin is extensively reabsorbed (> 95%) so that only miniscule amounts are excreted in the urine (Bourdeau *et al* 1972; Bourdeau and Carone 1974). The evidence strongly favors the idea that glycated albumin is much less efficiently reabsorbed. Studies with test proteins have shown that the reabsorbtion of macromolecules in the proximal tubule does correlate with the molecules positive charge (Christensen *et al* 1981, 1983).

3.   Age Related Attenuation of Editing:
Editing is diminished in consequence of age, diabetes and any other condition associated with an increase in GFR (Table I). There is however a striking difference between the attenuation of editing associated with age, and that loss of editing associated with diabetes mellitus or mannitol diuresis. In the case of diabetes or mannitol

diuresis, the loss of editing is sudden and reflects the rapid onset of a robust increase in GFR. This sudden reduction in the magnitude of editing reflects the dilution of urinary glycated albumin by non-reabsorbed unmodified albumin. Paradoxically, in this form of editing reduction, even though the relative amount of glycated albumin falls (as a percent of total albumin excreted) the actual quantity excreted in a 24 hour period increases by a factor of 2-4 (Table I).

In contrast, the attenuation of editing observed in mammals with age is very gradual and exhibits a smooth continuum in humans between the ages of 5 and 60 (Fig. 1). This gradual attenuation in the magnitude of editing is not associated with microalbuminuria, and is instead associated with a modest decline in GFR, which is characteristic of aging (Davies and Shock, 1950), and also a decline in the total quantity of glycated albumin excreted per diem. These declines are in part a reflection of the gradual decrease (with aging) in the number of surviving functional glomeruli (Anderson and Brenner, 1986).

4.   Editing and Diabetes:
We have found in our studies of diabetics that, in the presence of significant amounts of glucoalbumin, editing ratios are quite low. Glucoalbumin serves as an integrated, longer term (2 - 4 weeks) record of plasma glucose levels. In fact there is an inverse correlation between the magnitude of glucoalbumin levels and the magnitude of editing (Fig. 2).

In human diabetes, editing is strikingly reduced. E.g., we find ratios of 12 in age matched controls vs 3 in diabetic subjects. These data are the means of 10 non-diabetic (ages 10-35) and 25 diabetic (ages 10-37) subjects. The level of editing at any point in time does not correlate with the duration of diabetes or with the age or sex. Our data show a strong correlation between the elevation of the percent glucoalbumin, the amount of urinary albumin and the decline in editing (Kowluru et al, 1987).

Studies in human diabetics, however, do not allow an assessment of the rate at which editing is lost following the onset of hyperglycemia. We therefore studied the time course for the development of this process in rats following a streptozotocin injection (Fig. 3). We found that

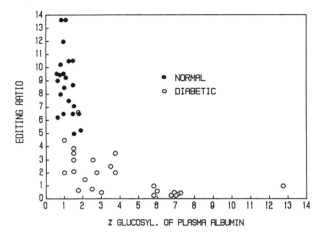

Fig. 2) Relationship Between Editing Ratio and Hyperglycemia:
Editing ratios were determined in nondiabetic (n = 22) and diabetic (n = 25) humans and were plotted against percent plasma glucoalbumin.

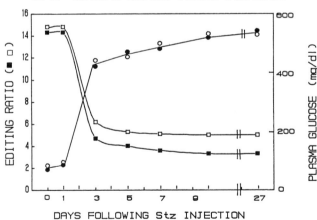

Fig. 3) Time course for onset of reduced editing in streptozotocin diabetic rats.
Editing ratios and hyperglycemia were measured at different time intervals in Sprague-Dawley rats (n = 4) treated with Stz. A separate group of Stz treated rats (n = 4) were given Sorbinil.

concomitant with the onset of hyperglycemia, or mannitol infusion, there is an associated attenuation of editing in the diabetic animal (Kowluru, et al, 1987). The aldose reductase inhibitor Sorbinil did not prevent the reduction in editing found with streptozotocin induced hyperglycemia.

5.   Increased GFR and Reduction in Editing:
      In Table I we show a comparison of the effects of mannitol diuresis, diabetes and age on the GFR and on editing ratios.   These data show that the attenuation of editing with age is accompanied by a decrease in the total amount of glycated protein excreted per 24 hours.   We found that the attenuation of editing seen with mannitol diuresis and diabetes is accompanied by increases in both GFR and the total amount of glycated albumin excreted (Table I).   Thus the rapid decline in the magnitude of the editing ratio seen with diabetes or mannitol infusion reflects the dilution of glycated albumin by unmodified albumin whose presence in increased quantities (because of the increase in GFR) appears to overwhelm the reabsorptive capacity of the proximal tubular epithelium (Kowluru et al, 1987). As might be expected, there is a clear correlation between the increase in GFR and the reduction in the magnitude of editing found in diabetes mellitus (r = -0.44, n = 30) (Kowluru et al, 1987).

6.   Editing, Ageing and Glomerular Charge:
      We have sought the explanation for the attenuation of editing with increased GFR, primarily in the differential handling of unmodified and glycated albumins by the proximal tubular epithelium.   How then explain the attenuation of editing with increasing age?   One attractive hypothesis proposes that the total negative charge on the glomerular filter increases with increasing age.   This charge is normally contributed by glycosaminoglycans as well as the sialoglycoprotein podocalyxin (Caulfield and Farquhar 1976; Kanwar 1984; Kerjaschki et al 1984).   We have utilized a simple and direct approach to measure putative differences in the amount of negative charge on the glomerular filter between older and younger rats.   We have prepared ^{35}S and ^{3}H labelled polysulfonated dextrans (Chang et al 1975; Woods and Mora 1958) which are quite homogeneous with respect to the Stoke's radius of the dextran polymer (22° A). We found (using iso-electric focussing) a "normal" range of values with regard to the quantity of sulfate attached to the dextran polymers.   Thus a population of dextrans which are

homogeneous with respect to size was found to exhibit a gaussian distribution with respect to its content of negative charge. These dextran polymers were infused into the jugular vein of both young and old rats. If in fact the glomerular filter is more negatively charged in older animals one would expect this to influence the ratio of [^{35}S] sulfate charge to the mass of excreted [^{3}H] dextran as compared to that ratio exhibited by the material infused into the plasma. An attractive feature of this approach is that the critical parameter (charge to mass ratio) varies independently of the total quantity of dextran excreted. In addition, interpretation of these data depends upon the prior demonstration that sulfonated and unmodified dextrans are not reabsorbed by the tubular epithelium (Chang et al, a,b 1975, 1976). The model would predict that in older animals the filtration bias is away from negative charge while in younger animals the less negatively charged filter would permit the escape of dextrans with increased amounts of sulfate. The data indicate in fact that this expectation is realized and reveal such an age and charge dependent prejudice. I. e, the sample population of excreted dextrans is skewed in the older animals toward dextrans with diminished sulfate content. The ratio of the quantity of negative charge to dextran polymer between younger and older animals is 1.4:1 (Kowluru et al, 1988b).

7.   Life Time Scenario for Editing:
     A somewhat simplistic "lifelong editing scenario" emerges from these data. Editing is most pronounced in young mammals. From youth onward, editing exhibits a gradual attenuation in magnitude, apparently in consequence of the gradual accumulation of increasing negative charge at the functional surface of the glomerular filter. Increased negative charge could reflect increased synthesis of glycosaminoglycans, sialic acid containing macromolecules (e.g.,podocalyxin) or possibly, NEG of basement membrane components (Schnider and Kohn 1980; Monnier et al 1984). Any increase in GFR sufficient to exceed the threshold of maximal tubular reabsorbtion for albumin (whether associated with diabetes mellitus or a mannitol induced diuresis) will cause an abrupt attenuation in editing since glycated albumin becomes increasingly diluted by non-reabsorbed unmodified albumin.

8.   The Pattern of Glycation:
We have examined glycation in a number of proteins in vitro including proteins with lysine content varying between 7 (calmodulin) and 57 (albumin). Albumin shows a pattern of glycation which is in agreement with the general idea that some lysines are slightly more available for glycation than others. With the exception of an "outlier" lysine at residue 525 which is extensively glycated, and in the absence of lipid binding, almost all of the lysines in albumin participate in the process of glycation equally in a non-specific way (Garlick and Mazer, 1983). Since a crystal structure has not been determined for albumin, the applicability of criteria assembled in our working model (see below) in explaining the increased rate of glycation for lysine residue 525 is not yet known.

We have also analyzed the glycation of calmodulin in some detail. These studies in which the pattern of glycation was analyzed in the four (of 8) CNBr fragments which contain one or more lysines, we found that among the 7 available lysines, glycation occurs in a relatively non-specific way with no single lysine dominating and none excluded from the glycation process (Kowluru et al, 1988).

There are a number of observations which suggest the possibility that adjacent positively charged domains would enhance the probability of encountering any given lysine in the unprotonated form which is (known to be) essential for the formation of the Schiff's base between lysine and a reducing sugar (Sykes, 1975).

9.   The Glycation Limit:
In general proteins appear to glycate up to a limit of two to four moles of glucose per mole of protein (Figs. 4, 5 and Table II). After attachment of this initial complement of glucose residues, the further glycation of lysine displays a rate which is less than 2% of the initial rate. All of the proteins we have studied thus far exhibit this phenomenon of a limit upon glycation and also exhibit an increase in negative charge associated with glycation (I. e., a lowering of their pI). A likely explanation for this change in charge is that the pKa of the ketoamines that are formed by rearrangement of the Schiff's base is lower than the pKa of the lysines from which they are formed. This is also likely to be true for the pKa's of advanced glycation end products. A role for positive charge clusters is

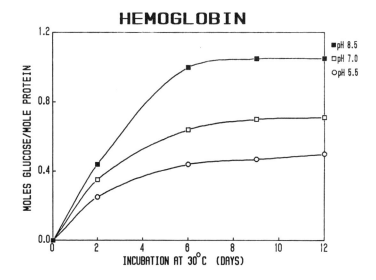

Fig. 4)   Time Course for Glycation of Hemoglobin as a
Function of pH:
200 mM glucose was used throughout. Both rate and extent of
glycation show the anticipated enhancement at higher pH's.

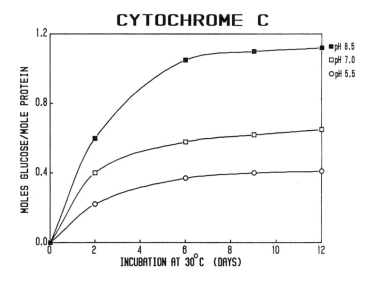

Fig. 5) Time Course for the Glycation of Cytochrome C as a
Function of pH: (Conditions as in Fig. 4).

attractive in initially permitting the pKa of participating lysines to exhibit a lower value at which glycation becomes more likely. The average pKa of protein lysines is about 10.4 (Tanford, 1962).

10. Glycation Rates:
     There are, in addition data to indicate that the Amadori rearrangement is catalyzed by acidic or basic groups adjacent to the cognizant lysine (Shapiro *et al* 1980; Garlick and Mazer 1983). Thus, lysines which reside within or adjacent to positive charge clusters, and which also have adjacent acidic or basic residues (E. g., the carboxylate anion) are the best candidates to form ketoamines. Although Schiff's base formation is rapid, it is rapidly reversible when not stabilized by rearrangement to the ketoamine. On the other hand, the Amadori rearrangement exhibits a far slower rate, but once formed, the ketoamines appear quite stable (Higgins and Bunn, 1981). Some factors which contribute to the relative slowness of NEG would include:
1)   The stepwise increase in negative charge associated with each glycation step produces a stepwise reduction in glycation rate culminating in a virtual cessation of glycation after 2 - 4 glycation steps.
2)   The fact that glycation's initial step depends upon the unprotonated form of lysine and the straight chain form of glucose, neither of which predominate (although glucose 6-PO_4 does predominantly exhibit the straight chain form).
3)   The ketoamine form is a stable end product whose formation is a function of the rate of Amadori rearrangement. The rearrangement appears as the slowest, i.e., the rate limiting step in protein glycation.

11. A Working Model for Protein Glycation:
     These considerations have been assembled into a working model to account for the limit upon and the observed rates and patterns of glycation. The model depends heavily upon the observation that the negative charge of the proteins will increase following each glycation step. The model also utilizes the concept that local clusters of positive charge serve as facilitators of initial Schiff's base formation as well as the idea that vicinal acidic (e. g., the carboxylate anion) or basic (e. g., the ammonium ions) groups facilitate the Amadori rearrangement.

     This model makes predictions with regard to the effects upon glycation of acidic and basic media, and the effects of salt, urea, amino- and phospho-sugars. The model predicts that amino- sugars glycate more rapidly and more extensively than phosphorylated sugars, that glycation occurs more rapidly and more extensively in a basic than in an acidic medium; that concentrated salt or urea solutions would interfere with glycation (in the former case by masking positive charge clusters and in the latter case, by relaxing folding forces (i. e., hydrogen bonds) which contribute to the assembly of positive charge clusters). Amino sugars would be expected to glycate more extensively and more rapidly since they would not increase negative charge. The amino group would also provide a locus for additional glycation. The only expectation which does not survive experimental scrutiny is the prediction that glycation with phosphorylated sugars would proceed more slowly and less extensively (Fig. 6). A possible explanation for this anomaly is that the linear forms of sugars can readily form Schiff's bases while the ring forms cannot. Phosphosugars predominantly exhibit the linear form while simple hexoses predominantly exhibit the ring form. A central concept of this model is that the functional pKa's of unmodified lysines (following the initial glycation steps) are actually increased by the increase in protein negative charge. Thus the probability of encountering such a lysine in the unprotonated state becomes increasingly small with incremental glycation steps, and hence the rate of subsequent glycation reactions approaches zero.

12. <u>Protein Glycation: Effects upon Protein Recognition</u>:
There are some non-trivial questions concerning the nature of the structure or entity recognized by the proximal tubular epithelium when it reabsorbs unmodified albumin and how this process of recognition is perturbed by glycation. Moreover, the finding has recently been reported that infusions of lysine will interfere with reabsorbtion of unmodified albumin by the mammalian nephron (Mogensen and Solling 1977; Mogensen et al 1981).

We have considered a number of possibilities. In the first, unprotonated lysines might be recognized by the tubular epithelium and would become progressively less available as the glycation process proceeds. In this view, "Limit" glycation of albumin (e. g., 3 moles of glucose/mole of albumin) would decrease the availability of an unprotonated lysine for recognition by tubular epithelium. This hypothesis is rendered implausible by reason of the

PROTEIN	PROTEIN : GLUCOSE (mole : mole)
Calmodulin	1 : 2.5
Albumin	1 : 2.3
Hemoglobin	1 : 0.7
Actin	1 : 3.7
Troponin	1 : 2.5
Tropomyosin	1 : 3.3
Spectrin	1 : 3.0
Cytochrome - C	1 : 0.68
Myoglobin	1 : 2.29

Table II) Extent of Protein glycation:
Proteins were glycated in the presence of 200 mM [^{3}H] glucose at 30°C for 9-12 days in the presence of trace Na$^+$ azide. The incorporation of glucose was quantitated by TCA precipitation.

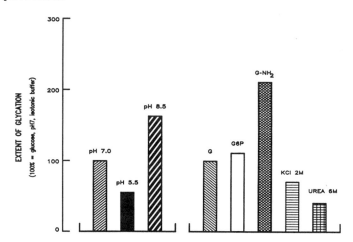

Fig. 6)   Albumin Glycation Under Varying Experimental Condtions:
The extent of albumin glycation was measured as a function of pH, salt concentration (2 M KCl), 6 M urea, and modified sugars, which were all present at (200 mM).

fact that the pKa of lysine in polypeptides is about 10.4, so that the fraction of time spent by any given lysine in the unprotonated state would be quite small. In this view, even unprotonated lysines adjacent to clusters of positive charge could not provide reliable signals for protein reabsorbtion and would be an unlikely candidate to emerge from an evolutionary selection process.

A second possibility would depend upon a constellation of protein specific steric features, one or more of which are perturbed by glycation. This possibility is not excluded but requires special recognition features for each of the macromolecules reabsorbed by the proximal tubule.

A third possibility is that one or more protonated lysines is required for recognition. This idea seems improbable since (for albumin) glycation modifies only 3 of some 57 available lysines and ought not to perturb such a recognition process. I. e, there remain an abundance of protonated lysines from which the tubule could choose.

A fourth (and to us most likely) possibility is that the increase in negative charge resulting from glycation can interfere with reabsorbtion. There are data to suggest that the proximal tubule does in fact show a generic preference for more positive proteins (Christensen et al 1981; 1983). In this view the discriminatory function shown by the epithelial cell surface is a general one, designed to function for many proteins on the basis of global charge rather than for individual proteins on the basis of sequence specificity.

III   Discussion:

These ideas in combination with our own data and those available in a solid (and growing) body of published observations on protein glycation are most consistent with the following interpretation: The process of nonenzymatic glycation consistently lowers the PI of the modified proteins including such examples as hemoglobin (Krishnamoorthy et al, 1976), albumin (Kowluru et al, 1987), calmodulin (Kowluru et al, 1988a), ferritin (Williams and Siegal, 1985) and carbonic anhydrase (Kondo et al, 1987). The reason for this is not identified but is likely to reflect lower pKa's for ketoamines (or advanced glycation end products) than for the lysines from which they are formed by glycation. Proximal tubular epithelium has been found to show a generic preference for the reabsorbtion of proteins which are (relatively) more positively charged (Christensen *et al*, 1981, 1983).

Editing of glycated albumins by the nephron seems best explained by the efficient reabsorbtion of unmodified albumin in contrast with the far less efficient reabsorbtion of glycated albumin. This differential in reabsorbtion rates is now being quantitated by micropuncture studies. The phenomenon of editing alters the ratio of glycated to unmodified albumin from < 1% in the plasma of a healthy 10 year old human to > 15% in the urine of the same individual. The fact that glycation of albumin diminishes its reabsorbtion by the proximal tubular epithelium requires explanation. A most parsimonious (but nonexclusive) view attributes this change in recognition to the increase in albumin's negative charge. In view of the negative charge of the normal glomerular filter, preferential filtration of glycated albumin (with a pI of 4.5 vs 4.7 for unmodified albumin) appears untenable as an explanation for editing.

In conclusion, this report reviews evidence for editing of glycated albumin by the nephron and the effects upon editing of diabetes and ageing. The increased negative charge of glycated albumin appears to dominate its interactions both with the proximal tubule and the ageing glomerulus. We do not yet know whether the increases in glomerular negative charge, suggested by the age dependent decline in editing, are specific for the very specialized glomerular structures or represent a more general biochemical reflection of ageing. The increasing negative charge associated with the process of glycation may play a significant role in the rather striking reductions observed in the rates of glycation of various proteins which follows upon addition of two to four hexose moieties. One of the important potential pathways for the development of the histopathology of diabetes mellitus associated with glycation is the perturbation of protein recognition by glycation. This creates opportunities for glycated proteins to enter "ectopic" domains where they are not normally encountered, and/or to fail to appear within specific subcellular or extracellular domains where they normally interact. This misdirection or impaired routing of glycated proteins will require systematic evaluation in order to properly assess its putative role in diabetic histopathology.

We thank S. Solomon, T. Whaley, C. Unkefer and M. Dembo for productive and seminal discussion of the material presented here, and Alexandra Vigil and Angela Martinez for expert manuscript preparation. The authors also thank the Journal of Experimental Medicine for allowing us to reproduce some data (Figs. 1, 2, 3 and Table I) published in JEM 166:1259-1279, 1987. This work was supported by Institutional Supporting Research award X81W.

IV   References:

Anderson S, Brenner BM (1986). Effects of ageing on the renal glomerulus. Amer. J. Med. 80:435-442.

Bernstein RE (1987). Nonenzymatically glucosylated proteins. Adv. Clin. Chem. 26:1-77.

Bourdeau JE, Carone FA, Ganote CE (1972). Serum albumin uptake in isolated perfused renal tubules. J. Cell. Biol. 54:382-398.

Bourdeau JE, Carone FA (1974). Protein handling by renal tubule. Nephron 13:22-34.

Brownlee M, Cerami A (1981). The biochemistry of the complications of diabetes mellitus. Ann. Rev. Biochem. 50:385-432.

Bunn HF (1981). Nonenzymatic glucosylation of protein: Relevance to diabetes. Amer. J. Med. 70:325-330.

Chang RLS, Ueki IF, Troy JL, Dean WM, Roberston CR, Brenner BM, (1975). Permselectivity of the glomerular capillary wall to macromolecules. II. Experimental studies in rats using neutral dextran. Biophys. J. 15:887-906.

Chang RLS, Dean WM, Robertson CR, Bennett CM, Glassock RJ, Brenner BM (1976). Permselectivity of the glomerular capillary wall. Studies of experimental glomerulonephritis in the rat using neutral dextran. J. Clin. Invest. 57: 1272-1286.

Chang RLS, Dean WM, Robertson CR, Brenner BM (1975). Permselectivity of the glomerular capillary wall: iii. Restricted transport of polyanions. Kidney Int. 8:212-218.

Caulfield JP, Farquhar MG (1976). Distribution of anionic sites in glomerular basement membranes: Their possible role in filtration and attachment. Proc. Natl. Acad. Sci. USA 73:1646-1650.

Christensen EI, Carone FA, Rennke HG (1981). Effect of molecular charge on endocytic uptake of ferritin in renal proximal tubule cells. Lab. Invest 44:351-358.

Christensen EI, Rennke HG, Carone FA (1983). Renal tubular uptake of protein: Effect of molecular charge. Am. J. Physiol. 266:F436-F441.

Davies DF, Shock NW (1950). Age changes in glomerular filtration rate, effective renal plasma flow and tubular excreting capacity in adult males. J. Clin. Invest. 29:496-507.

Ditzel J, Anderson H, Daugaard-Peters N (1975). Oxygen affinity of hemoglobin and red cell 2,3-diphosphoglycerate in childhood diabetes. Acta. Pediatr. Scand. 64:355-361.

Garlick RL, Mazer JS (1983). The principal site of nonenzymatic glucosylation of human serum albumin in vivo. J. Biol. Chem. 258:6142-6146.

Ghiggeri GM, Candiano G, Delfino G, Bianchini F, Queirolo C (1984). Glucosyl albumin and diabetic microalbuminuria: Demonstration of altered renal handling. Kidney Int. 25:565-570

Ghiggeri GM, Candiano G, Delfino G, Queirolo C (1985). Electricalcharge of serum albumin in normal and diabetic humans. Kidney Int. 28:168-174

Gonen B, Go R, Quinn T (1987). Nonenzymatic glucosylation of proteins: Possible relevance to microangiopathy. Front. Diabetes 8:1-15.

Higgins PJ, Bunn HF (1981). Kinetic analysis of the nonenzymatic glycosylation of hemoglobin. J. Biol. Chem. 256:5204-5208.

Kanwar YS (1984). Biophysiology of glomerular filtration and proteinuria. Lab. Invest. 51:7-21.

Kerjaschki D, Sharkey DJ, Farquhar MG (1984). Identification and characterization of podocalyxin. The major sialoprotein of the renal glomerular epithelial cell. J. Cell. Biol. 98:1591-1596.

Kondo T, Murakami K, Ohtsuka y, Tsuji M. Gasa S, Taniguchi N, Kawakami Y (1987). Estimation and charcterization of glucosylated carbonic anhydrase I in erythrocytes from patients with diabetes mellitus. Clin. Chim. Acta. 166:227-236.

Kowluru A, Kowluru R, Bitensky MW, Corwin EJ, Solomon S, Johnson JD (1987). Suggested mechanism for the selective excretion of glucosylated albumin. J. Exp. Med. 166:1259-1279.

Kowluru RA, Heidorn DB, Edmondson SP, Bitensky MW, Kowluru A, Downer NW, Whaley TW and Trewhella J (1988). Effects of Calmodulin Glycation. Biochemistry (submitted).

Kowluru A, Bitensky MW, Kowluru RA (1988). Manuscript in preparation.

Krishnamoorthy R, Wajcman H, Labie D (1976). Isoelectro focussing: A method of multiple applications for hemoglobin studies. Clin. Chim. Acta. 69:203-209.

Mogensen CE (1976). Renal function changes in diabetes. Diabetes 25:872-880.

Mogensen CE, Solling K (1977). Studies on renal tubular protein reabsorption: Partial and near complete inhibition by certain amino acids. Scand. J. Clin. Lab. Invest. 37:477-486.

Mogensen CE, Solling K, Vittinghus E (1981). Studies on mechanisms of proteinuria using amino acid induced inhibition of tubular reabsorption in normal and diabetic man. Contr. Nephrol. 26:50-65.

Monnier VM, Stevens VJ, Cerami A (1979). Nonenzymatic glucosylations sulfhydryl oxidation and aggregation of lens proteins in experimental sugar cataracts. J. Exp. Med. 150:1098-1107.

Monnier VM, Kohn RR, Cerami A (1984). Accelerated age related browning of human collagen in diabetes mellitus. Proc. Natl. Acad. Sci. USA 81:583-587.

Schnider SL, Kohn RR (1980). Glucosylation of human collagen in ageing and diabetes mellitus. J. Clin. Invest. 66:1179-1181.

Shapiro R, McManus MJ, Zalut C, Bunn HF (1980). Sites of nonenzymatic glucosylation of human hemoglobin. J. Biol. Chem. 255:3120-3127.

Sykes P (1975). A guide book to mechanism in organic chemistry (Fourth edition). Longman Group Ltd. Chapter 8.

Tanford C (1962). The interpretation of hydrogen ion titration curves of proteins. Adv. Protein Chem. 17:69-165.

Vlassara H, Brownlee M, Cerami A (1985). Recognition and uptake of human diabetic peripheral nerve myelin by macrophages. Diabetes 34:553-557.

Williams SK, Devenny JJ, Bitensky, MW (1981). Micropinocytic ingestion of glucosylated albumin by isolated microvessels: possible role in the pathogenesis of diabetic microangiopathy. Proc. Natl. Acad. Sci. USA 78:2393-2397.

Williams SK, Howarth NL, Devenny JJ, Bitenksy MW (1982). Structural and functional consequences of increased tubulin glucosylation in diabetes mellitus. Proc. Natl. Acad. Sci. USA 79:6546-6550.

Williams SK, Devenny JJ, Pinter G, Bitensky MW (1983). Preferential transendothelial transport of glucosylated albumin in the kidney. Microvasc. Res. 3:96a (abstract).

Williams SK, Pinter GG (1983). Selective permeability of kidney capillaries to glucosylated albumin. Physiologist 26:67a.

Williams SK, Siegal RK (1985). Preferential transport of nonenzymatically glucosylated ferritin across the kidney glomerulus. Kidney Int. 28:146-152.

Woods JW, Mora PT (1958). Synthetic polysaccharides III Polyglucose sulfates. J. Am. Chem. Soc. 80:3700-3702.

The Maillard Reaction in Aging,
Diabetes, and Nutrition, pages 205–218
© 1989 Alan R. Liss, Inc.

MACROPHAGE RECEPTOR-MEDIATED PROCESSING AND
REGULATION OF ADVANCED GLYCOSYLATION ENDPRODUCT
(AGE)-MODIFIED PROTEINS: ROLE IN DIABETES AND AGING.

Helen Vlassara, Michael Brownlee and Anthony Cerami

The Rockefeller University, New York, N.Y. 10021

ABSTRACT

Tissue and cell surface proteins modified nonenzymatically by
glucose are shown to be removed by macrophages through a recently
characterized high affinity receptor. Insulin appears to be a
potent suppressor of this macrophage AGE removal activity, while
TNF acts as a stimulant. Coupling of AGE-proteins to their AGE-
receptor results in TNF and IL-1 synthesis and secretion. This
suggests that AGE may act as a signal for growth-promoting
factor secretion in a coordinated replacement process during tissue
remodeling. A greater than 2-fold decrease in receptor number
and binding capacity found in cells from aged mice as compared to
young suggests that aging may adversely affect the AGE-receptor -
efficiency and by impeding crosslinked AGE-protein removal add to
ongoing aging tissue damage.

INTRODUCTION

In contrast to the short-term nonenzymatic reaction with
proteins of short half-life which results in reversible Amadori adduct
formation, prolonged glycosylation of proteins with long half-life
leads to the formation of irreversible adducts which can crosslink
proteins (Monnier et al., 1984). These products, called Advanced
Glycosylation Endproducts (AGE), forming on long-lived proteins,
such as collagen, myelin proteins, etc. *in vitro* or *in vivo*, have been
recently shown to be recognized and endocytosed by mouse peritoneal
macrophages (Vlassara et al., 1984) and human monocytes (Vlassara
et al., 1987).

RECEPTOR-MEDIATED RECOGNITION OF AGE'S

Macrophage recognition of glucose-modified proteins was first found using glycosylated myelin proteins (Vlassara et al., 1984) and mouse elicited macrophages and was shown to be specific for the Advanced Glycosylation Endproducts (AGE), as binding by the cells was effectively competed by AGE-modified albumin (AGE-BSA), while neither unmodified BSA nor unmodified myelin competed. In addition, macrophage recognition of AGE-myelin proteins was shown to be followed by endocytosis, as demonstrated by resistance of cell-associated radioactivity to removal by trypsin action, and by low temperature inhibition of ligand accumulation in the cellular fraction (Vlassara et al., 1985b). Furthermore, we were able to show that protein modification only by AGE formed *in vitro* or *in vivo* results in macrophage uptake, while Amadori product formation alone does not (Vlassara et al., 1984).

The relevance of these observations to the human physiology was evaluated in subsequent studies utilizing normal human peripheral monocytes and peripheral nerve myelin from normal and diabetic autopsy subjects (Vlassara et ai., 1985a). With increasing concentrations of labeled myelin from a diabetic subject, macrophage myelin uptake and accumulation increased in a saturable fashion, reaching levels 3-4 times higher than the age-matched nondiabetic (Vlassara et al., 1985a).

The relationship between subject age and myelin uptake by human monocyte/macrophages was also investigated with myelin samples prepared from normal and diabetic patients of different ages (Figure 1) (Vlassara, 1988).

A linear increase in the amount of normal myelin accumulation with age was observed, suggesting that a mechanism of protein removal may be functioning normally, based on macrophage recognition of AGE formed on senescent proteins. In addition, diabetic myelin uptake was uniformly increased regardless of age, implying that in disease states such as diabetes, where advanced glycosylation is accelerated, such a mechanism could contribute to tissue damage, i.e. segmental demyelination.

AGE-RECEPTOR CHARACTERIZATION

The important question as to whether there was a specific macrophage/monocyte receptor which recognized a distinct Advanced Glycosylation Endproduct (AGE) or family of Endproducts accumulating

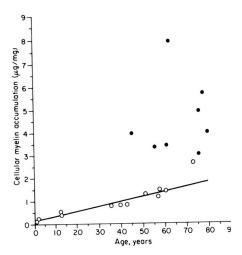

FIGURE 1. Intracellular accumulation of iodinated normal (open circles) and diabetic (solid circles) human peripheral nerve myelin by monocyte/macrophages as a function of subject age.

on long-lived proteins after prolonged exposure to glucose, was pursued using AGE-bovine serum albumin (AGE-BSA) as a probe (Vlassara et al., 1985b). Previous studies (Vlassara et al., 1984) had already shown AGE-myelin to be competed for uptake by AGE-BSA, suggesting that the receptor recognition was specific for AGE regardless of type of protein. Similarly, enzymatically digested AGE-BSA competed to more than 80% of the intact AGE-protein (unpublished data), further confirming the receptor specificity for the AGE moiety. AGE-BSA was specifically bound to cells at $4°C$, and taken up and degraded at $37°C$, in a concentration dependent saturable manner. Scatchard analysis of AGE-BSA binding data indicated that there are approximately 1.5×10^5 receptors per cell, with an affinity constant (K_a) of $1.75 \times 10^7 M^{-1}$ (Figure 2). In addition specific binding of AGE-BSA to the macrophage receptor was competitively inhibited by BSA which had been chemically coupled to a synthetic analogue of AGE, 2-furoyl-4(5)-furanyl-1H-imidazole (FFI-BSA) (Pongor et al., 1984). This suggested that the AGE-receptor recognizes a specific type of AGE structure having important homology with FFI. *In vivo* a whole family of AGE are

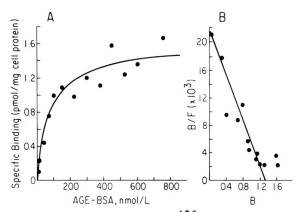

FIGURE 2. (A) Specific binding of ^{125}I-labeled AGE-BSA to
mouse peritoneal macrophages. (B) Scatchard analysis of binding
data in A. Units for the Scatchard plot are as follows: Bound,
pmol/mg of cell protein; Bound/free, pmol·nM^{-1}.

believed to form on proteins during long-term exposure to glucose
(Reynolds, 1963; Reynolds, 1965), and a number of these may bind
to the AGE receptor with specific individual affinities.

There has been considerable evidence over the past decade or
more that macrophage/monocyte-derived cells play an important
role in the regulation of extracellular matrix protein turnover,
which is crucial to the maintenance of connective tissue homeostasis
as organisms age (Krane, 1984; Mundy and Raisz, 1981). Receptor-
mediated endocytosis by macrophage/monocytes is also involved in
the removal of *in vivo* deposited lipoproteins from arterial intima
(Brown and Goldstein, 1983; Steinberg, 1983). This *in vivo* forming
ligand which is specifically recognized by macrophages however
has not yet been identified. Also, *in vitro*, covalent modification
of proteins such as low density lipoprotein (LDL) by chemical
reagents such as acetic anhydride or maleic anhydride results in
macrophage uptake of these proteins via the scavenger receptor
(Goldstein et al., 1979), while modification of albumin by formaldehyde
results in similar recognition by hepatic phagocytes (Horiuchi et
al., 1985). Although the AGE-receptor was shown to be distinct
from the mannose/fucose receptor (Vlassara et al., 1984), the
possibility that it was identical to one of the previously described
scavenger receptors could not be excluded. In a series of competition

and cross-competition studies between AGE-proteins and several scavenger receptor ligands, e.g. acetyl-LDL, maleyl-BSA, formaldehyde-treated albumin, and a number of negatively charged compounds, such as fucoidin, it was possible to demonstrate that the AGE-receptor was distinct from the other scavenger receptors (Vlassara et al., 1986). In addition inhibition of AGE-BSA binding caused by fucoidin, polyinosinic acid, polyadenylic acid and heparin probably reflected nonspecific membrane sensitivity to strong polyanionic competitors, shared equally by other macrophage receptors, e.g. acetyl-LDL, and beta-VLDL.

Using RAW 264.7 cells (a murine macrophage cell line) as a source of AGE-receptor we have recently been able to solubilize and study its ligand specificity (Radoff et al., 1988). Analogues of FFI that possessed the furan ring and the imidazole moiety had the highest affinity for the receptor.

Crosslinking studies of ^{125}I-BSA and RAW 264.7 cells, with the crosslinking agent suberimidate, revealed that the AGE-receptor complex has a molecular weight of approximately 90 kD (Figure 3) (Radoff et al., 1988). Addition of cold AGE-BSA prevented the crosslinking reaction, whereas unmodified BSA had no effect, further confirming the AGE-receptor specificity. We have subsequently isolated a 90 kD protein from the membrane fraction of RAW 264.7 cells, utilizing an FFI-affinity column that we have synthesized

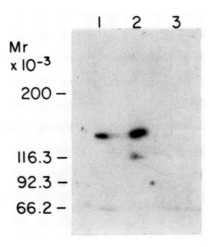

FIGURE 3. Chemical crosslinking of membrane binding protein on RAW 264.7 cells to [^{125}I]AGE-BSA.

(Radoff and Vlassara, submitted). By combining several sequential FPLC chromatographic steps we have been able to isolate the protein to homogeneity.

RECEPTOR-MEDIATED REMOVAL OF AGE-MODIFIED CELLS

Reasoning that certain cells have a long enough lifespan to allow AGE formation on their surface proteins, we hypothesized that the AGE-receptor may also mediate the removal of aging cells by selectively recognizing a cell surface alteration that accumulates over time. As shown in Figure 4, human erythrocytes having AGE attached to their surface were avidly bound and subsequently ingested by human monocytes (Vlassara et al., 1987). Percent binding and ingestion of *in vitro* glycosylated erythrocytes, as well as diabetic mouse RBC by macrophages was significantly greater than that of unmodified red cells, and specific for AGE recognition, as it was completely inhibited by the addition of excess AGE-BSA. In addition AGE-RBC survival *in vivo* was markedly shortened. These studies indicated that the AGE-receptor mechanism may be in part responsible for specific recognition and removal of cells with prolonged half-life, likely to be glucose-modified as they age.

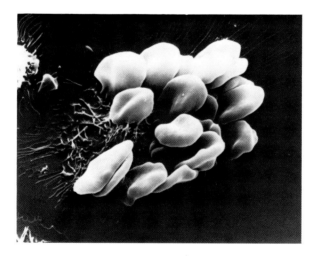

FIGURE 4. Electron scanning micrograph of human AGE (FFI)-modified RBC bound by human peripheral monocytes at 4°C. Micrograph made by David M. Phillips of the Population Council.

REGULATION OF AGE-RECEPTOR FUNCTION

The macrophage receptor for glucose-modified proteins defined by these studies has a unique biological significance, since it is the first such receptor which recognizes a ligand known to form extensively *in vivo*. Via this receptor, macrophages can selectively recognize a time-dependent signal of protein modification and thus degrade only senescent macromolecules. The AGE-protein receptor could by this mechanism have an important role in the regulation of extracellular protein turnover, importantly the vessel wall proteins. Furthermore, since AGE formed on extravascular matrix long-lived collagen can trap LDL (Brownlee et al., 1985) which can subsequently undergo sufficient AGE-modification, the AGE-receptor may normally play a role in the removal of atherogenic material. In various disease states however as well as in aging, the efficiency of this removal system is not complete, as indicated by the continuous increase of AGE formation with age and/or hyperglycemia (Brownlee et al, 1988). In both states, the rate at which aging-associated vascular changes take place may be profoundly affected by genetic and/or environmental factors which alter the efficiency of this receptor-mediated removal process. A number of macrophage receptors have been found to undergo modulation in response to a number of hormones and other physiological mediators (Warren and Vogel, 1985; Fox and DiCorleto, 1986). Since such factors might influence the net amount of crosslinking AGE-proteins in the tissues, we have begun to study the effects of diabetes on the macrophage AGE-receptor, particularly the effects of glucose and insulin levels (Vlassara et al., 1988a). It should be noted that exposure of macrophages from normal animals to either elevated glucose or insulin concentrations *in vitro* failed to demonstrate any short-term effect on the AGE-receptor number or function. Therefore, binding and degradation studies of radioiodinated AGE-BSA by resident peritoneal macrophages from experimentally-induced and genetically hypo- and hyperinsulinemic diabetic mice were carried out. The main difference between the two genetically diabetic animals is the occurrence of a severe hyperinsulinemia in the C57Bl/6J (*db/db*) mice; the KsJ diabetic mice had serum glucose and insulin of around 500 mg/ml and 8.4 μU/ml respectively compared to serum glucose (480 mg/ml) and insulin levels (420 μU/ml) of the 6J mice. Scatchard plot analysis of binding data obtained from macrophages of normal non-diabetic mice revealed 1.5×10^5 receptors/cell with a binding affinity of 1.7×10^7 M^{-1} (Figure 5a) (Vlassara et al., 1988a). Macrophages from hypoinsulinemic alloxan-induced diabetic animals, on the other hand, showed a two- to three-fold increase in AGE-receptor number per cell (Figure 5b). A similar increase was observed with macrophages from C57Bl/KsJ

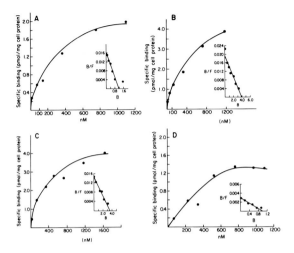

FIGURE 5. Specific binding and Scatchard analysis (inset) of data with ^{125}I-labeled AGE-BSA, unlabeled AGE-BSA, and (A) C57Bl/6J (*db/+*) nondiabetic, (B) C57Bl/KsJ (*db/db*) hypoinsulinemic, (C) C57Bl/6J (+/+) experimentally diabetic, and (D) C57Bl/6J (*db/db*) hyperinsulinemic mouse peritoneal macrophages.

mice (*db/db*) (Figure 5c). The binding constant for both of these groups of animals was approximately the same as the control animals. The increase in AGE-receptor number in these two diabetic models was accompanied by an increased (25-30%) degradation of the endocytosed AGE-BSA (Vlassara et al., 1988a).

   In contrast, macrophages from the hyperinsulinemic but equally hyperglycemic C57Bl/6J (*db/db*) mice were markedly different (Figure 5d). These macrophages had a distinct reduction in both the number of AGE-receptors (6×10^4/cell) and binding affinity (4×10^6 M^{-1}), with a fifty per cent reduction in the amount of AGE-BSA degraded. Thus, it appears that insulin and not high glucose, or the accumulation of AGE-proteins, is the causative agent for this modulation of the AGE-receptor. These observations have led us to the conclusion that the alteration of the AGE-receptor can be prompted by the exposure of the macrophage in vivo to the high or low insulin concentrations. It is not clear whether this reflects the necessity for exposure of an insulin-sensitive macrophage precursor or that hyperinsulinemia generates a more proximal regulatory signal *in vivo*. However, these studies provided evidence for a specific insulin-sensitive mechanism that may modulate the properties and function of the macrophage AGE-receptor. In certain cases of diabetes, such as in non-insulin-dependent diabetic patients with elevated peripheral insulin levels, and in most insulin-dependent patients whose high peripherally injected doses must compensate for hepatic requirements and extraction, a down-regulation of this removal mechanism for proteins modified by advanced glycosylation products may be critically important. Factors that reduce its efficiency would also play a major role in determining the total amount and rate of hyperglycemia-accelerated glucose-modified protein accumulation in diabetic blood vessel walls. In nondiabetic subjects, such a mechanism may explain the well-documented association between hypocaloric intake or fasting, where insulin levels are reduced, and retardation of aging in animal models (Harrison et al., 1984).

AGE-RECEPTOR MEDIATED INDUCTION OF MONOKINES

In the constant removal and resynthesis that takes place *in vivo* there obviously must be signals to orchestrate the orderly remodeling of tissue proteins. We have begun to examine the process by which removal of AGE-protein might be coordinated with its replacement by newly-synthesized material. We have found that in response to the binding of AGE-proteins the macrophage synthesizes and releases the monokines cachectin/tumor necrosis factor (TNF) and interleukin 1 (IL-1) (Figure 6) (Vlassara et al., 1988b).

The two monokines cachectin/TNF and IL-1 have diverse biological activities many of which are shared by both, and which have been extensively reviewed (Beutler and Cerami, 1987; Dinarello, 1987; Le and Vilcek, 1987). Of importance to the uptake of AGE-proteins is the fact that both have been reported to have growth factor-like (Sugarman et al., 1985), and angiogenic activities (Frater-Schröeder et al., 1987). In these studies, normal human peripheral blood monocytes were incubated in medium containing human interferon-γ (1ng/ml, 50 units/ml) and polymyxin (100ng/ml), in the presence of either normal BSA (Nl-BSA, 250 μg/ml), *in vitro* glycosylated BSA (Glu-BSA, 250 μg/ml or G6P-BSA, 250 μg/ml), or chemically synthesized FFI-BSA (150 μg/ml). Following incubation, cachectin/TNF was measured in the media by an enzyme-linked immunosorbant assay (ELISA) using a purified monoclonal anti-cachectin antibody. Figure 6 records the amount of material made by each of the experimental groups. Macrophages incubated with unmodified albumin (Nl-BSA) released only minimal levels of cachectin/TNF. In contrast, medium from macrophages incubated

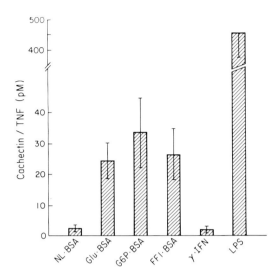

FIGURE 6. Detection of cachectin/TNF secretion by human monocytes in response to AGE proteins.

with each of the three types of AGE-BSA contained approximately 10 times the amount of cachectin/TNF found with Nl-BSA. In the absence of interferon-γ, human monocyte supernatants contained approximately one-half the amount of cachectin/TNF in response to AGE-protein. This difference presumably reflects the ability of interferon-γ to exert a priming effect on human monocytes, which augments their subsequent cachectin/TNF secretory response (Nathan et al., 1983; Pace et al., 1983). In order to determine whether the observed appearance of cachectin/TNF was associated with the induction of new mRNA or translation of cryptic cachectin/TNF message (Beutler et al., 1986), Northern blot analysis of monocyte mRNA for cachectin/TNF was performed. A small background amount of message was detected in the monocyte preparations that had been incubated with Nl-BSA, while cells incubated with the three AGE-BSA preparations had significantly increased amounts of message (Vlassara et al., 1988b). These results suggested that the AGE-proteins increase both the cellular levels of cachectin/TNF mRNA and the amount of secreted cytokine in non-cytotoxic amounts. AGE-proteins are the first endogenously produced materials that, although not inflammatory in origin, can induce this potent cytokine.

Under identical experimental conditions, the amount of cell-associated and extracellular IL-1 released by macrophages in response to AGE-BSA was measured (Vlassara et al., 1988b). Total IL-1β was significantly higher in the AGE-BSA preparations than the Nl-BSA or the interferon-γ controls. Since cachectin/TNF can prompt the release of IL-1, it is not clear whether the AGE-BSA is acting directly or through the release of the cachectin/TNF. Even if its production represents a secondary response to cachectin/TNF, IL-1 still shares and would therefore amplify the activities of cachectin/TNF relating to tissue growth and remodeling.

The finding of cytokine release by macrophages in response to AGE-proteins is of great significance since it offers an explanation to several observations noted previously in association with these cytokines. The ability of cachectin/TNF and IL-1 to stimulate mesenchymal cells to synthesize and release collagenase and other extracellular proteases could reflect their role in initiating local degradative events. Similarly the ability of cachectin/TNF and IL-1 to prompt a synthetic/proliferative response in cells such as fibroblasts, and the release of other growth factors might be viewed as their role in the repair process. Such a role for cachectin/TNF and IL-1 might further explain why these genes have been so highly conserved in mammals.

The *in vivo* modification of matrix proteins by time-dependent formation of glucose-derived AGE's may thus constitute a unique biologic time-clock which signals macrophages to secrete cachectin/TNF, IL-1, and possibly other cytokines, which in turn influence both the degradation as well as the proliferation of tissue components (Figure 7). Since the macrophage has been found to produce a number of monokines (Nathan, 1987), the coordinated response of this remodeling system is of critical importance. An imbalance of this system in certain states such as in diabetes, where accelerated AGE formation occurs as a result of high glucose concentration, or in aging where AGE accumulation is increased as a function of time, may explain in part the excessive proliferative response characteristic of several diabetic and aging tissues.

A four- to six-fold increase in maximum binding and degradation of nonenzymatically glycosylated albumin (AGE-BSA) by macrophage/monocytes previously exposed to TNF was also demonstrated as compared to non-exposed cells, while there was no effect on the binding and degradation of unmodified BSA. These effects were completely blocked in the presence of an anti-TNF antibody (Vlassara et al., submitted). These data suggest that

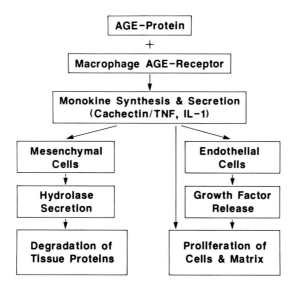

FIGURE 7. Schematic representation of potential mechanisms by which AGE-mediated synthesis and secretion of cachectin/TNF and IL-1 might contribute to the regulation of normal tissue remodelling.

AGE-induced TNF may normally play an important regulatory role in the macrophage removal of glucose modifications forming on long-lived tissue proteins, such as in vessel walls.

Finally, the effect of aging on the macrophage AGE-receptor was recently evaluated in young (six-months old) and old (2.5-years old) mice. A greater than two-fold decrease in both receptor number and binding affinity was found in cells from the old group as compared to the young group of animals. These data suggest that aging in itself may adversely affect the AGE-receptor efficiency, which may compound the tissue damage by preventing the removal of crosslinked glycosylated proteins (Vlassara et al., submitted).

REFERENCES

Beutler B, Cerami A (1987). Cachectin: more than a tumor necrosis factor. New Engl J Med 316:379-385.

Beutler B, Krochnin N, Milsark IW, Luedke C, Cerami A (1986). Control of cachectin (tumor necrosis factor) synthesis: mechanisms of endotoxin resistance. Science 232:977-980.

Brown MS, Goldstein JL (1983). Lipoprotein metabolism in the macrophage: implications for cholesterol deposition in atherosclerosis. Ann Rev Biochem 52:223-261.

Brownlee M, Vlassara H, Cerami A (1985). Nonenzymatic glycosylation products on collagen covalently trap low density lipoprotein. Diabetes 34:938-941.

Brownlee M, Cerami A, Vlassara H (1988). Advanced glycosylation end products in tissue and the biochemical basis of diabetic complications. N Engl J Med 318:1315-1321.

Dinarello CA (1987). Interleukins, tumor necrosis factors (cachectin), and interferons as endogenous pyrogens and mediators of fever. In Pick E (ed): "Lymphokines," New York: Academic, pp 1-27.

Fox PL, DiCorleto PE (1986). Modified low density lipoproteins suppress production of a platelet-derived growth factor-like protein by cultured endothelial cells. Proc Natl Acad Sci USA 83:4774-4778.

Frater-Schröeder M, Risau W, Hallman R, Gautschi P, Böhlen P (1987). Tumor necrosis factor type α, a potent inhibitor of endothelial cell growth *in vitro*, is angiogenic *in vivo*. Proc Natl Acad Sci USA 84:5277-5281.

Goldstein JL, Ho YK, Basu SK, Brown MS (1979). Binding site on macrophages that mediates uptake and degradation of acetylated low density lipoprotein, producing massive cholesterol deposition. Proc Natl Acad Sci USA 76:333-337.

Harrison DE, Archer JR, Astle CM (1984). Effects of food restriction on aging: separation of food intake and adiposity. Proc Natl Acad Sci USA 81:1835-1838.

Horiuchi S, Takata K, Maeda H, Morino Y (1985). Purification of a receptor for formaldehyde-treated serum albumin from rat liver. J Biol Chem 259:53-56.

Krane SM (1984). Collagen degradation. In Berk PD, Castro-Malaspina H, Wasserman LR (eds): "Myelofibrosis and the Biology of Connective Tissue," New York: Alan R. Liss, vol 54, pp 89-102.

Le J, Vilcek J (1987). Tumor necrosis factor and interleukin 1: cytokines with multiple overlapping biological activities. Lab Invest 56:234-248.

Mundy GR, Raisz LG (1981). Disorders in mineral metabolism. In Bronner F, Coburn JW (eds): "Calcium Physiology," New York: Academic, vol III, pp 1-5.

Nathan CF (1987). Secretory products of macrophages. J Clin Invest 79:319-326.

Nathan CF, Murray HW, Wiebe ME, Rubin BY (1983). Identification of interferon-γ as the lymphokine that activates human oxidative metabolism and antimicrobial activity. J Exp Med 158:670-689.

Pace JL, Russell SW, Schreiber RD, Altman A, Katz DH (1983). Macrophage activation: priming activity from a T-cell hybridoma is attributable to interferon-γ. Proc Natl Acad Sci USA 80:3782-3786.

Pongor S, Ulrich PC, Bencsath FA, Cerami A (1984). Aging of proteins: isolation and identification of a fluorescent chromophore from the reaction of polypeptides with glucose. Proc Natl Acad Sci USA 81:2684-2688.

Radoff S, Vlassara (1988). Isolation of advanced glycosylation endproduct cell membrane-binding protein from murine RAW 264.7 cells. *Submitted.*

Radoff S, Vlassara H, Cerami A (1988). Characterization of a solubilized cell surface binding protein on macrophages specific for proteins modified nonenzymatically by advanced glycosylation end products. Arch Biochem Biophys 263:418-423.

Reynolds TM (1963). Chemistry of nonenzymatic browning: I. Adv Food Res 12:1-52.

Reynolds TM (1965). Chemistry of nonenzymatic browning: II. Adv Food Res 14:167-283.

Steinberg D (1983). Lipoproteins and atherosclerosis. Arteriosclerosis 3:283-301.

Sugarman BJ, Aggarwal BB, Hass PE, Figari IS, Palladino Jr MA, Shepard HM (1985). Recombinant human tumor necrosis factor-α: effects on proliferation of normal and transformed cells *in vitro.* Science 230:943-945.

Vlassara H, Brownlee M, Cerami A (1984). Accumulation of diabetic rat peripheral nerve myelin by macrophages increases with extent and duration of nonenzymatic glycosylation. J Exp Med 160:197-207.

Vlassara H, Brownlee M, Cerami A (1985a). Recognition and uptake of human diabetic peripheral nerve myelin by macrophages. Diabetes 34:553-557.

Vlassara H, Brownlee M, Cerami A (1985b). High-affinity receptor-mediated uptake and degradation of glucose-modifed proteins: a potential mechanism for the removal of senescent macromolecules. Proc Natl Acad Sci USA 82:5588-5592.

Vlassara H, Brownlee M, Cerami A (1988a). Specific macrophage receptor activity for advanced glycosylation end products inversely correlates with insulin levels in vivo. Diabetes 37:456-461.

Vlassara H, Brownlee M, Manogue KR, Dinarello CA, Pasagian A (1988b). Cachectin/TNF and IL-1 induced by glucose-modified proteins: role in normal tissue remodeling. Science 240:1546-1548.

Warren MK, Vogel SN (1985). Opposing effects of glucocorticoids on interferon-γ-induced murine macrophage Fc receptor and Ia antigen expression. J Immmunol 134:2462-2469.

The Maillard Reaction in Aging,
Diabetes, and Nutrition, pages 219–234
© 1989 Alan R. Liss, Inc.

METABOLIC AND IMMUNOLOGICAL CONSEQUENCES OF GLYCATION OF
LOW DENSITY LIPOPROTEINS

Joseph L. Witztum and Theodore Koschinsky

Department of Medicine, University of Calif.,
San Diego, La Jolla, CA 92093

INTRODUCTION

Nonenzymatic Glycation (NEG) of a variety of plasma
and structural proteins is known to occur in euglycemic
individuals and to an advanced degree in hyperglycemic,
diabetic subjects. In addition, long-lived structural
proteins undergo "browning reactions" that result in the
generation of complex glucose mediated crosslinking of
proteins termed "advanced glycosylation endproducts (AGE)
(Brownlee et al., 1984). A number of years ago our laboratory sought to determine if NEG occurred on plasma lipoproteins and if such modifications would have biological
relevance. In this report we will summarize our results
which demonstrate that glycation of low density lipoprotein
(LDL) may indeed affect its biological properties. In
addition, we will review evidence that both short- and
long-term glycation modifications of LDL render LDL immunogenic and that autoantibodies may result. The potential
implications of these findings will be discussed.

METABOLIC CONSEQUENCES OF NONENZYMATIC GLYCATION OF LDL

The rationale for determining the metabolic consequences of NEG of LDL derived from the studies of Weisgraber et al. (1978), which documented that lysine residues
of apo B, the major protein of LDL and the ligand for the
LDL receptor (Brown and Goldstein, 1986), were critical for
the specific recognition of LDL by its receptor. It was
demonstrated that a number of different modifications of

lysine residues, such as methylation, inhibit the ability of LDL to bind to the LDL receptor. The degree of inhibition was proportional to the extent of lysine modification and even when as few as 3% of lysine residues of apo B were modified, inhibition of LDL binding was demonstrated. Because NEG is known to involve the covalent binding of glucose to the epsilon amino group of lysine, we sought to determine if such glycosylation of LDL-apo B would also interfere with its ability to bind to its receptor. Extensive glycosylation of LDL was achieved by incubating LDL with glucose in the presence of cyanoborohydride, yielding a modified LDL in which greater than 30% of lysines residues were modified. This modification abolished the ability of LDL to bind to the LDL receptor and when injected intravenously into guinea pigs, its disappearance from plasma was greatly delayed, consistent with the predicted importance of the LDL receptor in mediating LDL clearance in vivo (Witztum et al., 1982).

At the time these studies were performed the extent of the LDL receptor pathway in man was not defined. Because heavily glycated LDL did not bind to the LDL receptor, its plasma clearance was accounted for solely by non LDL receptor-dependent mechanisms (Steinbrecher et al., 1983). Consequently, it was possible to estimate the extent of the LDL receptor pathway in man by the simultaneous injection of native LDL (which would trace both receptor-dependent and receptor-independent pathways) and glycated LDL (which would trace only receptor-independent pathways). The difference in rate of clearance between the two tracers would then represent that portion of the LDL clearance mediated by the LDL receptor. When such studies were performed in a number of normal subjects, we found that approximately 75% of LDL clearance was mediated by the LDL receptor (Kesaniemi et al., 1983), consistent with the predictions of Brown and Goldstein. These studies were important for they demonstrated the essential importance of the LDL receptor in mediating the clearance of LDL in man, and suggested that even minor alterations in the "affinity" of LDL for its receptor might be reflected in delayed clearance of LDL and increased plasma LDL levels. In other studies we determined that in normal individuals only 2 to 3% of LDL-lysine residues were modified, while in diabetics the values were approximately 3 to 5% (as determined by amino acid analysis of reduced apo B protein) (Witztum et al., 1982). To determine if modification of only 3-5% of

LDL lysine residues could slow LDL clearance from plasma, LDL was modified by in vitro incubation with glucose so as to produce glycated LDL preparations with varying degrees of lysines derivatized. Both native and glycated LDL were differentially labeled with radioiodine and injected simultaneously into guinea pigs. In our experience this in vivo assay is a far more sensitive technique to detect changes in LDL structure than is an in vitro assay measuring fibroblast binding. For each guinea pig the fractional catabolic rate (FCR) of the glycated LDL was expressed as a function of the simultaneously determined FCR of native LDL. Fig. 1 displays the extent of lysine modification

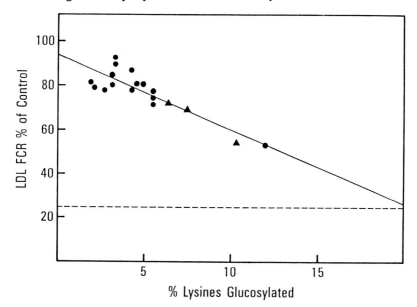

versus the extent to which the glycated LDL was cleared more slowly than the simultaneously determined native LDL. It can be readily appreciated that even minor degrees of modification, in the range of 3 to 6% of lysine residues glycated, inhibited LDL clearance from plasma by 5 to 20% (Steinbrecher and Witztum, 1984). Higher degrees of modification yielded much greater degrees of inhibition. Similar results have been seen in studies in rabbits (Wiklund et al., 1987). It is of considerable interest that this degree of inhibition of LDL clearance is compatible with previous reports by a number of investigators who have treated diabetic patients intensively with insulin therapy and found that plasma LDL levels fell approximately 5 to 20%, irrespective of the initial plasma LDL levels (reviewed in ref. 8). Of course in the studies with patients a number of metabolic parameters were affected by the intensive insulin therapy, including the actual level of LDL receptor activity (Chait et al., 1979), which in turn would also have a profound influence on LDL catabolism and LDL plasma levels.

Lopes-Virella et al. (1982) evaluated the effects of hyperglycemia to affect the ability of LDL to be a ligand for the LDL receptor. She compared the ability of LDL, isolated from diabetic patients during a period of very poor glycemic control, to LDL isolated from the same patient after intensive insulin therapy for their ability to bind to the LDL receptor of cultured fibroblasts. She showed that the LDL isolated during the intensive insulin therapy period wasa taken up and degraded by fibroblast LDL receptors 20-25% more efficiently than the LDL isolated during the period of poor control. It is important to note that her patients were Type I diabetics who were grossly hyperglycemic during the baseline studies. In our laboratory, we have performed similar studies in a number of patients and have confirmed these findings. Figure 2 shows a representative study. LDL was isolated from a Type

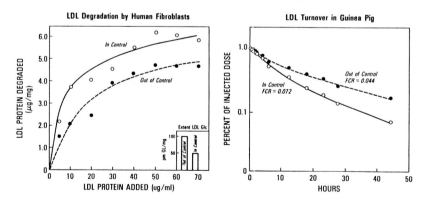

COMPARISON OF METABOLISM OF LDL ISOLATED
DURING "OUT OF CONTROL" AND "IN CONTROL"
PERIODS FROM A DIABETIC SUBJECT

I diabetic subject during a period of poor glucose control, and then subsequently, 10 days later, after intensive insulin therapy to correct his hyperglycemia.

Both LDL samples were iodinated and studied in vitro in cell culture for their ability to be taken up and degraded by human fibroblasts and were also simultaneously injected into guinea pigs to allow for an in vivo comparison of their ability to be cleared by LDL receptor pathways. As shown in the left panel, the LDL sample obtained during the improved control period had increased uptake and degradation compared to the LDL isolated during the out-of-control period, and this correlated inversely with the extent of NEG as shown in the inset. In confirmation of these findings, when injected in vivo into the guinea pig, the out-of-control LDL was cleared approximately 25% slower (Fig. 2, right panel). Similar studies have been seen in several other diabetic subjects confirming the data of Lopes-Virella et al.

These data suggest that LDL isolated from poorly controlled Type I diabetic patients may have a lower affinity for the LDL receptor than when LDL is isolated from the same patients during a period of more normal glycemia. The studies presented above suggest that, in part, this might be explained by the extent of NEG. However, the situation is far more complicated because, in general, poorly controlled diabetic subjects have hypertriglyceridemia, and as shown by Chait and colleagues, the triglyceride content of LDL greatly influences LDL binding to the LDL receptor (Aviram et al., 1988). Thus, in the studies of Hiramatsu et al. (Hiramatsu et al., 1985), LDL isolated from hyperglycemic diabetic subjects had decreased binding to LDL receptors in vitro, but only if LDL was isolated from plasma in which triglyceride levels were above 500 mg/dl. In their study, however, they did not prospectively follow individual patients. In the study shown in Figure 2, the plasma triglyceride level of the patient was below 300 mg/dl at baseline and thus it is likely that the change in affinity of his LDL for the LDL receptor was predominantly influenced by the extent of NEG. However, in most of the other subjects that we studied, hypertriglyceridemia was clearly an important factor. Thus, it is our current impression that in hyperglycemic diabetic subjects, LDL is inherently a less effective ligand for the LDL receptor and that this is accounted for by both NEG, as well as by significant compositional changes caused by hypertriglyceridemia. As noted above, a decreased ability of LDL to bind to its receptor, coupled with downregulation of the LDL receptor due to insulin deficiency, would lead to increased plasma LDL levels. Such an increase in LDL levels in and of itself is likely to be more atherogenic.

LDL may be more atherogenic in diabetics by still other mechanisms. Using a sensitive radioimmunoassay, we have shown that LDL isolated from diabetics is more extensively glycated than LDL isolated from euglycemic individuals (Curtiss and Witztum, 1983). Lopes-Virella et al. (Lyons et al., 1987) have reported that such LDL have enhanced uptake in human monocyte-macrophages. Furthermore, they demonstrated that LDL incubated with glucose in vivo to mimic diabetic LDL also have enhanced macrophage uptake, although the mechanism by which this uptake occurs has not yet been defined (Lopes-Virella et al., 1988). Thus, the generation of Amadori products on LDL may lead to enhanced macrophage uptake and by such a mechanism be more atherogenic. It should be noted that LDL is known to accumulate in the aortic wall, bound to extracellular matrix. In this setting it would be exposed to high glucose concentrations for an extended period of time. Not only would this permit it to undergo extensive NEG, but undoubtedly it also would undergo AGE reactions as well. Vlassara et al. (Vlassara et al., 1985) have recently demonstrated that macrophages possess a specific receptor that recognizes certain AGE complexes. AGE-modified LDL, formed in the intima of the aorta, could be taken up by macrophages by this process as well. Finally, it should be noted that diabetics have been reported to have increased amounts of lipid peroxides in plasma and, in particular, that LDL, and other lipoproteins, have been reported to have higher degrees of lipid peroxidation (Morel and Chisolm, 1987). Our laboratory has previously shown that oxidative modification of LDL renders it highly atherogenic, since it greatly enhances its uptake in macrophages by the acetyl LDL receptor pathway (Steinbrecher et al., 1984). Any process which prolongs the half-life of LDL in plasma might lead to such increased modification and any increase in its half-life within the artery wall, such as might occur by the binding to matrix proteins via glucose adducts (Brownlee et al., 1984), would theoretically also make LDL more susceptible to oxidative modification. While proof for all of these possibilities in humans is lacking at present, evidence for the presence of oxidatively modified LDL within the artery wall of hypercholesterolemic rabbits has recently been obtained (Haberland et al., 1988; Palinski et al., 1989). It is a reasonable hypothesis that a variety of post-secretory modifications of LDL occur in diabetic subjects that cumulatively, and potentially inter-actively, serve to increase its atherogenicity.

IMMUNOLOGICAL CONSEQUENCES OF GLYCATION OF LDL

As noted above, we demonstrated that in euglycemic men up to 75% of the clearance of plasma LDL was mediated by the LDL receptor pathway. In this experiment, native LDL was used as a tracer of receptor-dependent and recep-tor-independent clearance, while glycated LDL was used as the tracer of the receptor-independent pathway. In subse-quent studies, we sought to determine the extent of the LDL receptor pathway in diabetic subjects and repeated this ex-periment in the same manner (Witztum et al., 1984). How-ever, in 3 of the first 4 diabetic subjects tested, there was a greatly enhanced rate of removal of the glycosylated LDL tracer from plasma, as compared to the native tracer. A representative plasma decay curve is shown in Figure 3.

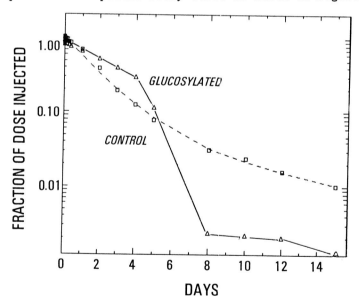

It should be noted that even the initial rate of plasma disappearance of the glycated tracer is more rapid than occurred in euglycemic individuals and that after 3-4 days, there was a sudden break in the plasma decay curve with an extremely rapid plasma removal occurring over the subsequent 24-48 hours. The shape of this curve was reminiscent of an immune-mediated removal. Traditional immunologic theory suggested that the simple covalent attachment of one glucose molecule to an autologous protein would not be immunogenic. Nevertheless, we designed an experiment to test the possibility that glycation of LDL was immunogenic. Guinea pig LDL was isolated and incubated with glucose for 7 days in the presence or absence of cyanoborohydride to produce "reduced glycated LDL" (GLC_{RED} LDL) or "nonreduced glycated LDL" (GLC_{NR} LDL), respectively (Witztum et al., 1983). These products, together with appropriate controls, were then used to immunize guinea pigs. Subsequent studies revealed that animals immunized with GLC_{RED} LDL developed high titered antisera that specifically recognized GLC_{RED} LDL. Furthermore, these antisera recognized specifically the glucitollysine residue when present on any one of a variety of similarly modified proteins (Figure 4). However, this antiserum did not recognize glucose attached to lysine residues when present in

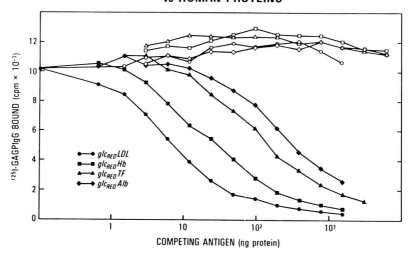

COMPETITION OF GUINEA PIG glc_{RED} LDL vs HUMAN PROTEINS

the Amadori form (the open symbols in Figure 4). However, if the Amadori form of glycated LDL was first subjected to sodium borohydride, which is known to convert such adducts to glucitollysine, then immunoreactivity was observed. In response to immunization with GLC_{NR} LDL, a much lower

titered antiserum resulted, and interestingly, this antiserum recognized not only the Amadori type product, but
the reduced, glycosylated product, i.e., glucitollysine, as
well. However, this antiserum recognized Amadori products
only when present on guinea pig LDL (Witztum et al., 1984).
It should be noted that when guinea pig albumin was subject
to reductive glycosylation and used to immunize guinea
pigs, antisera were also generated, but in this case, the
antiserum recognized glucitollysine only when present on
modified guinea pig albumin. This latter point illustrates
a generalized phenomenon which we have observed repeatedly,
namely, that LDL appears to be an extremely potent vehicle
for presenting an immunogen and that the immune system
readily recognizes even the most minor modifications of
lysine residues on even autologous LDL (Steinbrecher et
al., 1984). For example, if one methylates lysine residues
on guinea pig LDL and uses this to immunize guinea pigs, an
antiserum is produced that recognizes methyllysine not only
on guinea pig LDL, but when present on any one of a variety
of similarly modified proteins. However, if one used
methylated guinea pig albumin as immunogen in a guinea pig,
the resulting antiserum appears far more specific for the
modified albumin, i.e., it recognizes methyllysine residues
in other proteins very poorly, or not al all. As a result
of this generalized observation, we have utilized
homologous LDL as an immunological tool to develop region-
specific antibodies (Curtiss and Witztum, 1983). For
example, using glycated mouse LDL as an immunogen in mice,
and then utilizing the spleens of these mice to produce
monoclonal antibodies, we were able to generate a large
number of murine monoclonal antibodies that specifically
recognized the glucitollysine residue without concern that
antibodies were being generated against the carrier. The
availability of murine monoclonal antibodies that recognize
glucitollysine when present on any one of a variety of
proteins has proven useful in studies of protein glycation.
Such antibodies can be used to develop radioimmunoassays
(Curtiss and Witztum, 1983), to detect glucitollysine in
proteins by Western blot techniques (Curtiss and Witztum,
1985) and, recently, have been used in immunocytochemical
studies of human tissues to directly visualize Amadori
products (Kelly et al., 1989).

A second and potentially more profound implication of
the observation that the simple covalent attachment of
glucose to autologous proteins renders them immunogenic is

the potential that such modifications could generate autoantibodies in people. As noted above, modifications of
autologous LDL appear to be a particularly potent immunogen
and the resulting antibodies recognize the modification not
only on LDL, but on other similarly modified proteins as
well. For example, LDL, found in the arterial wall in
rather high concentrations, bound to extracellular matrix
proteins, likely has a very prolonged halflife and may well
undergo extensive glycation. Autoantibodies formed against
such glycated LDL could bind not only to the modified LDL
but other similar glycated tissue proteins as well, such as
glycated collagen.

We have previously shown the presence of autoantibodies in human plasma that recognize reductively glycated
LDL and that such autoantibodies appear to have the same
specifity as that found in the immunized guinea pigs, i.e.,
they recognize glucitollysine residues when present not
only on LDL but on a number of similarly modified proteins.
Nakayama et al. (Nakayama et al., 1985) have also demonstrated the presence of autoantibodies to glucitollysine.
In our initial studies we found such autoantibodies only in
diabetic subjects (in those subjects who participated in
the original turnover studies that demonstrated the rapid
plasma removal of a glycated tracer) but in more recent
studies, using more sensitive techniques, we hasuch
autoantibodies in normal as well as in diabetic subjects
(table). In these studies, we found autoantibodies
that recognize both GLC_{RED} LDL as well as GLC_{NR} LDL (i.e.,
both glucitollysine as well as Amadori forms of the
glucose-lysine adduct). This was true whether such adducts
were present on LDL or on albumin (Koschinsky et al.,
1988). While these preliminary studies did not reveal any
significant difference in titers between normal and Type I
and Type II diabetics, further studies are indicated using
more appropriately matched populations of control and
diabetic subjects.

As noted above, even the simple covalent attachment
of glucose to lysine residues in LDL, and other proteins,
renders the autologous proteins immunogenic. It is now
well recognized that glycation of proteins, particularly
structural proteins, undoubtedly leads to far more advanced
chemical reactions, termed the "browning reactions" that
have been designated "advanced glycosylation endproducts"
(AGE). Because AGE have been observed in vitro and in vivo

Table 1. Antibody Titers in Human Sera to NGE and AGE

Plated Antigen	Serum Source	Number Tested	Antibody Titer					
			<4	4	16	64	256	>256
Glc$_{NR}$ LDL	Type I DS	12				2	4	6
	NS	11	3	1		4	2	1
	Type II DS	11			2	3	3	3
	NS	11	5	1		2	2	1
Glc$_{RED}$ LDL	Type I DS	12	1		1	3	1	6
	NS	11	3		3	2	1	2
	Type II DS	11			1	3	4	3
	NS	11	2	1	2		5	1
AGE-LDL	Type I DS	12	9	2	1			
	NS	11	5	4	2			
	Type II DS	10			1	8	1	
	NS	11	3			3	5	
AGE-Alb	Type I DS	12	10	1	1			
	NS	11	9	1	1			
	Type II DS	10	3	3	3		1	
	NS	11	8		1	2		

A titer is defined as the reciprocal of highest dilution of serum that has immunoglobulin binding to indicted antigen at a level twice that of controls. DS = diabetic sera; NS = normal sera.

(reviewed in Cerami et al. 1988) and because such complicated adducts are much more extensive and more complicated
than simple glucose-lysine adducts, one would predict that
they, too, should be immunogenic. For example, LDL found
within the artery wall, with its prolonged half-life,
undoubtedly undergoes such AGE reactions, causing LDL-LDL
polymerization, as well as LDL-matrix polymerizations
mediated by such AGE products. To test the possibility
that AGE were also immunogenic, guinea pig LDL was
incubated with glucose (80 mM) for periods up to 3 months
and the AGE-modified LDL used to immunize guinea pigs.
Antisera were obtained that specifically reacted with such
AGE-modified LDL, but not with native LDL. In addition,
such antisera also recognized guinea pig albumin that had
been incubated with glucose for three months. Thus,
clearly, even these more complicated adducts are immunogenic. To determine if autoantibodies also existed in the
plasma of humans to such adducts, we utilized AGE-modified
LDL as an antigen and determined the titer of autoantibodies to this antigen in a select series of normal and
diabetic subjects. As shown in the table, there were low
titered autoantibodies to this adduct present in serum of

both normal and diabetic subjects and similar antibodies
were also found to AGE-albumin as well. Again, the finding
that such antibodies were present in apparently equal
titers in both normal and diabetic subjects should not be
taken as indicative of a true prevalence study, since these
populations were not appropriately matched. However, these
data demonstrate that such autoantibodies exist. Furthermore, it should be appreciated that incubation of LDL (or
other proteins) with glucose for 3 months to produce an
AGE-protein will not give a reproducible antigen that would
allow for systematic testing of large numbers of sera in a
reproducible fashion. To this end, it will be useful to
have specific adducts, that presumably are components of
the AGE complexes, to use as specific antigens. FFI has
been proposed as one such component of the AGE complex
(Cerami et al., 1988). In preliminary studies, we have
utilized FFI conjugated to LDL as the target antigen to
test for autoantibodies in both normal and diabetic subjects. In both groups of subjects, much higher titered
antisera were observed than when AGE-LDL was the antigen,
with titers frequently exceeding 1:256. In part such high-
titered antisera might reflect the presence of specific
autoantibodies, and/or in part, an increased sensitivity of
the assay which contains large amounts of a single antigen
for testing. As the chemistry of the AGE complex is unrav-
eled, and specific AGE components are delineated, our
ability to detect autoantibodies should be greatly
enhanced.

As noted above, we have documented that subtle
modifications of LDL render LDL highly immunogenic. LDL
bound within the arterial wall may well undergo numerous
other types of post-translational modifications that result
in conjugation of fragments to lysine residues of apo B.
As noted earlier, lipoproteins from diabetic subjects have
been reported to have enhanced lipid peroxidation. During
the process of lipid peroxidation of LDL, highly reactive
aldehyde fragments are formed from the peroxidation of the
polyunsaturated fatty acids. These aldehydes, in turn, can
form covalent bonds with apo B, principally with lysine
residues. For example, malondialdehyde (MDA), and 4-
hydroxynonenal (4-HNE) are products that form as a result
of the lipid peroxidation of LDL lipids (Esterbauer et al.,
1987). In turn, they condense with lysine residues of apo
B. We recently reported that these products are also immunogenic and have generated antisera that recognize these

lysine adducts. Using immunocytochemical techniques, we
have also demonstrated that such MDA-lysine adducts, and
4-HNE-lysine adducts, exist in the artery wall in atherosclerotic plaque and that LDL extracted from the artery
wall contains such adducts. In addition, we have demonstrated that there are high titered autoantibodies to MDA-
lysine residues in human (and animal) plasma as well as
autoantibodies to 4-HNE lysine adducts (Palinski et al.,
1989). Thus, in addition to the autoantibodies that might
form against both short- and long-term glycated products of
LDL (and other glycated tissues), autoantibodies that might
react with antigens resulting from oxidative modification
of LDL also might occur in diabetic subjects. As noted
elsewhere in this symposium, glycation of proteins might
actually enhance the possibility of oxidative damage and
increase the subsequent generation of such immunogenic
epitopes. Thus a variety of autoantibodies could form
immune complexes with the modified LDL within the artery
wall. These immune- complexes may then have enhanced
uptake by macrophages, mediated by the F_c receptor. In
this way such modifications might further serve to be
atherogenic. It is well known that large amounts of
immunoglobulins accumulate in the atherosclerotic artery
wall (Parums and Mitchinson, 1981). In part, this may
represent nonspecific trapping of immunoglobulins, mediated
by crosslinking through AGE complexes (Brownlee et al.,
1984). However, we suggest the hypothesis that in
addition, such antibodies are specifically directed against
modified LDL (and modified structural proteins). By
forming such immune complexes, they further contribute to
the atherogenic process. It should be mentioned that such
a process might also be involved in the accumulation of
large amounts of immunoglobulins found in other tissues in
diabetics, such as in the kidney.

CONCLUSION

In this report, we have briefly summarized the potential complications that may occur from both short- and
long-term glycation of lipoproteins. This review has
concentrated on the metabolic and immunological consequences that may occur when LDL is modified. A number of these
mechanisms may contribute to increasing the atherogenicity
of LDL. In addition, we have previously shown that all of
the lipoprotein classes have enhanced degrees of NEG. In a

similar manner, such modifications of other lipoproteins may also interfere with normal lipoprotein metabolism and also may be immunogenic. Obviously much work needs to be done to validate these concepts. However, it is likely that both short- and long-term glycation of LDL, and possibly other lipoproteins, contributes to the increased incidence and severity of atherosclerosis that characterizes the hyperglyemic, diabetic patient.

REFERENCES
1. Aviram M, Lundkatz S, Phillips MC, Chait A (1988). The influence of the triglyceride content of low density lipoproteins on the interaction of apoprotein B-100 with cells. J Biol Chem 263:6842-6848.
2. Brown MS, Goldstein JL (1986). A receptor-mediated pathway for cholesterol homeostasis. Science 232:34-47.
3. Brownlee M, Vlassara H, Cerami A (1984). Nonenzymatic glycosylation and the pathogenesis of diabetic complications. Ann Intern Med 101:527-537.
4. Cerami A, Vlassara H, Brownlee M (1988). Role of advanced glycosylation products in complications of diabetes. Diab Care 11:73-79.
5. Chait A, Bierman EL, Albers JJ (1979). Low density lipoprotein receptor activity in cultured human skin fibroblasts. Mechanism of insulin induced stimulation. J Clin Invest 64:1309-1319.
6. Curtiss LK, Witztum JL (1983). A novel method for generating region-specific monoclonal antibodies to modified proteins: Application to the identification of human glucosylated low density lipoproteins. J Clin Invest 72:1427-1438.
7. Curtiss LK, Witztum JL (1985). Plasma apolipoproteins A-I, A-II, B, C-I and E are glucosylated in hyperglycemic diabetics. Diabetes 34:452.
8. Esterbauer H, Jurgens G, Quehenberger O, Keller E (1987). Autooxidation of human low density lipoprotein: Loss of polyunsaturated fatty acids and vitamin E and generation of aldehyde. J Lipid Res 28:495-509.
9. Haberland ME, Fong D, Cheng L (1988). Malondialdehyde-altered protein occurs in atheroma of Watanabe heritable hyperlipidemic rabbits. Science 241:215-218.
10. Hiramatsu K, Bierman EL, Chait A (1985). Metabolism of low-density lipoprotein from patients with diabetic hypertriglyceridemia by cultured human skin fibroblasts. Diabetes 34:8-14.

11. Kelly SB, Olerud JE, Witztum JL, Curtiss LK, Gown AM, Odland GF (1989). A method for localizing the early products of nonenzymatic glycosylation in fixed tissue. Investigative Dermatology (in press).

12. Kesaniemi YA, Witztum JL, Steinbrecher UP (1983). Receptor-mediated clearance of LDL in man -- new estimates using glucosylated LDL. J Clin Invest 71:950-959.

13. Koschinsky T, Lai D, Vlassara H, Brownlee M, Witztum JL (1988). Immunogenicity of advanced glucosylation endproducts (AGE) in guinea pigs and man. Diabetes 37:784 (abstract).

14. Lopes-Virella MF, Klein RL, Lyons TJ, Stevenson HC, Witztum JL (1988). Glucosylation of low density lipoprotein enhances cholesteryl ester synthesis in human monocyte-derived macrophages. Diabetes 37:550-557.

15. Lopes-Virella MF, Sherer GK, Lees AM, Wohltmann H, Mayfield R, Sagel J, LeRoy EC, Colwell JA (1982). Surface binding, internalization and degradation by cultured human fibroblasts of low density lipoproteins isolated from type 1 (insulin-dependent) diabetic patients: Changes with metabolic control. Diabetologia 22:430-436.

16. Lyons TJ, Klein RL, Baynes JW, Stevenson HC, Lopes-Virella MF (1987). Stimulation of cholesteryl ester synthesis in human monocyte-derived macrophages by low-density lipoproteins from Type 1 (insulin-dependent) diabetic patients: the influence of non-enzymatic glycosylation of low-density lipoproteins. Diabetologia 30:916-923.

17. Morel DW, Chisolm GM (1987). Vit E treatment decreases in vivo oxidation and in vitro cytotoxicity of lipoproteins from rats with experimental diabetes. Fed. Proc. 46:416.

18. Nakayama H, Taneda S, Aoki S, Komori K, Kuroda Y, Misawa K, Tsushima S, Nakagawa S (1985). Antibodies to nonenzymatic glucosylated albumin in the human serum. Biochem Biophys Res Comm 131:720-725.

19. Palinski W, Rosenfeld ME, Ylä-Herttuala S, Gurtner GC, Socher SS, Butler SW, Parthasarathy S, Carew TE, Steinberg D, Witztum JL (1989). Low density lipoprotein undergoes oxidative modification in vivo. Proc Natl Acad Sci USA (in press).

20. Parums D, Mitchinson MJ (1981). Demonstration of immunoglobulin in the neighborhood of advanced

atherosclerotic plaques. Atherosclerosis 38:211-216.

21. Steinbrecher UP, Fisher M, Witztum JL, Curtiss LK (1984). Immunogenicity of homologous low density lipoprotein after methylation, ethylation, acetylation or carbamylation: Generation of antibodies specific for derivatized lysine. J Lipid Res 25:1109-1116.

22. Steinbrecher UP, Parthasarathy SM, Leake DS, Witztum JL, Steinberg D (1984). Modification of low density lipoprotein by endothelial cells involves lipid peroxidation and degradation of low density lipoprotein phospholipids. Proc Natl Acad Sci USA 81:3883-3887.

23. Steinbrecher UP, Witztum JL (1984). Glucosylation of low density lipoproteins to an extent comparable to that seen in diabetes slows their catabolism. Diabetes 33:130-134.

24. Steinbrecher UP, Witztum JL, Kesaniemi YA, Elam R (1983). Comparison of glucosylated LDL with methylated or cyclohexandione-treated LDL in the measurement of receptor-independent LDL catabolism. J Clin Invest 71:960-964.

25. Vlassara H, Brownlee M, Cerami A (1985). High-affinity receptor-mnediated uptake and degradation of glucose-modified proteins: a potential mechanism for the removal of senescent macromolecules. Proc Natl Acad Sci USA 82:5588-5592.

26. Weisgraber KH, Innerarity TL, Mahley RW (1978). Role of the lysine residues of plasma lipoproteins in high affinity binding to cell surface receptors on human fibroblasts. J Biol Chem 253:9053-9062.

27. Wiklund O, Witztum JL, Carew TE, Pittman RC, Elam RL, Steinberg D (1987). Turnover and tissue sites of degradation of glucosylated low density lipoprotein in normal and immunized rabbits. J Lipid Res 28:1098-1109.

28. Witztum JL, Mahoney EM, Branks MJ, Fisher M, Elam R, Steinberg D (1982). Nonenzymatic glucosylation of low-density lipoprotein alters its biological activity. Diabetes 31:283-291.

29. Witztum JL, Steinbrecher UP, Fisher M, Kesaniemi A (1983). Nonenzymatic glucosylation of autologous LDL, and albumin, render them immunogenic in the guinea pig. Proc Natl Acad Sci 80:2757-2761.

30. Witztum JL, Steinbrecher UP, Kesaniemi YA, Fisher M (1984). Autoantibodies to glucosylated proteins in the plasma of patients with diabetes mellitus. Proc Natl Acad Sci USA 81:3204-3208.

The Maillard Reaction in Aging,
Diabetes, and Nutrition, pages 235–248
© 1989 Alan R. Liss, Inc.

PHARMACOLOGICAL MODULATION OF THE ADVANCED GLYCOSYLATION
REACTION

Michael Brownlee

Anita and Jack Saltz Professor of Medicine
Co-Director, Diabetes Research Center
Albert Einstein College of Medicine
Bronx, New York 10461

CHEMICAL BASIS FOR ACCELERATED ADVANCED GLYCOSYLATION
PRODUCT ACCUMULATION IN DIABETES

Advanced products of nonenzymatic glycosylation appear
to play a critical role in the evolution of diabetic
complications because of their characteristic chemical
properties. As discussed below, these slowly-formed
glucose-derived compounds are chemically irreversible, and
thus accumulate continuously with time as a function of
glycemic level. The degree of this accumulation in
patients' dermal collagen has been shown to correlate with
the severity of diabetic retinopathy present (Monnier, et
al., 1986). These products participate in the critical
process of glucose-derived cross-link formation (Reynolds,
1963, Reynolds, 1965, Monnier et al., 1983), and by so doing
alter the structure and function of the vascular wall. In
addition, these products are recognized by specific cell
surface receptors, an event that stimulates local cytokine
growth factor production. Finally, formation of these
products on DNA results in altered structure and function of
genetic elements.

The formation of advanced glycosylation products begins
with the formation of the more familiar early glycosylation
products (Fig. 1).

Nonenzymatic glycosylation begins with glucose attachment to amino groups via nucleophilic addition (Gottschalk, 1972, Beswick, et al., 1985). This addition reaction of glucose with either epsilon-amino groups of lysine residues, alpha-amino groups of N-terminal amino acid residues, or the amines of nucleic acid bases, first results in the formation of unstable Schiff base adducts. It is likely, although unproven, that Schiff base adducts exist both in an open-chain aldimine form, and a more stable glycosylamine ring form. The rate of Schiff base formation (k_1) is approximately equal to the rate of dissociation (k_{-1}). Levels of the labile Schiff base increase rapidly, and equilibrium is reached in a matter of hours (Baynes, et al., 1984). Ambient glucose concentration over that brief period determines the steady-state level of Schiff base adducts.

Once formed, Schiff base adducts of glucose and protein amino groups undergo a slow chemical rearrangement over a period of weeks to form a more stable, but still chemically reversible sugar-protein adduct, the Amadori product (Higgins, et al., 1981, Mortensen, et al., 1983). This product, like the Schiff base adduct, may also exist in both an open chain and a ring form, but current evidence suggests that the beta pyranose conformation is preferred. The chemistry of Amadori products has been extensively studied using hemoglobin and albumin as model proteins. Until recent kinetic studies became available, however, it was not widely appreciated that Amadori glycosylation products, like the Schiff base adducts from which they form, are also chemically reversible equilibrium products. It has now been determined that the rate constant for formation of Amadori products on hemoglobin at 37^0 (k_2) is 14.2×10^{-6} s^{-1}, and the rate constant for dissociation (k_{-2}) is 1.7×10^{-6} s^{-1}. These values give a calculated equilibrium constant (K) of 8.4 (Mortensen, et al., 1983).

Equilibrium of Amadori glycosylation products is reached over a period of approximately 28 days. Thus, even on very long-lived proteins, the total amount of Amadori product is only proportional to the integrated glucose concentration of the preceding four weeks. After the relatively brief period of time necessary to attain equilibrium, measured levels of Amadori products reach a constant steady-state value which does not increase as a function of time beyond that point.

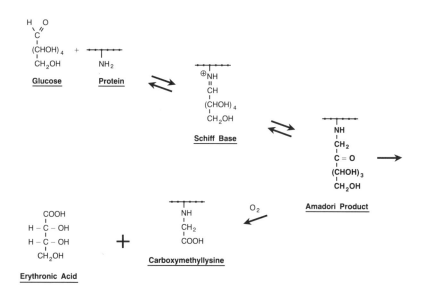

Fig. 1. Formation of reversible, early nonenzymatic glycosylation products, and their oxidative degradation by a recently proposed mechanism.

This has been experimentally confirmed by measuring Amadori products on diabetic tissue proteins exposed to similar levels of hyperglycemia for widely differing periods of time. A two- to three-fold increase in the level of Amadori product is consistently observed, whether diabetic samples are compared to normals after 18 weeks (Yue, et al., 1983) or after many years (Vogt, et al., 1982). These values represent the same equilibrium levels of Amadori productsreached relatively quickly on all proteins whose survival time is longer than the time required for equilibrium to be achieved. Since these early glycosylation products increase when blood glucose is high, return towards normal when blood glucose levels are optimized, and do not continue to accumulate on stable tissue molecules over years of chronic diabetes, it is not surprising that their concentration does not correlate with either the presence or severity of diabetic retinopathy (Vishwanath, et al., 1986).

Within a given protein, the amino groups most susceptible to Amadori product formation appear to be those in proximity to groups that can participate in local acid-base catalysis of the Amadori rearrangement (Iberg, et al., 1986). The variable susceptibility of different proteins to Amadori product formation probably reflects the same type of differences in amino group microenvironment (Shapiro, et al., 1980, Garlick, et al., 1983, Ahmed, et al., 1986).

The two determinants of nonenzymatic glycosylation in vivo are glucose concentration and duration of macromolecule exposure to glucose. As glucose concentrations rise, the rate of Amadori product accumulation increases proportionately via mass action. Opposing this process may be a newly described pathway for the oxidative degradation of Amadori products (Fig. 1). This reaction cleaves the Amadori productinto peptide-bound carboxymethyllysine and free erythronic acid (Ahmed, et al., 1986). Both compounds have been measured in urine, and thus appear to form in vivo. Such a pathway could reduce the amount of Amadori product available to serve as a precursor for advanced glycosylation product formation.

Genetic variability in the regulatory elements of this pathway could account for some of the well-documented differences in individual patient's susceptibility to hyperglycemia-mediated tissue damage (Knowles, et al, 1965, Deckert, et al., 1981, Dornan et al, 1982, Chan, et al., 1985).

Advanced glycosylation products form on molecules having low physiologic turnover rates, such as matrix protein components and DNA interminally differentiated cells. Here, Amadori products slowly undergo an extensive series of dehydrations, reactions, and rearrangements to form complex advanced glycosylation endproducts (Sell, D.R., et al., in press). Advanced glycosylation endproducts are frequently pigmented or fluorescent, and most importantly for diabetic complications, they participate in glucose-derived cross-link formation (Reynolds, 1963, Reynolds, 1965). In contrast to the Amadori product, which is in equilibrium with glucose, these advanced glycosylation products are irreversibly attached to proteins. Consequently, the level of advanced glycosylation endproducts in diabetic tissue does not return to normal levels when hyperglycemia is corrected, but instead continue to accumulate over the lifetime of the vessel wall (Monnier, et al., 1984, and Brownlee, M, et al., unpublished data).

Specific chemical characterization of AGE-proteins has been difficult, since Amadori products can theoretically undergo a large number of potential rearrangements, and many AGE's may be unstable to hydrolysis. To date, evidence has been obtained for two general types of glucose-derived advanced glycosylation product cross-links (Pongor, et al., 1984, Chang, et al., 1985, Njoroge, et al., 1987, Farmar, et al., 1988, Sell, et al., in press, Kato, et al., in press, Dyer et al., in press, Hayashi, et al., 1986).

One type closely resembles the heterocyclic imidazole derivative, 2-furoyl-4(5)-(2-furanyl)1-H-imidazole (Figure 2). This yellow-brown compound, abbreviated FFI, has a fluorescence spectrum that is characteristic of AGE-proteins and has been found to exist in enzymatically hydrolyzed tissue (Chang, J.C.F. et al., 1985). This type of AGE appears to form from the condensation of two Amadori products. The other type of AGE crosslink appears to form from the reaction of an Amadori product with the Amadori-derived compound 3-deoxyglucasone (Njoroge, et al., 1987, Farmar, et al., 1988). This highly reactive dicarbonyl compound cyclizes to form electrophilic pyrrole intermediates with reactive OH groups in benzylic positions. These then react with amino groups to form pyrrole-based crosslinks. Examples of this type of AGE include the 1-alkyl-2-formyl-3,4-diglycosyl pyrroles (AFGPs), an arginine-ribose-lysine crosslink called "pentosidine", a fluorescent HPLC peak designated "peak L1", and the newly identified Maillard Fluorescent Product 1 (MFP-1) (Farmar, et al., 1988, Sell, et al., in press, Kato, et al., in press, Dyer, et al., in press). Formation of other AGEs appears to involve generation of glycolaldehyde from Schiff bases via a reverse aldol condensation reaction. This product is an even more reactive cross-linking agent than 3-deoxyglucasone (Hayashi, et al., 1986). The kinetics of AGE formation with respect to glucose concentration have not been rigorously characterized, but preliminary experiments suggest that AGE formation over time is exponential.

It has been known for some time that early (and presumably advanced) nonenzymatic glycosylation products can also form when proteins are incubated with a variety of non-glucose sugars, including most of the glycolytic intermediates that are elevated in diabetic target tissues (Stevens, et al., 1977). However, systematic investigations of non-glucose-derived AGEs have been reported only recently (McPherson, et al., 1988). In these studies, fructose was shown to form early glycosylation products at the same rate as glucose, but the rate of advanced glycosylation product cross-link formation was nearly 10 times more rapid. In vivo fructosylation was also demonstrated by analysis of human lens proteins. Since intracellular concentrations of fructose are elevated in some diabetic tissues with activated polyol pathway enzyme activity, a partial link may exist between these particular reversible and irreversible consequences of hyperglycemia.

THE PATHOLOGIC CONSEQUENCES OF ADVANCED GLYCOSYLATION ENDPRODUCT FORMATION

It has been known for many years that the incidence and prevalence of diabetic vascular complications correlate strongly with disease duration and cumulative level of hyperglycemia, although there is clearly significant variability in the response of different individuals to comparable levels of chronic hyperglycemia (Diabetes in America: Diabetes Data Compiled, 1984, 1985). Ultimately, however, progression of these lesions becomes independent of blood glucose level. In patients whose glycemia is completely normalized by successful pancreas transplantation, for example, proliferative diabetic retinopathy continues to progress (Ramsay, et al., 1988). Similarly, continued progression of background retinopathy is observed in diabetic dogs with a prior history of chronic hyperglycemia, despite three years of normalized glycemic control (Engerman, et al., 1987). Together, these old and new observations suggest that permanent modifications have occurred in long-lived molecules of diabetic tissues chronically exposed to hyperglycemia, which perpetuate the development of further pathology in the absence of blood glucose elevation.

The central features of the chemistry and consequences of advanced glycosylation endproduct formation are strikingly congruent with these characteristics of the natural history of diabetic complications. Advanced glycosylation products also accumulate continuously in patients as a function of time and glucose concentration, and eventually AGEs will continue to form on glucose-modified proteins in the absence of glucose (McPherson, et al., 1988, Eble, et al, 1983). Once formed _in_ _vivo_, the irreversibility of AGEs on long-lived macromolecules would promote continued progression of diabetic complications, even in patients whose blood glucose levels have been normalized.

The consequences of AGE formation that contribute to the development and progression of micro- and macrovascular insufficiency in diabetic patients can be subdivided into those involving crosslinks on extracellular matrix proteins, those involving interactions with cellular AGE receptors, and those involving nucleic acid and nucleoprotein cross-links inside terminally differentiated insulin-independent cells.

On extracellular matrix proteins, AGE formation causes deposition of immobilized extravasated plasma proteins via glucose-derived crosslinks; accumulation of matrix proteins due to reduced susceptibility of crosslinked proteins to enzymatic degradation; increased matrix pore size due to permanent changes in the physical association of matrix components; and cellular hypertropy/hyperplasia due to an irreversible decrease in binding affinity for growth-inhibiting heparan sulfate proteoglycans.

Interactions of AGEs with specific cellular receptors stimulate the proliferation of several cell types, synthesis of matrix components, and the induction of procoagulatory /prothrombotic changes in endothelial surfaces. A number of these responses are mediated by growth-promoting cytokines produced by macrophages and endothelial cells in response to AGE binding.

Inside cells which do not require insulin for glucose transport, elevated concentrations of glucose and of even more reactive glycolytic intermediates can promote AGE formation on nucleotide base amino groups, and probably also between DNA and protein. Formation of AGEs on

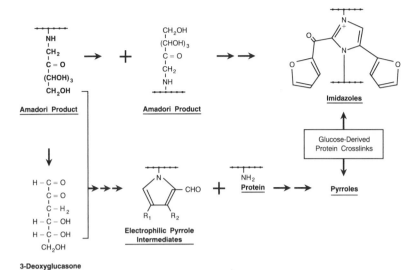

Fig. 2. Formation of irreversible advanced glycosylation endproducts (**AGE**) from Amadori products. Through a complex series of chemical reactions, Amadori products can form families of imidazole-based and pyrrole-based glucose-derived crosslinks.

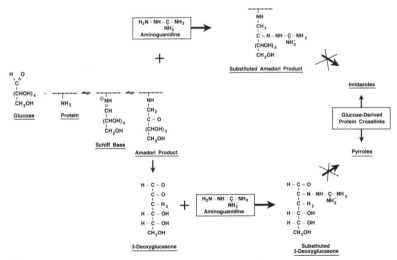

Fig. 3. Prevention of **AGE**-protein crosslink formation by aminoguanidine. Aminoguanidine binds preferentially to reactive **AGE** crosslink precursors, forming unreactive substituted products which can no longer participate in **AGE** crosslink formation.

DNA is associated with mutations and decreased gene expression which may alter the balance between normal cell maintenance and excessive cell proliferation in the diabetic vascular wall.

PHARMACOLOGIC INHIBITION OF ADVANCED GLYCOSYLATION PRODUCT FORMATION

Since the chemical determinants and the biological consequences of AGE formation appear to explain so many of the features of diabetic complications, pharmacologic agents were sought that could inhibit this process by selectively blocking reactive carbonyls on early glycosylation products and on their derivatives 3-deoxyglucasone and glycolaldehyde. The essentially non-toxic nucleophilic hydrazine compound aminoguanidine HCl (LD50=1800 mg/kg in rodents) was selected as the prototype inhibitor (shown schematically in Fig. 3). Importantly, this compound does not interfere with the formation of normal, enzymatically-derived collagen crosslinks, as determined both indirectly (Brownlee, et al., 1986) and by direct quantitation of lysyl oxidase-dependent crosslink products (Reiser,K.M., Yamin, M., et al., unpublished data).

In vitro, aminoguanidine effectively inhibits the formation of AGEs, and inhibits AGE-crosslinking of soluble proteins to matrix. In addition, this compound inhibits AGE-crosslinking of collagen, and prevents crosslink-induced defects of heparin binding to collagen/fibronectin and crosslink-induced defects of heparan-sulfate proteoglycan binding to basement membrane (Brownlee, et al., 1986,Brownlee, et al., 1987,Brownlee, et al., 1986, and Brownlee, M, et al., unpublished data).

In vivo, the effect of aminoguanidine on early vascular lesions has been examined in aorta and kidney. In untreated diabetic rats, matrix AGE content and the quantity of plasma proteins crosslinked to diabetic matrix are four-fold higher in both aorta and kidney than in comparable samples from non-diabetics by sixteen weeks of diabetes. In contrast, these same parameters are nearly normal in tissues from aminoguanidine-treated diabetic animals. Preliminary data from ongoing long-term studies examining the effect of aminoguanidine on glomerular morphology suggest that diabetes-induced irreversible thickening of glomerular basement membrane and AGE-derived collagen crosslink formation is also prevented by aminoguanidine treatment (Brownlee, M., Steffes, M., et al., unpublished data). Concurrent studies in humans are also in progress focusing on the pharmacokinetics and potential toxicity of aminoguanidine HCl.

The therapeutic potential of aminoguanidine and its chemically related analogs is currently being evaluated in several animal models of different diabetic complications, in preparation for future clinical efficacy trials in patients.

REFERENCES

Ahmed M U, Thorpe S R, Baynes J W (1988) Identification of Carboxymethyllysine as a degradation product of fructosyllysine in glycated protein. J Biol Chem 261, 4889-94.

Baynes, J W, Thorpe, S R & Murtiashaw, M H (1984) Nonenzymaticglucosylation of lysine residues in albumin. In Methods in Enzymology: Posttranslational Modifications (Wold, F. & Moldave, K., eds.), Vol. 106, Academic Press, Inc., New York, pp.88-98.

Beswick H T, Harding, J J Aldehydes (1985) or dicarbonyls in non-enzymic glycosylation of proteins. Biochem J 226, 385-389.

Brownlee M, Vlassara H, Cerami A (1987) Aminoguanidine prevents hyperglycemia-induced defect in binding of heparin by matrix molecules. Diabetes 36:85A.

Brownlee M, Vlassara H, Kooney A, Cerami A (1986) Inhibition of glucose-derived protein crosslinking and prevention of early diabetic changes in glomerular basement membrane byaminoguanidine. Diabetes 35 (Suppl 1).

Brownlee M, Vlassara H, Kooney T, Ulrich P, Cerami A (1986) Aminoguanidine prevents diabetess-induced arterial wall protein cross-linking. Science, 232:1629-32.

Chang, J Y C, Cole, E & Hanna (1985) Diabetic nephropathy and proliferative retinopathy with normal glucose tolerance. Diabetes Care 8, 385-390.

Chang, J C F, Ulrich, P C, Bucala, R & Cerami (1985) A Detection of an advanced glycosylation product bound to protein **in situ**. J. Biol. Chem. **260**, 7970-7974.

Deckert, T & Poulsen, J E (1981) Diabetic nephropathy: fault or destiny? Diabetologia **21**, 178-183.

Diabetes in America: Diabetes Data Compiled 1984. (1985) NIH Publication No. 85-1468.

Dornan, T L, Ting, A, McPherson, C K, Peckar, C O, Mann, J I, Turner, R C & Morris, P J (1982) Genetic susceptibility to the development of retinopathy in insulin-dependent d-iabeticsDiabetes **31**, 226-231.

Dyer, D, Thorpe, S, and Baynes, J W Identification of a fluorescent Maillard product in human lens in Proceedings of the NIH Conference on the Maillard Reaction in Aging, Diabetes and Nutrition, Baines, J W, and Monnier, V M, eds. Elsevier, in press.

Eble, A S, Thorpe, S R & Baynes, J W (1983) Nonenzymatic glucosylation and glucose-dependent cross-linking of proteins. J Biol Chem **258**, 9506-9512.

Engerman R L, Kern T S (1987) Progression of incipient diabetic retinopathy during good glycemic control. Diabetes 36:808-12.

Farmar, J, Ulrich, P, and Cerami (1988) A Novel pyrrole from sulfite-inhibited Maillard reaction: insight into the mechanism of inhibition. J Org Chem 53:2346-49.

Garlick, R L & Mazer, J S (1983) The principal site of nonenzymatic glycosylation of human serum albumin **in vivo**. J Biol Chem **258**, 6142-6146.

Garlick, R L, Mazer, J S, Higgins, P J & Bunn, H F (1983) Characterization of glycosylated hemoglobins: relevance to monitoring of diabetic control and analysis of other proteins. J Clin Invest **71**, 1062-1072.

Gottschalk, A (1972) Interaction between reducing sugars and amino acids under neutral and acid conditions. In The Glycoproteins (Gottschalk, A., ed.), Am. Elsevier, New York, pp. 141-157.

Hayashi, T W, and Namiki, M in Proceedings of the 3rd International Symposium on the Maillard Reaction, eds. Fujimaki, M, Namiki, M, and Kato, H Elsevier (1986).

Higgins, P J & Bunn, H F (1981) Kinetic analysis of the nonenzymatic glycosylation of hemoglobin. J Biol Chem **256**, 5204-5208.

Iberg N, Fluckiger R. (1986) Nonenzymatic glycosylation of albumin **in vivo**. J Biol Chem **261**, 13542-45.

Kato, H, Hayase, F, Shin, D B, Oimomi, M, and Baba, S 3-Deoxyglucasone, an intermediate product of the Maillard reaction, in Proceedings of the NIH Conference on the Maillard Reaction in Aging, Diabetes and Nutrition, Baines, J W, and Monnier, V M, eds. Elsevier, in press.

Knowles, H C, Guest, G M, Lampe, J, Kessler, M & Skillman, T G (1965) The course of juvenile diabetes treated with un-measured diet. Diabetes **14**, 239-273.

McPherson, J D, Shilton, B H, and Walton, D J (1988) Role of fructose in glycation and cross-linking of proteins. Biochemistry 27:1901-7.

Monnier, V M & Cerami (1983) A Nonenzymatic glycosylation and browning of proteins **in vivo**. In The Maillard Reaction in Foods and Nutrition (Waller, G R & Feather, M S, eds.), pp. 431-439, The American Chemical Society, Symposium Series # 215, Washington, D.C.

Monnier V M, Vishwanath V, Frank K E, et. al. (1986) Relation between complications of type I diabetes mellitus and collagen-linked fluorescence. N Engl J Med **314**, 403-8.

Monnier, V M, Kohn, R R & Cerami (1984) A Accelerated age-related browning of human collagen in diabetes mellitus. Proc Natl Acad Sci USA **81**, 583-587.

Mortensen, H B & Christophersen, C (1983) Glucosylation of human haemoglobin A in red blood cells studied **invitro**. Kinetics of the formation and dissociation ofhaemoglobin A_{1c}. Clinica Chimica Acta **134**, 317-326.

Njoroge, F G, Sayre, L M, Monnier, V M (1987) Detection of D-glucose-derived pyrrole compounds during maillard reaction under physiological conditions. Carbohydrate Research **167**, 211-220.

Pongor, S, Ulrich, P C, Bencsath, F A & Cerami, (1984) A Aging of proteins: isolation and identification of a fluorescent chromophore from the reaction of polypeptides with glucose. Proc Natl Acad Sci USA **81**, 2684-2688.

Ramsay, R C, Goetz, F C, Sutherland, D E R, Mauer, S M, et al (1988) Progression of diabetic retinopathy after pancreas transplantation for insulin-dependent diabetes mellitus. New Engl J Med **318**, 20[8-214.

Reynolds, T M (1963) Chemistry of nonenzymatic browning: I Adv Food Res **12**, 1-52.

Reynolds, T M (1965) Chemistry of nonenzymatic browning: II Adv Food Res **14**, 167-283.

Sell, D R, and Monnier, V M Structural elucidation of a fluorescent Maillard crosslink from aging human collagen. in Proceedings of the NIH Conference on the Maillard Reaction in Aging, Diabetes and Nutrition, Baines, J W, and Monnier, V M, eds. Elsevier, in press.

Stevens, V D, Vlassara, H, Abati, A, and Cerami, A (1977) Nonenzymatic glycosylation of hemoglobin. J Biol Chem 252:2998-3004.

Shapiro, R, McManus, M J, Zalut, C & Bunn, H F (1980) Sites of nonenzymatic glycosylation of human hemoglobin A. J Biol Chem 255, 3120-3127.

Vishwanath V, Frank K E, Elmets C A, et al (1986) Glycation of skin collagen in type I diabetes mellitus: correlation with long-term complications. Diabetes 35, 916-21.

Vogt, B W, Schleicher, E D & Wieland, O H (1982) Epsilon- -amino-lysine-bound glucose in human tissues obtained at autopsy: increase in diabetes mellitus. Diabetes 31, 1123-1127.

Yue, D K, McLennan, S & Turtle, J R (1983) Non-enzymatic glycosylation of tissue protein in diabetes in the rat. Diabetologia 24, 377-381.

The Maillard Reaction in Aging,
Diabetes, and Nutrition, pages 249–257
© 1989 Alan R. Liss, Inc.

SENESCENCE OF T CELLS: A POTENTIAL CONSEQUENCE OF THE
MAILLARD REACTION?

Richard A. Miller

Department of Pathology, Boston University
School of Medicine, Boston, MA 02118

ABSTRACT. The immune system of old mice is
heterogeneous, containing a mixture of long
and short-lived T cells, some of which respond
to activating mitogens, amid others that do
not. Studies of T cell activation have revealed defects in calcium signal generation
and oncogene expression, among others, that
are gradually revealing the molecular basis
for immunosenescence. New evidence suggests
that the proportion of longer lived cells, detectable with antibodies to the PGP-1 surface
glycoprotein, increases with age in mice, and
that it is the PGP-1^{hi} T cell subpopulation
that is least responsive to mitogens. It is
now possible to test the idea that the
longest-lived T cells may contain stable
components whose nonenzymatic glycosylation
contributes to their poor T cell function.

It has been known for decades that aging leads to a
decline in most measures of immune function, both in the
intact animal and in in vitro culture models, and that
declines in the function of the thymus-derived T
lymphocyte are particularly pronounced (Gottesman, 1987;
Housman and Weksler, 1985; Miller, 1988). The last few
years have brought substantial progress in our understanding of the biochemical basis for T cell dysfunction, and first hints about the developmental origin
of the defective cells. This position paper will

summarize this newer work, which implicates a mitogen-
nonreactive, long lived memory T cell subset as a major
contributor to immunosenescence. The ability to purify the
long-lived, functionally deficient cells will allow us to
compare them biochemically to functionally competent T
cells in the same individual.

Peripheral T cells in the blood, spleen and lymph
nodes are largely derived from immunocompetent thymus
emigrants, which are in turn the product of intense intra-
thymic selection among the progeny of bone marrow-derived
prothymocytes. The rate at which thymic emigrants seed
the periphery is very high in fetal life, and still
considerable throughout childhood, but declines
dramatically as the thymus involutes during the early part
of adult life (Scollay et al., 1980). So goes the
textbook version: less generally appreciated, however, is
the enormous capacity of the peripheral immune system for
self-renewal even in the absence of thymic emigration
(Rocha et al., 1983; Rocha, 1987). Experimental thymectomy of adult mice, or therapeutic thymectomy (e.g. for
myasthenia) in humans, produces an immune system that
differs in subtle ways from the normal, but that is in
most respects well populated and quite immunocompetent
(Taylor, 1965; Miller, 1965; Metcalf, 1965; Kappler et
al., 1974; Simpson and Cantor, 1975). Direct measures of
T cell turnover by thymidine uptake kinetics (reviewed by
Sprent, 1977) show that while some proportion (10% to 50%
by various estimates) of the peripheral T cells turn over
within days to a few weeks of their previous mitosis, the
majority seem to turn over at a much slower rate. Studies
of chromosomal morphology after therapeutic irradiation
similarly suggest the presence of a T lymphocyte subset
that survives, in G_0, for months to years in humans
(Buckton et al., 1962; Goh et al. 1976). One practical
consequence of the presence of long-lived memory T cells
is the retention of long-lasting immunity after deliberate
vaccination.

The decline in T cell proliferative responses to
polyclonal activators (e.g. plant mitogens or antibodies
to the T cell receptor complex), the most commonly used in
vitro model of immunosenescence, has in recent years been
shown to reflect a loss in both the production of T cell
derived growth factors (e.g. interleukin 2, IL-2), and in
responsiveness to these factors (Gillis et al., 1981,

Gottesman et al., 1985, Miller, 1984). Since secretion of IL-2, and expression of the p55 chain of the high affinity IL-2 receptor both begin a full 4 - 8 hours after the exposure of a resting T cell to an activator, several labs have begun to study still earlier events in the activation process whose failure might lead to a loss in IL-2 and IL-2 receptor expression. Defects have so far been documented in the accumulation of c-myc mRNA (about 1 - 4 hrs after Con A addition; Buckler et al., 1988), and even in mitogen-induced increases in cytoplasmic Ca^{2+} concentration seen within the first 1 - 3 minutes of mitogen exposure (Miller et al., 1987; Proust et al., 1987).

Many of these studies have been consistent with a "mosaic" model of the aging immune system, which in its simplest form would postulate that old individuals have two kinds of T cells: some that function as well as T cells in young controls, and others that fail to participate in immune responses at all. Thus limiting dilution techniques have shown (Nordin and Collins, 1983; Miller, 1984) a decline with age in the proportion of mouse T cells that can respond to mitogen or alloantigen to produce IL-2, proliferate in the presence of IL-2, or develop into a clone of cytotoxic effectors under IL-2's influence. In these functional assays, the amount of response (e.g. IL-2 secretion, clone size, etc.) generated per responding cell was shown not to change with age, even as the number of responding cells declined. Cell cycle analyses, whether by ^{3}H-thymidine uptake or by flow cytometric methods, have generally produced consistent results, suggesting a decline, with age, in the number of T cells that will leave G_0 to enter the mitotic cycle (Abraham et al., 1977; Staiano-Coico et al., 1984; Kubbies et al., 1985). The number of murine T cells that express the IL-2 receptor after Con A addition also declines with age (Vie and Miller, 1986).

Can one identify a biochemical basis for the failure of many T cells in old mice (and humans) to respond to activating agents? Flow cytometric analysis of intracytoplasmic Ca^{2+} concentrations ("$[Ca]_i$") reveal an age-related decline in the number of T cells that increase $[Ca]_i$ after Con A addition (Miller et al., 1987). Recent work from our lab (Philosophe and Miller, submitted) has suggested that this heterogeneity in calcium signal generation may indeed explain the parallel heterogeneity of functional competence seen in limiting dilution analyses, by showing that cells selected (on the flow cytometer) for poor calcium signal generation immediately after mitogen addition are indeed dramatically depleted in cells able to produce IL-2, proliferate in response to IL-2, or mature into clones of cytotoxic effectors. The defects in calcium signal generation seem to be multifactorial. On the one hand, we can show an age-dependent decline in the rate at which ^{45}Ca is taken up from the extracellular medium in the first 60 seconds after Con A addition (Lerner et al., submitted). On the other hand, declines in calcium influx rates are not likely to be the sole cause of deficits in calcium signal generation, since aged T cells are resistant to alterations in $[Ca]_i$ even when these are induced by ionomycin, a lipophilic ionophore that bypasses the receptor-linked calcium influx channels and transports calcium into aged T cells at a rate not lower than the corresponding rate of influx into young T cells (Miller et al., 1988). The resistance to ionomycin strongly implicates changes in the plasma membrane ATP-dependent calcium extrusion pump as a key element in age-associated deficits in T cell activation.

Until very recently, the developmental origin of these calcium resistant, hyporeactive T cells was obscure. In principle, deficient T cells might represent the most recent thymic emigrants -- perhaps the dysfunctional products of a thymus no longer able to select competent cells for emigration. Alternatively, the defective T cells might prove to be the stale remnants of the original cohorts of thymic emigrants, so long out of the mitotic cycle to have accumulated a degree of genetic, oxidative, or glycosylative damage sufficient to render them inoperative. Further insight has come from the identification of the PGP-1 surface glycoprotein as a marker for memory cells.

PGP-1 is a 95 kilodalton molecule of unknown function found on a wide range of tissues, including brain, liver, cultured fibroblasts, phagocytes (PGP stands for "phagocyte glycoprotein"), and subsets of cells within the bone marrow and thymus (Trowbridge et al., 1982). Budd and his co-workers (1987a,b) have recently shown that PGP-1 serves to discriminate, within the mouse T cell immune system, virgin lymphocytes (i.e. those that have not yet encountered antigen) from "memory" T cells that have undergone at least one round of antigen-induced clonal expansion. Exposure of PGP-1^{lo} T cells to mitogens or antigens converts them within a day or so to the PGP-1^{hi} phenotype; the PGP-1^{hi} phenotype, once acquired, seems to remain stable even after the cells revert from blast transformation to the stable, resting state typical of memory T cells. In animals primed to an environmental antigen, antigen-specific T memory cells seem to be found almost exclusively within the PGP-1^{hi} group. The observation that adult thymectomy leads (within weeks) to the development of an immune system containing mostly PGP-1^{hi} T cells is consistent with the model in which all PGP-1^{lo} cells are derived from recent thymus emigration, and, once converted by antigen to the PGP-1^{hi} state, rarely if ever revert to the PGP-1^{lo} phenotype. Other labs have identified, in the human T cell immune system, a series of surface antigens, including human PGP-1, that seem to discriminate virgin from memory cells, have shown mitogen-driven conversion of PGP-1^{lo} to PGP-1^{hi} cells, and have identified the PGP-1^{hi} compartment as the locus for nearly all antigen-specific memory T cell reactivity (Sanders et al., 1988).

Since the rate of thymic emigration declines with age, while the rate of antigen-driven conversion of virgin to memory cells is likely to continue unabated, we postulated that the ratio of PGP-1^{hi} to PGP-1^{lo} cells was likely to increase with age in mice. Lerner et al. (submitted) have shown that this is indeed the case: the proportion of T cells with the PGP-1^{hi} phenotype increases from about 25% in young mice (3 - 5 months old) to about 70% in old mice (18 - 24 months old). The increase affects cells in both the CD4 helper and CD8 cytotoxic classes, and applies to blood, spleen and lymph node T cell populations.

We have also shown that the shift, with age, from PGP-1^{lo} to PGP-1^{hi} cells has functional implications. Limiting dilution analyses (Lerner et al., submitted) showed that _functional_ precursors for helper, cytotoxic, and proliferative function were much enriched in the PGP-1^{lo} T cell subsets compared to the PGP-1^{hi} T cell set. PGP-1^{hi} T cells were also shown to be deficient in production of calcium signals in response to Con A, antibody to the CD3 component of the T cell receptor, and even the receptor-independent ionophore ionomycin (Philosophe and Miller, submitted). Thus the shift from an immune system made up primarily of responsive $PGP-1^{lo}$ virgin cells to one containing a majority of $PGP-1^{hi}$, mitogen-hyporesponsive T cells could well make a major contribution to immune dysfunction in aging.

This developmental model for age-associated defects in the immune response is probably oversimplified. For one thing, the $PGP-1^{hi}$ population is likely to contain a mixture of recently stimulated cells and others that have not undergone mitosis for months (in mice) to years (in humans), and it is plausible to predict a higher level of function in the former cell population. Indeed, both our limiting dilution and calcium data provide some support for the idea that $PGP-1^{hi}$ cells in old mice are not only more numerous than in young mice, but also less functional (Miller, Philosophe, and Yamada, unpublished data.)

Much additional work needs to be done to define the ontogeny, immunology, and cell biology of memory T cells. In the context of a symposium on the Maillard reaction, however, a model that postulates accumulation of very long lived T cells as a proximate cause of immunosenescence, and the availability of the PGP-1 marker to enrich for these dysfunctional cells, together provide both a rationale for a search for advanced glycosylation products in T cells of old mice and humans, and a method for comparing "old" and "new" T cells from donors of any age. If indeed T cells gradually lose the ability to respond to stimuli as a function of the time since their last encounter with antigen, it becomes very important to define the biochemical differences between the "fresh" reactive T cells and their "stale" nonresponsive companions that predominate in old age. There are few clues yet as to which molecules, or even which organelles, are responsible for the functional deficits in the latter cell type, although the defects in very early signal transduction (calcium influx, calcium concentration changes) argue that changes in the cell membrane and associated juxta-membranal machinery are more likely to be involved than are changes in gene regulation. The development of new chromatographic methods for detection of glycosylation products, and of antibodies with specificity for these products, will shortly allow us to compare T cells from old and young donors, and to compare "fresh" and "stale" T cells within old donors, in a search for the molecular basis for deficient T cell function in aging.

ACKNOWLEDGMENTS:

This research was supported by NIH grants AG-07114 and AG-03978, by a Research Career Development Award from the National Institute on Aging, and by a Scholar Award from the Leukemia Society of America. I wish to acknowledge Adam Lerner, Ben Philosophe, and Takatsugu Yamada for their contributions to the work described in this review.

REFERENCES:

Abraham C, Tal Y, Gershon H (1977). Reduced in vitro response to concanavalin A and lipopolysaccharide in senescent mice: a function of reduced number of responding cells. Eur. J. Immunol. 7:301-304.

Buckler A, Vie H, Sonenshein G, Miller RA (1987). Defective T lymphocytes in old mice: diminished production of mature c-myc RNA after mitogen exposure not attributable to alterations in transcription or RNA stability. J. Immunol. 140:2442-2446.

Buckton KE, Jacobs PA, Court Brown WM, Doll R (1962). A study of the chromosome damage persisting after X-ray therapy for ankylosing spondylitis. Lancet 2:676-682.

Budd RC, Cerottini JC, Horvath C, Bron C, Pedrazzini T, Howe RC, Macdonald HR (1987a). Distinction of virgin and memory T lymphocytes. Stable acquisition of the Pgp-1 glycoprotein concomitant with antigenic stimulation. J. Immunol. 138:3120-3129.

Budd RC, Cerottini JC, MacDonald HR (1987b). Phenotypic identification of memory cytolytic T lymphocytes in a subset of Lyt-2[+] cells. J. Immunol. 138:1009-1013.

Gillis S, Ferm MM, Ou W, Smith KA (1978). T cell growth factor: parameters of production and a quantitative microassay for activity. J. Immunol. 120:2027-2032.

Goh K, Reddy MM, Hempelmann LH (1976). Chromosomal aberrations in lymphocytes of normal adults long after thymus irradiation. Radiation Research 67:82-85.

Gottesman SRS (1987). Changes in T-cell-mediated immunity
with age: an update. Rev. Biol. Res. in Aging 3:79-111.
Gottesman SRS, Walford RL, Thorbecke GJ (1985).
Proliferative and cytotoxic immune functions in aging
mice. III. Exogenous interleukin-2 rich supernatant
only partially restores alloreactivity in vitro.
Mechanisms of Ageing and Development 31:103-113.
Hausman PB, Weksler ME (1985). Changes in the immune
response with age. In Finch CE, Schneider, EL (eds):
"Handbook of the Biology of Aging," 2nd edition, New
York: Van Nostrand Reinhold, pp. 414-432.
Kappler JW, Hunter PC, Jacobs D, Lord E (1974).
Functional heterogeneity among the T-derived lymphocytes
of the mouse. I. Analysis by adult thymectomy. J.
Immunol. 113:27-38.
Kubbies M, Schindler D, Hoehn H, Rabinovitch PS (1985).
BrdU-Hoechst flow cytometry reveals regulation of human
lymphocyte growth by donor-age-related growth fraction
and transition rate. J. Cell. Physiol. 125:229-234.
Metcalf D (1965). Delayed effect of thymectomy in adult
life on immunological competence. Nature 208:1336.
Miller JFAP (1965). Effect of thymectomy in adult mice on
immunological responsiveness. Nature 208:1337-1338.
Miller RA (1984). Age-associated decline in precursor
frequency for different T cell-mediated reactions, with
preservation of helper or cytotoxic effect per precursor
cell. J. Immunol. 132:63-68.
Miller RA (1988). The cell biology of aging:
immunological models. J. Gerontology, in press.
Miller, RA, Philosophe B, Ginis I, Weil G, Jacobson B.
(1988). Defective control of cytoplasmic calcium
concentration in T lymphocytes from old mice. J.
Cellular Physiol., in press.
Miller RA, Jacobson B, Weil G, Simons ER (1987).
Diminished calcium influx in lectin-stimulated T cells
from old mice. J. Cell. Physiol. 132:337-342.
Nordin AA, Collins GD (1983). Limiting dilution analysis
of alloreactive cytotoxic precursor cells in aging mice.
J. Immunol. 131:2215-2218.
Proust JJ, Filburn CR, Harrison SA, Buchholz MA, Nordin AA
(1987). Age-related defect in signal transduction
during lectin activation of murine T lymphocytes. J.
Immunol. 139:1472-1478.
Rocha B, Freitas AA, Coutinho AA (1983). Population
dynamics of T lymphocytes. Renewal rate and expansion

in the peripheral lymphoid organs. J. Immunol. 131:2158-2163.

Rocha BB (1987). Population kinetics of precursors of IL 2-producing peripheral T lymphocytes: evidence for short life expectancy, continuous renewal, and post-thymic expansion. J. Immunol. 139:365-372.

Sanders ME, Makgoba MW, Sharrow SO, Stephany D, Springer TA, Young HA, Shaw S (1988). Human memory T lymphocytes express increased levels of three cell adhesion molecules (LFA-3, CD2, and LFA-1) and three other molecules (UCHL1, CDw29, and Pgp-1) and have enhanced IFN-gamma production. J. Immunol. 140:1401-1407.

Scollay RG, Butcher EC, Weissman IL (1980). Thymus cell migration. Quantitative aspects of cellular traffic from the thymus to the periphery in mice. Eur. J. Immunol. 10:210-218.

Simpson E, Cantor H (19). Regulation of the immune response by subclasses of T lymphocytes. II. The effect of adult thymectomy upon humoral and cellular responses in mice. Eur. J. Immunol. 5:337-343.

Sprent J (1977). Migration and lifespan of lymphocytes. In Loor F, Roelants GE (eds): "B and T Cells in Immune Recognition," New York: John Wiley, pp. 59-82.

Staiano-Coico L, Darzynkiewicz Z, Melamed MR, Weksler ME (1984). Immunological studies of aging. IX. Impaired proliferation of T lymphocytes detected in elderly humans by flow cytometry. J. Immunol. 132:1788-1792.

Taylor RB (1965). Decay of immunological responsiveness after thymectomy in adult life. Nature 208:1334-1335.

Trowbridge IS, Lesley J, Schulte R, Hyman R, Trotter J (1982). Biochemical characterization and cellular distribution of a polymorphic, murine cell-surface glycoprotein expressed on lymphoid tissues. Immunogenetics 15:299-312.

Vie H, Miller RA (1986). Decline, with age, in the proportion of mouse T cells that express IL-2 receptors after mitogen stimulation. Mech. Ageing and Dev. 33:313-322.

The Maillard Reaction in Aging,
Diabetes, and Nutrition, pages 259–275
© 1989 Alan R. Liss, Inc.

"AUTOXIDATIVE GLYCOSYLATION": FREE RADICALS AND GLYCATION
THEORY

Simon P. Wolff, Zainab A. Bascal and James V. Hunt

Toxicology Laboratory,
University College London,
5 University St.,
LONDON WC1E 6JJ, UK

ABSTRACT   Studies have shown that
glycation in vitro is complicated by the
ability of glucose to oxidise, in the presence
of trace amounts of transition metal, generating
protein-reactive ketoaldehydes, hydrogen
peroxide and diverse free radicals. Protein
exposed to glucose undergoes fragmentational and
conformational alterations, and these, as well
as thiol oxidation, appear to be caused by
hydroxyl radicals. Glycofluorophore formation is
dependent upon ketoaldehyde formation. It is
suggested that glucose autoxidation contributes
to oxidative stress in pathophysiology
associated with diabetes and ageing via this
newly described process of "autoxidative
glycosylation".

INTRODUCTION

Protein Glycation: Relevance to Diabetes and Ageing

Protein glycation, a factor possibly contributing to
tissue damage in diabetes mellitus and ageing, has been
extensively modelled by the exposure of protein to glucose
for extended periods in vitro [Cerami, 1986]. This
treatment often results in substantial alterations in
protein structure and function, changes which are generally

presumed to result from the covalent attachment of the glucose to protein lysyl, and other, amino groups [Harding, 1985]. Amadori products, first described from a food and sugar chemical viewpoint, are believed to be the primary glycation adducts formed, but later rearrange and undergo dehydrational reactions to form the so-called advanced glycosylation adducts [Pongor et al., 1984]. These contribute to the generation of new chromo- and fluorophores on the protein, and stimulate protein crosslinking reactions [Eble et al., 1983; Ahmed et al., 1986]. These reactions are believed to be of pathophysiological significance in that long-lived and low-turnover proteins such as collagen tend to be increasingly "browned" with age, and more so in diabetic individuals, particularly those with secondary disease [Monnier et al.; Brownlee et al., 1988].

Glucose Autoxidation

It appears to be assumed that the covalent attachment of glucose to amino groups via the Amadori pathway, and subsequent rearrangement and dehydration reactions, during such glycation studies, are sufficient to account for the structural changes observed [Cerami, 1986; Pongor et al., 1984; Harding, 1985]. Glucose, however, in common with other α-hydroxyaldehydes [Wolff et al., 1984], is prone to transition metal-catalysed oxidation (via its enediol) generating hydrogen peroxide, reactive intermediates, such as the hydroxyl radical, as well as ketoaldehydes [Wolff and Dean, 1987a]. Oxidative chemistry of glucose could well contribute to macromolecular alterations associated with experimental glycation.

Autoxidation-Derived Ketoaldehydes and Protein Glycation

It has been shown previously, consistent with this possibility, that the ketoaldehyde products of glucose autoxidation contribute substantially to total monosaccharide covalently attaching to protein during the exposure of protein to glucose in vitro [Wolff and Dean, 1987a;b]. Glucose autoxidation is slow, but the amounts of ketoaldehyde formed over the typical time courses of glycation studies are in the range consistent with some contribution to total protein-attached monosaccharide and also contribute to chromo- and fluorophoric alterations [Wolff and Dean, 1987a;b; Wolff and Dean, 1988]. This suggests a role for transition metal-catalysed enediol oxidation in tissue damage associated with age and diabetes [Wolff et al., 1987].

RESULTS

Glucose Induced Protein Fragmentation and Benzoate Hydroxylation

The glucose-induced fragmentation of ^{14}C-radiomethylated bovine serum albumin, (assessed by the release of radiolabel into a trichloracetic acid-soluble fraction [Hunt et al., 1988]), and the corresponding hydroxylation of benzoate [Gutteridge, 1987] during exposure to glucose, under various conditions, are illustrated in Figure 1. The addition of Cu^{2+} ions, which form oxidising/hydroxylating agents in the presence of hydrogen peroxide, stimulated these processes (by 1.8 and 4.6-fold respectively), whereas DETAPAC, which sequesters the trace amounts of transition metal necessary for glucose enediol oxidation [Wolff and Dean, 1987a;b], inhibited them (by 90.4% and 96.8%, respectively). The polyhydric alcohol, sorbitol, considered a selective hydroxyl radical scavenger similarly inhibited benzoate hydroxylation and protein cleavage (96% and 75.3%).

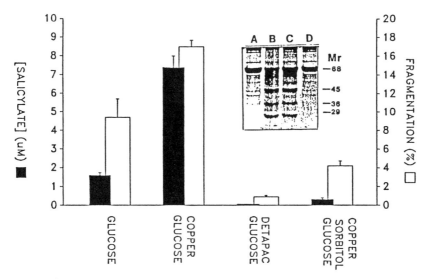

FIGURE 1

Glucose induces protein fragmentation which correlates with
its ability to hydroxylate benzoate, under various
conditions.

^{14}C-radiomethylated BSA (1mg/ml) or benzoate (1mM) were
incubated with 25mM glucose alone, or in the presence of
100uM Cu^{2+}, 1mM DETAPAC or 250mM sorbitol together with
100uM Cu^{2+} in 100mM potassium phosphate buffer, pH 7.4, for
8 days at 37°C. The hydroxylation of benzoate by glucose
was measured by fluorescence (308nm excitation; 410nm
emission), using a salicylate standard [Gutteridge, 1987]
and appropriate controls. SDS PAGE of albumin (1mg/ml)
exposed to glucose under analogous conditions was performed
as described previously [Hunt et al., 1988]. Track A:
Control-incubated albumin; B: Cu^{2+} (100uM), glucose (25mM);
albumin; C: glucose, albumin; D: glucose, DETAPAC (1mM),
albumin. Reprinted with permission from Hunt et al.,1988b.

Confirmation of Fragmentation by SDS PAGE and the Effect of Other Monosaccharides

SDS PAGE analysis of albumin exposed to glucose under similar conditions (Figure 1;inset) confirmed that true fragmentation occurred and produced a limited fragmentation pattern strongly reminiscent of the normoxic exposure of albumin to hydroxyl radicals generated by the gamma-radiolysis of water [Dean et al., 1986], or peroxide in the presence of Cu^{2+} [Hunt et al., 1988]. Fragmentation of protein was produced by glucose in the presence and absence of added Cu^{2+} (Figure 1; inset, Tracks B and C respectively) but was inhibited by DETAPAC in both cases (Track D).

Hydroxyl Radicals and Protein Fragmentation

The role of oxidising agents in protein structural change induced by glucose was further investigated in competition experiments using benzoic acid and deoxyribose (which reacts with the hydroxyl radical to form malonaldehyde [Halliwell and Gutteridge, 1981]) as hydroxyl radical scavenger/detectors (Figure 2). Both agents inhibited protein fragmentation (by 53.5% and 35.3% respectively, at 1mM;Figure 2) and this protection was associated with simultaneous hydroxylation of the benzoate and oxidation of deoxyribose to malonaldehyde (Figure 2;insets a and b). Given that the hydroxyl radical scavenger sorbitol was a potent inhibitor of glucose-induced protein fragmentation (Figure 1) it can be concluded that the hydroxyl radical (or a similarly reactive hydroxylating/oxidising species [Rush and Koppenol, 1987]) is responsible for a substantial part of the structural damage experienced by protein exposed to glucose in vitro. The contribution of superoxide radical production to protein structural change induced by exposure to glucose can, in contrast, be ignored since superoxide ($O_2 \cdot^-$), and its conjugate acid the hydroperoxyl radical ($HO_2 \cdot$) react poorly with protein [Wolff and Dean, 1986;Dean et al., 1986].

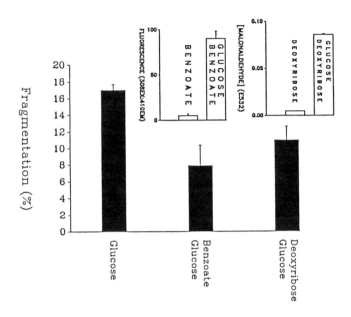

FIGURE 2

Hydroxyl radical scavenger/detectors protect against glucose-induced fragmentation and reveal hydroxyl radical formation.

Fragmentation by 25mM glucose in the presence of 100uM Cu^{2+} was assessed using radiomethylated albumin (1mg/ml). Benzoate and deoxyribose were added at a concentration of 1mM. Fluorescence of benzoate hydroxylation products (Inset A) was assessed after precipitation of protein with TCA and retitration to pH 7.2 using concentrated potassium phosphate buffer. Malonaldehyde formed as a result of deoxyribose oxidation was estimated by incubation of a 5% TCA-treated reaction aliquot with an equal volume of 50mM thiobarbituric acid (TBA) for 30 minutes at 100°C. Reprinted with permission from Hunt et al, 1988b.

The Role of Hydrogen Peroxide and "Site-Specific Radical Attack"

The role of hydrogen peroxide in the generation of the fragmenting agent could be demonstrated by the inhibitory effect of catalase (Figure 3).

CATALASE INHIBITS PROTEIN FRAGMENTATION

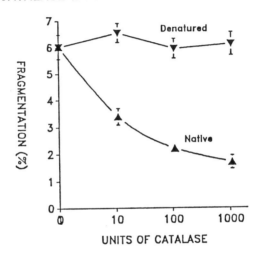

FIGURE 3

Catalase protects against glucose-induced protein degradation.

1mg/ml radiomethylated albumin was incubated with 25 mM glucose and 100uM Cu^{2+} in the presence of catalase (Sigma; 11000 units/mg) over a 3 day period. Denatured catalase was prepared by incubation of the protein at $100^{o}C$ for 15 minutes. Reprinted with permission from Hunt et al, 1988b.

Increasing concentrations of catalase produced increasing extents of inhibition of fragmentation, which approached a maximum of circa 75% (72.2% at 1100u/ml, relative to a heat-inactivated control), comparable to the 75.3% inhibition of fragmentation shown by sorbitol, at a 2 x 10^5-fold excess (Figure 1). This absence of total inhibition may be explained in the context of "site-specific radical attack" [Czapski, 1978] in which antioxidants cannot interrupt the local attack of oxidants at the site in which they are generated; for example, in the case of hydroxyl radicals produced by the reaction of hydrogen peroxide with transition metal at protein surfaces [Gutteridge and Wilkins, 1983]. A maximal inhibition of considerably less than 100% for a radical-mediated biological reaction is thus not unexpected. In contrast, the possibility that protein fragmentation occurs by peptide hydrolysis, or some other non-oxidative autolytic mechanism, subsequent to the covalent attachment of monosaccharide to amino groups, is not consistent with the observation that sorbitol, deoxyribose and benzoate significantly inhibited fragmentation (Figures 1 & 2) whilst having an insignificant effect on the incorporation of monosaccharide into protein (Table 1). Structural change induced by the exposure of protein to glucose can thus be dissociated from the incorporation of monosaccharide into protein per se.

MODIFIERS OF FRAGMENTATION: EFFECTS ON GLYCATION?

COVALENT ATTACHMENT
(Moles Monosaccharide/Mole Protein)

Control	6.24 ± 0.33
Sorbitol	5.95 ± 0.45
Benzoate	5.75 ± 0.66
Deoxyribose	5.81 ± 0.39
DETAPAC	4.43 ± 0.30

(n = 4)

TABLE 1

Incorporation of monosaccharide into protein

The incorporation of label from D-[U-^{14}C]-glucose into protein (1mg/ml), after 8 days of incubation in 100mM potassium phosphate buffer at 37°C was measured as described previously [Wolff and Dean, 1987a]. The concentrations of agents used to attempt to modify the incorporation of monosaccharide into protein, were 1mM for deoxyribose, benzoate and DETAPAC. The final concentration of glucose was 25mM, containing 2.5 uCi D-[U-^{14}C]-Glucose/ml.

Monosaccharide Oxidation and Glycofluorophore Development; The Role of Transition metal

The effect of agents modifying protein fragmentation by glucose upon the development of novel fluorophores (Figure 4) was particularly revealing and strengthened the hypothesis that autoxidation-derived ketoaldehydes contribute to "glycofluorophore" development [Wolff and Dean, 1987a;b]. DETAPAC inhibited ketoaldehyde formation, chromophore and glycofluorophore production to an extent observed previously [Wolff and Dean, 1987a;b], confirming that autoxidation-derived ketoaldehydes play a role in glycofluorophore development.

FLUORESCENCE AND KETOALDEHYDE FORMATION

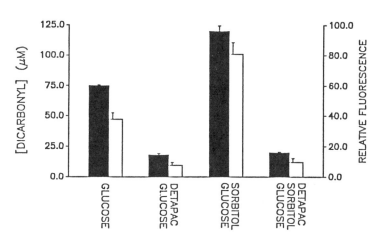

FIGURE 4

Glycofluorophores and Ketoaldehyde Formation

Ribonuclease (10mgs/ml) was exposed to glucose (25mM) in the presence of sorbitol (250mM) and/or DETAPAC (1mM) for 12 days. Ketoaldehydes were measured using the Girard-T reagent as described previously [Wolff and Dean, 1987a] after 5% TCA-precipitation of protein. "Glycofluorophores" (novel fluorophores formed as result of the exposure of protein to glucose) were measured using excitation at 350nm and emission at 415 nm [Wolff and Dean, 1987a].

Sorbitol Oxidation: Dissociation of Protein Damage from Glycofluorophore Development

Sorbitol, in contrast, substantially increased ketoaldehyde and glycofluorophore formation (Figure 4). This was a surprising result and we speculated that sorbitol, when reacting with hydroxyl radicals produced by glucose autoxidation, could generate open-chain α-hydroxyaldehydes (subsequent to HO_2. elimination from α-hydroxyalkylperoxyl radicals [Bothe et al., 1978]), which were subject to facile autoxidation, generating further ketoaldehydes. Sorbitol was thus exposed to hydroxyl radicals (generated by the gamma-radiolysis of water) and incubated under analogous conditions to those used for the study described in Figure 4. Table 2 shows that sorbitol subjected to attack by hydroxyl radicals is indeed prone to ketoaldehyde formation, compared with non-irradiated sorbitol. The ketoaldehydes generated by the autoxidation of sorbitol oxidation products contribute to glycofluorophore development.

SORBITOL AUTOXIDATION POST HYDROXYL RADICAL ATTACK

[KETOALDEHYDE] (μM)

	Pre—Incubation	Post—Incubation
Control Sorbitol	0.0	0.0
Irradiated Sorbitol	1.2	26.3

TABLE 2

(C.O.V. = 5%)

Generation of ketoaldehydes from hydroxyl radical oxidised sorbitol

100mM sorbitol was exposed (in deionised water) to 100nmoles/ml of hydroxyl radical generated by the gamma-radiolysis of water in the 2000Ci ^{60}Co source at Brunel (described previously [Wolff and Dean, 1986]), diluted with an equal volume of 100mM potassium phosphate buffer, pH 7.4 and incubated at 37°C for 3 days. The content of ketoaldehydes in the irradiated and incubated sample was then assessed using the Girard T reagent as described previously, using non-irradiated, or non-incubated samples as comparisons. Reprinted with permission from Hunt et al, 1988b.

The result with sorbitol also indicates that glycofluorophore formation cannot be simply equated with structural damage when protein is exposed to high levels of monosaccharide, but is dependent upon the chemistry of other components in the system since sorbitol inhibits protein fragmentation (Figure 1), but stimulates glycofluorophore development (Figure 4). This observation may be of relevance to studies of tissue fluorescence in human diabetes [Monnier et al., 1986], although we do not wish to suggest that sorbitol acts as an antioxidant in vivo.

Profound Inhibition of Crystallin Glycation by Chelating Agents

DETAPAC, EDTA and N-hydroxyethylethylenediamine-triacetic acid (HEDTA) produced substantial inhibition of crystallin glycation (Figure 5). The extent of inhibition was far in excess (> 80% at day 10) of inhibition observed in the case of albumin (ca. 50%) [Wolff and Dean, 1987a,b]. It is clear that transition metal chelators of appropriate affinity are powerful inhibitors of crystallin glycation. DETAPAC produced an inhibition of ca 50% at only 10uM (Figure 6). Inhibition of glycation was somewhat diminished as the protein concentration was increased (not shown), but the extent of the inhibitory effect, together with the interest in inhibition of glycation in the diabetic complications, suggests that chelating agents might be of some therapeutic potential. Thiol oxidation stimulated by glucose [Stevens et al., 1978], and the role of transition metal in this process was studied indirectly using a simple turbidimetric technique (Figure 6 inset). Glucose is known to stimulate crystallin thiol oxidation in vitro resulting in the formation of high-molecular weight bodies capable of scattering light [Monnier et al., 1979]. DETAPAC inhibited this process greatly [Figure 5;inset]. EDTA, HEDTA, o-phenanthroline and bipyridyl also inhibited the process in rough proportion to their ability to inhibit glycation (not shown).

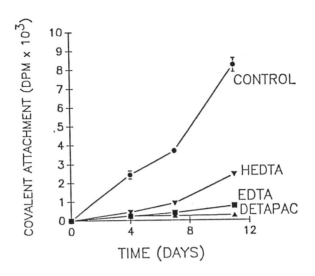

FIGURE 5

Time-Dependence of Inhibition of Crystallin Glycation

Crystallins were exposed to 25mM glucose at a final concentration of 10mgs/ml. The concentration of metal chelating agents was 1mM.

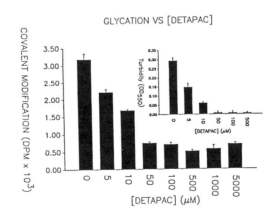

FIGURE 6

Dose-Response for Inhibition of Crystallin Glycation by DETAPAC

Glycation was permitted to proceed as above but for only 48 hours. Inset shows parallel effect of DETAPAC on crystallin aggregation.

DISCUSSION

Protein Fragmentation, Tissue Damage and Glycation

The widespread study of glycation in relation to diabetes and ageing is based on the explicit or implicit assumption that functional and structural alterations resulting from the exposure of macromolecules to hyperglycaemic levels of glucose are caused by the covalent attachment of glucose to protein amino groups, with resultant changes in surface charge, hydrogen bonding capacity, cellular recognition and/or the formation of complex products capable of crosslinking [Cerami, 1986;Pongor et al., 1984; Harding, 1985]. In fact, the incorporation of monosaccharide into protein can be dissociated from structural change associated with the exposure of protein to glucose.

Glucose Autoxidation, Hydroxyl Radical Production and Protein Structural Damage

The structural alterations observed when protein is exposed to glucose appear to be largely dependent upon hydroxyl radicals produced by glucose autoxidation (see Scheme). DETAPAC inhibits protein damage by inhibiting the underlying process of glucose autoxidation, and by inhibiting hydroxyl radical production from hydrogen peroxide, generated as a result of glucose oxidation [Wolff et al., 1984; Wolff and Dean, 1987a;b]. In contrast, sorbitol, benzoate and deoxyribose compete with protein for hydroxyl radicals produced by glucose autoxidation as a result of the reaction of transition metal with hydrogen peroxide, but do not inhibit glucose autoxidation per se. Cu^{2+} stimulates protein structural change by stimulating hydroxyl radical production from accumulated hydrogen peroxide.

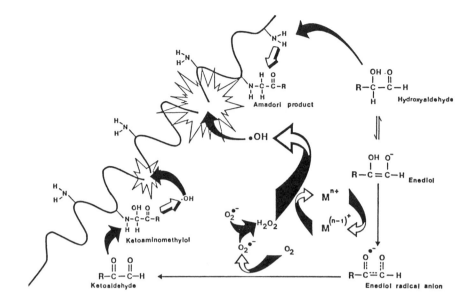

SCHEME

Protein damage by free radicals. The contribution of ketaminomethylol autoxidation to site-directed radical damage is suggested. Reprinted with permission from Hunt et al., 1988b.

Covalent Attachment of Glucose to Ribonuclease and Crystallin

Using ribonuclease and crystallins, it has been observed that the contribution of glucose autoxidation to covalent modification is very substantial. A maximal inhibition of monosaccharide attachment of only 45% was achievable with BSA using DETAPAC [Wolff and Dean, 1987a]. In the case of BSA, it was considered that the maximum achievable inhibition of 45% was indicative of two routes of attachment: that occurring via the autoxidative pathway, and that proceeding via the conventional, Amadori route [Wolff and Dean, 1987a,b]. In addition, we speculated that the ability of BSA to bind Cu^{2+} [Halliwell, 1988] could be a complicating factor preventing the complete removal, by extrinsic chelating agents, of transition metal able to catalyse autoxidation. With ribonuclease and crystallins, however, inhibition of attachment of greater than 80% was observed. These data indicate that the vast majority of monosaccharide may, in fact, attach in a transition metal-dependent manner; in the case of proteins which do not possess high-affinity Cu^{2+}-binding sites. This suggests that autoxidative glycosylation may be a dominant process in glycation; at least in vitro.

Glycation Studies Suggest Antioxidant Therapy

The possibility of autoxidative glycosylation and associated free radical and peroxide production have to be considered in any circumstance in which biological structures are exposed to elevated levels of monosaccharide. If experimental glycation studies are an appropriate model for the sequelae of diabetes and ageing, then monosaccharide autoxidation and inappropriate oxidation must play a role in their pathophysiology, consistent with the evidence for increased oxidative stress in these circumstances [Wolff, 1987]. This would seem to provide further support for the potential of agents which minimize biological autoxidative processes and their consequences in the therapy of non-malignant diseases associated with diabetes mellitus and ageing [Wolff, 1987].

ACKNOWLEDGEMENTS

We thank the Juvenile Diabetes Foundation International, The Medical Research Council and the Sir Jules Thorn Trust for financial support, Alison Woollard for artwork and Lyn Robinson for computational assistance.

REFERENCES
Ahmed, M.U., Thorpe, S.R. and Baynes, J.W. (1986) Identification of N-carboxymethyllysine as a degradation product of fructoselysine in glycated protein. J. Biol. Chem. 261, 4889-4894
Bascal, Z.A. and Wolff, S.P. (1988) Glucose autoxidation, crystallin glycation, transition metals and cataract. (submitted to Biochem. J.)
Beswick, H.T and Harding, J.J. (1984) Conformational changes induced in bovine lens alpha-crystallin by carbamylation. Biochem. J. 223, 221-227
Beswick, H.T. and Harding, J.J. (1987) Conformational changes induced in lens alpha- and gamma-crystallin by modification with glucose-6-phosphate. Biochem. J. 246, 761-769

Bothe, E., Schuchmann, M.N., Schulte-Frohlinde, D. and von Sonntag, C. (1978) HO_2. elimination from alpha-hydroxyalkylperoxyl radicals in aqueous solution. Photochem. Photobiol. 28, 639-644

Brownlee, M., Vlassara, H. and Cerami, A. (1984) Non-enzymatic glycosylation and the pathogenesis of diabetic complications. Ann. Int. Med. 101, 527-537

Brownlee, M., Cerami, A. and Vlassara, H. (1988) Advanced glycosylation end products in tissue and the biochemical basis of diabetic complications. New Engl. J. Med. 318, 1315-1321

Cerami, A. (1986) Aging of proteins and nucleic acids. What is the role of glucose? Trends Bio. Sci. 11, 311-314

Czapski, G. (1978) On the generation of the hydroxylation agent from superoxide radical: can the Haber Weiss reaction be the source of hydroxyl radicals? Photochem. Photobiol. 28, 651-653

Dean, R.T., Thomas, S.M., Vince, G. and Wolff, S.P. (1986) Oxidation-induced proteolysis and its restriction by some secondary protein modifications. Biomed. Biochim. Acta 45, 11-21

Eble, A.S., Thorpe, S.R. and Baynes, J.W. (1983) Non-enzymatic glycosylation and glucose-dependent cross-linking of protein. J. Biol. Chem. 258, 9406-9412

Gutteridge, J.M.C. (1987) Ferrous salt promoted damage to deoxyribose and benzoate. Biochem. J. 243, 709-714

Gutteridge, J.M.C. and Wilkins, S. (1983) Copper salt dependent hydroxyl radical formation. Biochim. Biophys. Acta 759, 38-41

Halliwell, B. (1988) Albumin: an important extracellular antioxidant. Biochem. Pharm. 37, 569-571

Harding, J.J. (1985) Post-translational covalent modification of protein. Adv. Prot. Chem. 37, 247-334

Harman, D. (1981) The ageing process. Proc. Natl. Acad. Sci. 78, 7124-7128

Hunt, J.V., Simpson, J.A. and Dean, R.T. (1988a) Hydroperoxide-mediated protein fragmentation. Biochem. J. 250, 87-93

Hunt, J.V., Dean, R.T. and Wolff, S.P. (1988b) Hydroxyl radical production and autoxidative glycosylation. Biochem J 256:205-212.

Monnier, V.M., Stevens, V.J. and Cerami, A. (1979) Non-enzymatic glycosylation, sulfhydryl oxidation, and aggregation of lens proteins in experimental sugar cataract. J. Exp. Med. 150, 1098-1107

Monnier, V.M., Vishwanath, V., Frank, K.E., Elmets, C.A., Dauchot, P. and Kohn, R.R. (1986) Collagen-linked fluorescence is associated with increased complications in Type I diabetes mellitus. N. Engl. J. Med. 314, 403-408

Pongor, S., Ulrich, P.C., Bencsath, F.A. and Cerami, A. (1984) Aging of proteins isolation and identification of a fluorescent chromophore from the reaction of polypeptides with glucose.Proc. Natl. Acad. Sci. 81, 2684-2688

Rush, J.D. and Koppenol, W.H. (1987) The reaction between ferrous polyaminocarboxylate complexes and hydrogen peroxide: an investigation by stopped flow spectrophotometry. J. Inorg. Biochem. 29, 199-215

Stevens, V.J., Rouzer, C.A., Monnier, V.M. and Cerami, A. (1978) Diabetic cataract formation: potential role fo glycosylation of lens crystallins. Proc. Natl. Acad. Sci. USA 75, 2918-2922

Wolff, S.P. (1987) The potential role of oxidative stress in diabtes and its complications: novel implications for theory and therapy. In "Diabetic Complications" (Ed. M.J.C.Crabbe) pp 167-220 Churchill-Livingstone, Edinburgh

Wolff, S.P. and Dean, R.T. (1986) Fragmentation of proteins by free radicals and its effect on their susceptibility to enzymatic hydrolysis. Biochem. J. 234, 399-403

Wolff, S.P. and Dean, R.T. (1987a) Glucose autoxidation and protein modification: the potential role of "autoxidative glycosylation" in diabetes mellitus. Biochem. J. 245, 243- 250

Wolff, S.P. and Dean, R.T. (1987b) Monosaccharide autoxidation: a potential source of oxidative stress in diabetes? Model reactions with nucleotides and protein. Bioelectrochem. Bioenerg. 18, 283-293

Wolff, S.P. and Dean, R.T. (1988) Aldehydes and dicarbonyls in the non-enzymatic glycosylation of proteins. Biochem. J. 249, 617-619

Wolff, S.P., Crabbe, M.J.C. and Thornalley, P.J. (1984) The autoxidation of simple monosaccharides. Experientia 40, 244-246

Wolff, S.P., Garner, A. and Dean, R.T. (1986) Free radicals, lipids, and protein degradation. Trends Biochem. Sci. 11, 27-31

Wolff, S.P., Wang, G-M. and Spector, A. (1987) Pro-oxidant activation of ocular reductants. I. Copper and riboflavin stimulate ascorbate oxidation causing lens epithelial cytotoxicity in vitro. Exp. Eye Res. 45, 777-789

The Maillard Reaction in Aging,
Diabetes, and Nutrition, pages 277–290
© 1989 Alan R. Liss, Inc.

INACTIVATION OF ERYTHROCYTE Cu-Zn-SUPEROXIDE DISMUTASE THROUGH NONENZYMATIC GLYCOSYLATION

Naoyuki Taniguchi [1], Noriaki Kinoshita [1],
Katsura Arai [1], Susumu Iizuka [2], Masamichi
Usui [3] and Takafumi Naito [3]
[1] Department of Biochemistry, Osaka
University Medical School, Nakanoshima,
Osaka 530, Japan, [2] Kucchan Kousei Hospital,
Kucchan 057, Hokkaido, Japan and [3] Department
of Orthopedics, Sapporo Medical College,
Sapporo 010

ABSTRACT. Human erythrocyte
Cu-Zn-superoxide dismutase undergoes
glycation reaction in vitro and in vivo
(Arai et al., 1987a; Arai et al., 1987b).
In addition, an increase in the glycation
of the superoxide dismutase was observed
in aged erythrocytes, indicating that the
glycation reaction is an age-related
change under physiological conditions.
In the cases of crude extracts as well as
pure enzyme preparations obtained from
erythrocytes of patients with Werner's
syndrome, the specific activity of the
glycated form expressed as units per mg
Cu-Zn-superoxide dismutase protein as
determined by both enzymatic assay and
immunoenzymatic assay was significantly
lower and the enzyme was unstable as
compared to the normal form.

INTRODUCTION

Werner's syndrome is an autosomal recessive
condition and is sometimes referred to as adult
progeria (Fleischmajer and Nedwick, 1973; Smith
et al., 1955). The disease is clinically
characterized by accelerated aging and an

increased frequency of malignant tumors. At the
cellular and molecular levels, cultured
fibroblasts have a markedly decreased replicative
life span (Martin, 1970; Goldstein et al., 1975),
and increased proportions of several enzymes in
the fibroblasts have been reported to be
heat-labile (Goldstein and Moerman, 1975;
Holliday and Porterfield, 1975), as found in old
fibroblasts. The etiology of the disease is
unknown, but an involvement of the free radical
scavenging system has been suggested (Nordenson,
1977). An age-related reduction of the Cu-Zn-SOD
has been reported by Reiss and Gershon (1976).

In this study, we recognized that the
erythrocyte Cu-Zn-superoxide dismutase from
Werner's syndrome had a large amount of glycated
form due to glycation at multiple sites and the
properties of the enzyme were found to be
immunochemically active but enzymatically
inactive. Therefore, the specific activity was
much lower than in controls. Moreover, the
enzyme was more unstable at 37°C as compared to
in the controls. These facts suggested that
glycation of the Cu-Zn-superoxide dismutase
occurs remarkably in patients with Werner's
syndrome, irrespective of glycermia, and these
results may provide an insight into the aging
process and of age-related diseases.

EXPERIMENTAL PROCEDURES

MATERIALS--A boronate affinity column (Glyco-Gel
B) was purchased from Pierce. N^{ε}-Glucitol
lysine was synthesized according to the method
described (Garlick and Mazer, 1983).

Blood was obtained from two male patients with
Werner's syndrome, aged 37 and 36 years. The
clinical picture in the patients was
characterized by typical symptoms such as a small
stature, premature baldness and graying of the
hair. One of the patients had diabetes mellitus
(case 1) but the other (case 2) did not.
Erythrocytes were obtained from venous blood (10

ml) of the two patients with Werner's syndrome and of the aged-matched controls.

Purification of Cu-Zn-superoxide dismutase from erythrocytes.--The enzyme was purified from one patient who had no diabetes mellitus according to the method described previously (Arai et al., 1986). Glycated and nonglycated Cu-Zn-superoxide dismutases were separated by boronate affinity (Glyco-Gel B) chromatography as described previously (Arai et al., 1987a).

Assay of Cu-Zn-superoxide dismutase activity and ELISA.--Superoxide dismutase activity was assayed by the method described by Beauchamp and Fridovich (1971) with a Gilford "Response" Spectrophotometer. Protein concentrations were determined according to the method described by Lowry et al. (1951) using bovine serum albumin as the standard. Enzyme-linked immunosorbent assay (ELISA) was performed essentially as the same procedure used for manganese superoxide dismutase as described previously (Iizuka et al., 1984). In brief, fractions of each aliquot (50μl) obtained from a Glyco-Gel B column were diluted with 50 μl of 50 mM $NaHCO_3$, pH 9.6 and the mixture was added to each well of the Microtiter plates. The plates were incubated overnight and washed three times with 50 mM phosphate buffered-saline, pH 7.4 containing 0.05 % Tween 20 and 0.1 % bovine serum albumin (washing buffer). The remaining protein-binding sites were blocked with 100 μl of 10 mM Tris-HCl buffer, pH 8.0 containing 1% bovine serum albumin for 1 hr at 4°C and the wells were treated thoroughly with the washing buffer. Fifty μl of goat anti-human Cu-Zn-superoxide dismutase IgG solution (15 μg/ml) in washing buffer was added to the antigen-coated well. After incubation 3 hr at 37°C, unbound antibody was removed by being washed three times with the washing buffer. To each well was then added 50 μl of rabbit anti-goat IgG-horseradish peroxidase conjugate that had been diluted 1:1,000 with the washing buffer. After 3 hr at 37°C, unbound second antibody was removed and the wells were washed six times with the same buffer. The peroxidase activity was detected with a freshly made solution of 30 mg of o-phenylenediamine in 50 ml of 0.1 M citrate buffer, pH 5.0 mixed with 0.003% H_2O_2. The purified human erythrocyte Cu-Zn-superoxide dismutase (Iizuka et al., 1984) was used as the standard. The glycated Cu-Zn-SOD was detected by the thiobarbituric acid method (Flückiger and Winterhalter, 1976).

Thermostability experiments.--In an experiment on the enzyme stability test, approximately 0.25 mg of the purified superoxide dismutase from one the patients with Werner's syndrome was dissolved in 100 mM potassium phosphate buffer, pH 7.2, followed by incubation at 37°C for 60 hr under sterile conditions. The same amounts of the enzymes purified from the normal healthy controls were used as controls. Ten µl aliquots were taken every 12 hr and used for assaying of the enzyme activity.

Isolation of glycated peptides.--Tryptic peptides derived from the glycated enzyme was isolated by high performance liquid chromatography on a C18 reverse phase column as described previously (Arai et al., 1987b). The peptides were detected on the basis of the absorbance at 215 nm. The peaks of peptides were collected and then subjected to amino acid analysis.

Amino acid analysis.--Glucitol-lysine in the superoxide dismutase was identified by the hydrolysis in 6 N HCl in the presence of sodium borohydride in sealed tubes under vacuum at 110°c for 24 h with a Hitachi-835 amino acid analyzer.

RESULTS

Nonglycated and glycated erythrocyte Cu-Zn-superoxide dismutases from a non-diabetic patient with Werner's syndrome.

As shown in Fig. 1, nonglycated and glycated forms of the crude enzyme extract from erythrocytes of a non-diabetic patient with Werner's syndrome were clearly separated on a boronate affinity column as judged by assaying the enzyme activity as well as thiobarbituric acid reaction, and we found that the enzyme activity of the glycated forms which bound to the column was very low. However, the amount of immunoreactive Cu-Zn-superoxide dismutase as determined by ELISA was significantly high. This indicates that the specific activity of the glycated form as expressed as units/mg of Cu-Zn-superoxide dismutase was found to be very low as compared to that of the nonglycated form. This suggests that the glycated forms in the erythrocytes of the patient were immunoreactive but enzymatically low active.

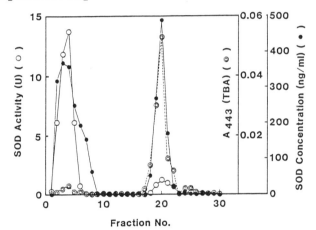

Figure 1. Separation of the glycated and nonglycated Cu-Zn-superoxide dismutases from crude extracts of erythrocytes of a patient with Werner's syndrome. Crude extracts from erythrocytes of a patient with Werner's syndrome were subjected to a column (0.8 X 5 cm) of Glyco-Gel B which had been equilibrated with 0.25 M ammonium acetate, pH 8.5 containing 0.01 M MgCl₂, and washed with 5 volumes of the starting buffer. Elution was started at the point indicated by an arrow, using 0.1 M sodium acetate

buffer, pH 5.5. Fractions of 1 ml each were
assayed for superoxide dismutase activity, the
thiobarbituric acid reaction and immunoreactive
superoxide dismutase by ELISA.

Low active forms of Cu-Zn-superoxide dismutase in the Werner's syndrome.

The erythrocyte Cu-Zn-superoxide dismutases
purified from two patients with diabetic (case 1)
and non-diabetic (case 2) Werner's syndrome were
separately loaded on the boronate affinity
column. A typical elution pattern is shown in
Fig. 2. The enzymes which had been purified from
the normal control and a patient (case 2) were
separated into two peaks. Twenty μl aliquots of
each fraction was used for the determination of
enzyme activity and protein concentration, and
100 μl aliquots were used for the thiobarbituric
acid reaction.

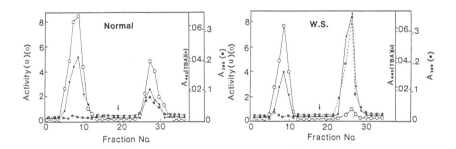

Figure 2. Separation of the glycated and
nonglycated Cu-Zn-superoxide dismutases purified
from erythrocytes of a normal healthy control
(Normal) and a patient with Werner's syndrome
(W.S.). The purified enzymes were applied to a
column (1 x 7 cm) of Glyco-Gel B which had been
equilibrated with the buffer as described under
"EXPERIMENTAL PROCEDURES", and washed with 5
volumes of the starting buffer. Elution was

started at the point indicated by an arrow, using
0.1 M sodium acetate buffer, pH 8.5 containing
0.1 M sorbitol.
Fractions of 2 ml each were assayed for
protein, superoxide dismutase activity and the
thiobarbituric acid reaction as described under
"EXPERIMENTAL PROCEDURES".

The specific activity of the nonglycated
fraction, which passed through the boronate
column was almost the same as that previously
reported from our laboratory (Arai et al.,
1987a). On the other hand, the enzyme activity
of the glycated form, which bound to the boronate
commn in both diabetic and nondiabetic patients
with Werner's syndrome was found to be very low.

From these results we could conclude that
the superoxide dismutase in patients with
Werner's syndrome underwent the glycation
reaction as that in normal controls did.
However, the amount of the inactive form
corresponding to the glycated form was remarkably
increased as compared to in controls.
Furthermore, the amount of the thiobarbituric
acid reactive product of the glycated enzyme in
Werner's syndrome was significantly increased as
compared to in the normal controls (Figures 1 and
2). This also supports that the amount of the
glycated form of Cu-Zn-superoxide dismutase in
Werner's syndrome was increased and that the
specific activity was very low.

Specific activity of the glycated forms of the
normal control and Werner's syndrome cases.
Table 1 shows the summarized data for the
specific activities of nonglycated and glycated
forms of Cu-Zn-superoxide dismutase. The
specific activity of the nonglycated form of the
superoxide dismutase from the normal control and
the Werner's syndrome cases were comparable. On
the other hand the specific activity of the
glycated form of the patients with Werner's

syndrome was found to be extremely low and less than 10% that of the normal healthy control.

Table 1. The specific activities of the glycated and nonglycated Cu-Zn-superoxide dismutases as determined on a Glyco-Gel B column.

Subject	Specific activity (units/mg protein)	
	Nonglycated form	Glycated form
Normal controls (8)	11,900 ± 1272	8,200 ± 1551
Werner's syndrome		
case 1	14,100	620
case 2	11,100	590

The nonglycated and glycated forms denote the fractions which passed through and bound to the Glyco-Gel B column, respectively. The specific activities of the glycated and nonglycated forms were determined by determining the total enzyme activity recovered in each fraction. The values represent the mean ± S.E.. The numbers in parentheses indicate the numbers of samples. p <0.001 (Student's t-test)

Peptide mapping and amino acid analysis of the purified enzyme.
        Our previous study indicated that glycation of Cu-Zn-superoxide dismutase led to gradual inactivation of the enzyme due mainly to the glycation of Lys 122 and Lys 128 through a Schiff base adduct between ε-lysine residues and glucose (Arai et al., 1987b). In order to confirm the glycation reaction in the Cu-Zn-superoxide dismutase of non-diabetic Werner's syndrome (case 2), peptide mapping analysis and amino acid analysis were carried out. As shown in Fig. 3, the tryptic peptide mapping pattern of normal blood was found to be

different from that of normal erythrocytes as
described (Arai et al., 1987b). Each peak was
collected and subjected to amino acid analysis.

Glycated sites and the amino acid anlaysis.

In our previous study on in vitro glycation
of Cu-Zn-superoxide dismutasewe we found that
major in vitro glycated sites are Lys 3, Lys 9,
Lys 30, Lys 36, Lys 122 and Lys 128. Among them
Lys 122 and Lys 128 are supposed to be a major
glycated sites and the glycation of these sites
are considered to be major role in the
inactivation of Cu-Zn-superoxide dismutase. In
the present study on the peptide mapping analysis
and amino acid analysis of the glycated enzymes,
several peaks corresponded to glycated peptides
as reported previously (Arai et al., 1987b), were
also found in normal and Werner's syndrome cases.
In each major peak a small amount of the glucitol
lysine was identified in each peptide (data not
shown). In the Werner's syndrome case, however
there was a peak which is deleted in the normal
control case (see Fig. 3 indicated by an arrow.)
This peak was subjected to amino acid analysis
and found to have a large amount of
glucitol-lysine (Fig. 4).

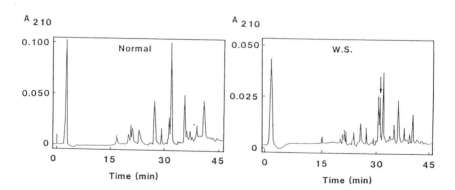

Figure 3. Peptide mapping analysis of
TPCK-trypsin digested peptides.
The glycated peptides were separated by HPLC as
described under "EXPERIMENTAL PROCEDURES". The

eluent was monitored for peptide by absorbance at
215 nm. Each fraction was pooled and subjected
to amino acid analysis. Normal, a peptide
mapping of Cu-Zn-superoxide dismutase from normal
healthy control; W.S, a peptide mapping of
Cu-Zn-superoxide dismutase from a patient with
Werner's syndrome.
An <u>arrow</u> indicates the peptide which is subjected
to amino acid analysis as shown in Fig. 4.

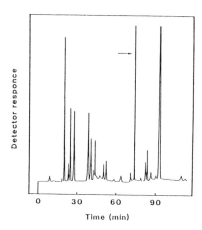

Figure 4. Demonstration of glucitol-lysine in
the TPCK-trypsin treated peptide of
Cu-Zn-superoxide dismutase from a patient with
Werner's syndrome. A pooled fraction as
indicated by an <u>arrow</u> in the Fig. 3 was subjected
to amino acid analysis. A peak indicated by an
<u>arrow</u> was identifed as glucitol-lysine. The
peptide was found to correspond to residues 1-13
as judged by the amino acid composition. This
indicated that major glycated sites are Lys 3 and
Lys 9. The glucitol-lysine was also found in the
Lys 122 and Lys 128 as was observed in the <u>in</u>
<u>vitro</u> glycated sites by our previous study (Arai
et al., 1987b).

Thermostability of the enzyme

Holliday and Porterfield (1974) reported that heat-labile glucose 6-phosphate dehydrogenase was present in cultured skin fibroblasts from patients with Werner's syndrome. In the present study, we also found that the superoxide dismutase purified from Werner's syndrome cases is thermo-labile, as shown in Fig. 5.

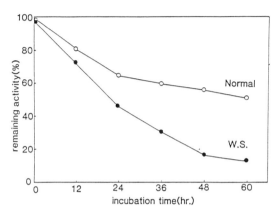

Figure 5. Thermo-stability of the glycated forms of Cu-Zn-superoxide dismutase from a normal control and a Werner's syndrome case. After treatment of the superoxide dismutases from a normal healthy control (Normal) and a Werner's syndrome case 2 (W.S.) at 37°C for various times, the remaining activities were determined as described under "EXPERIMENTAL PROCEDURES".

DISCUSSION

It is still unknown that the mechanism by which increased glycation of Cu-Zn-superoxide dismutase occurs in Werner's syndrome, irrespective of the presence of hyperglycemia. There are several factors influencing extent of glycation in vivo. Cohen (1986) described that those factors are 1) degree and duration of hyperglycemia, 2) half-life of the protein in the circulation or in tissue, 3) permeability of tissue to free glucose, 4) number of free amino

groups and 5) accessibility and pK of the amino
groups within the structure of the protein. In
fact old erythrocytes contain more glycated
hemoglobin (Hb Alc) than do young ones
(Fitsgibbons, 1976) and decreased content of the
Hb Alc was reported in erythrocytes of patients
with hemolytic anemia and a shortened red cell
life span, and erythrocytes of normal subjects
who have sustained an acute blood loss. These
observations suggest that the extent of glycation
reaction is regulated by reduction in the
half-life of a protein or in its residence time
in the circulation even without a correspondent
change in blood glucose levels. In the present
study we found that non-diabetic and diabetic
patients with Werner's syndrome had increased
glycated Cu-Zn-superoxide dismutase with
heat-labile properties. One possible explanation
is that the turnover of the glycated SOD is very
slow in the patients with Werner's syndrome
because of the impairment of degradating process
of glycated proteins.

It has been proposed that the glycation of
an enzyme protein may alter some of its
functions. In the present study we found that
the superoxide dismutase from Werner's syndrome
case was found to be thermolabile. We have found
that the nonenzymatic glucosylation (glycation)
occurs in several lysine residues including Lys
122 and Lys 128 which are located in an active
site liganding loop of the superoxide dismutase
(Arai et al., 1987a). The glycation leads to
gradual inactivation of the enzyme (Arai et al.,
1987a). Glycation is one of the
post-translational protein modification reactions
and is likely to be one of the causes of the
inactivation of the superoxide dismutase in
Werner's syndrome. Moreover, the glycation
reaction is one of the age-related changes of the
protein molecules. Nordensson reported the
increased rate of chromosome damage in vitro in
lymphocytes in Werner's syndrome and the
protection by exogeneously added superoxide
dismutase and catalase (Nordenson, 1977). The

question of whether or not this phenomenon can be explained by the glycation reaction requires further study for an answer. However, the process of degradation of the glycated enzyme, involving Amadori rearrangement in the molecule, might be different.

Acknowledgements

*This work was supported in part by a Grant-in Aid for Cancer Research from Ministry of Education, Science and Culture, Japan., and by the following foundations: Mochida Mutural Life Foundation, Takeda Medical Research Foundation, Health Sciecne Foundation and Chiba-Geigy Foundation for the Promotion of Science.

REFERENCES

Arai K, Iizuka S, Makita A, Oikawa K, Taniguchi N (1986). Purification of Cu-Zn-superoxide dismutase from human erythrocytes by immunoaffinity chromatographgy: Evidence for the presence of isoelectric heterogeneity. J Immunol Methods 91: 139-143.
Arai K, Iizuka S, Oikawa K, Taniguchi N (1987a). Increase in the glucosylated form of erythrocyte Cu-Zn-superoxide dismutase in diabetes and close association of the nonenzymatic glucosylation with the enzyme activity. Biochim Biophys Acta 924: 292-296.
Arai K, Maguchi S, Fujii S, Ishibashi H, Oikawa K Taniguchi N (1987b). Glycation and inactivation of human Cu-Zn-superoxide dismutase: Identification of the in vitro glycated sites. J Biol Chem 262: 16969-16972.
Beauchamp C, Fridovich I (1971). Superoxide dismutase: Improved assays and an assay applicable to acryulamide gels. Anal Biochem 44: 276-287.
Cohen, MP (1986). In Daibetes and Protein Glycosylation P1-4 Springer-Verlag, New York.
Fitsgibbons JF, Koler RD, Jones RT (1976). Rec cel age-related changes of hemoglobin Ala+b and Alc in normal and diabetic subjects. J Clin

Invest 58: 820-824.

Fleischmajer R, Nedwick A (1973). Werner's syndrome. Am J Med 54: 111-118.

Flückiger R, Winterhalter KH (1976). In vitro synthesis of hemoglobin Alc. FEBS Lett 71: 356-360.

Garlick RL, Mazer JS (1983). The principal site of nonenzymatic glycosylation of human serum albumin in vivo. J Biol Chem 258: 6142-6146. Goldstein S, Moerman, EJ (1975). Heat-labile enzymes in Werner's syndrome fibroblasts. Nature 255: 159.

Goldstein S, Niewiarowski S, Singal DP (1975). Pathological implications of cell aging in vitro. Fed Proc 34: 56-63.

Holliday R, Porterfield JS (1974). Premature aging and occurrence of altered enzyme in Werner's syndrome fibloblasts. Nature 248: 762-763.

Iizuka S, Taniguchi N, Makita (1984). A Enzyme-linked immunosorbent assay for human manganese-containing superoxide dismutase and its content in lung cancer. J Natl Cancer Inst 72: 1043-1049.

Lowry OH, Rosebrough NJ, Farr A, Randall RJ (1951). Protein measurement with the Folin phenol reagent. J Biol Chem 193: 265-275.

Martin GM, Sprague CA, Epstein CJ (1970). Replicatiotive life span of cultivated human cells. Laboratory Invest 23: 86-92.

Nordenson I (1977). Chromosome breaks in Werner's syndrome and their prevention in vitro. Hereditas, 87: 151-154.

Reiss U, Gershon D (1976). Rat liver superoxide dismutase: Purification and age-related modification. Biochem Biophys Res Commun 73: 255-262.

Smith RC, Winer LH, Martel S (1955). Werner's syndrome: Report of two cases. Arch Dermatol 71: 197-204.

The Maillard Reaction in Aging,
Diabetes, and Nutrition, pages 291–299
© 1989 Alan R. Liss, Inc.

NONENZYMATIC GLYCOSYLATION OF DNA BY REDUCING SUGARS

Annette T. Lee and Anthony Cerami

Laboratory of Medical Biochemistry,
The Rockefeller University
New York, New York 10021

ABSTRACT. The process of nonenzymatic glycosylation has proven to be not only of interest to
food chemists in the preservation of foodstuffs,
but has become of increasing interest to
biologists. The nonenzymatic glycosylation
of biologically relevant proteins has become
an important factor in explaining some of the
posttranslational modifications of proteins
observed in diabetes and aging. Using *in vitro*
and *in vivo* models, we describe in this paper
the implications that the nonenzymatic glycosylation of DNA may have in the biological aging
process.

For a number of years the nonenzymatic glycosylation
of proteins has become increasingly important in the study
of aging and the complications arising from diabetes. The
nonenzymatic glycosylation of proteins in foodstuffs was first
described by L.C. Maillard in 1912 and has since become a
model reaction for the modification of proteins *in vivo* by
reducing sugars such as glucose. The Maillard process
(Maillard, 1912) begins with the reaction of an amino
group on the protein and the aldehyde group of the reducing
sugar to form a Schiff base that can rearrange to form a
more stable Amadori product. The resulting Amadori product
can with time undergo a series of rearrangements and
dehydrations to form an array of advanced glycosylation
endproducts. These endproducts are characteristically

yellow-brown, fluorescent pigments that constitute stable crosslinks between long-lived proteins *in vivo*.

The formation of these crosslinks has been observed to occur and accumulate on proteins such as collagen (Monnier, Kohn and Cerami, 1984) lens crystallins (Monnier and Cerami, 1982) and other long-lived proteins (Brownlee, Vlassara and Cerami, 1984; Monnier and Cerami, 1983; Monnier, Stevens and Cerami, 1981). It has only been recently realized that the nonenzymatic glycosylation of DNA could also occur. This reaction was first investigated by Bucala et al. (1984) in model reactions using DNA or nucleotides and the reducing sugars, glucose and glucose-6-phosphate. It was hypothesized that amino groups on DNA bases could also participate in the Maillard reaction with reducing sugars thereby resulting in DNA modifications and subsequent DNA damage. Studies revealed that the reaction of glucose-6-phosphate with the primary amino groups of DNA or nucleotides leads to changes in absorbance and fluorescence spectra which are similar to those observed with nonenzymatically glycosylated proteins (Monnier and Cerami, 1981).

Further model experiments were carried out *in vitro* to better understand the requirements necessary to form stable crosslinks with DNA molecules. These experiments focused on the reaction of glucose-6-phosphate with amino groups of lysine and DNA (Lee and Cerami, 1987). The incubation of genomic *E.coli* DNA in the presence of glucose-6-phosphate and radiolabeled lysine resulted in a time and sugar concentration dependent accumulation of radiolabel onto the DNA. This accumulation is dependent on the presence of glucose-6-phosphate in the incubation solution, since no significant accumulation of radiolabeled lysine was detected when glucose-6-phosphate was omitted from the incubation. Of particular interest was the observation of the formation of a reactive intermediate when glucose-6-phosphate and lysine or putrescine were incubated in solution in the absence of DNA. This preincubation of glucose-6-phosphate and lysine or putrescine leads to the formation of reactive intermediates which accumulate over time and can react completely with added DNA within one hour (table 1). These additions to DNA are stable, covalent adducts of unknown structure. The amount of adduct formed is dependent on sugar and amino acid concentration as well as the length of time of the preincubation. The reaction of these intermediates involves the amino groups of the DNA bases since significant amounts of adduct formation only occurred with polynucleotides [poly (dA), poly d(C-G), poly d(A-T)] that contained amino groups on the DNA bases.

TABLE 1. The presence of glucose-6-phosphate and lysine in the preincubation mixture is necessary for the formation of reactive intermediates (From Lee and Cerami, 1987b.)

4-day preincubation at 37°C[a]	60 min incubation at 37°C[b]	(μmoles [^{3}H]lysine per μmoles DNA bases) X 10[9]
G-6-P	+ (DNA + [^{3}H]lysine)	3.6
[^{3}H]lysine	+ (G-6-P + DNA)	2.2
DNA	+ (G-6-P + [^{3}H]lysine)	2.8
G-6-P + [^{3}H]lysine +	(DNA)	100.0

[a] A 1ml solution of 1M G-6-P, 20 μCi of [^{3}H]lysine (97Ci/mmole) in 0.1M HEPES buffer, *E.coli* DNA (643μg/ml) or 1M G-6-P and 20 μCi of [^{3}H]lysine were incubated at 37°C for 4 days.
[b] 1ml of *E.coli* DNA (643μg/ml) and 20 μCi of [^{3}H]lysine (97Ci/ml) in 1M G-6-P, or 643 μg of *E.coli* DNA was added as indicated to the 4 day preincubation mixture prior to TCA precipitation.

In an attempt to characterize this reactive intermediate, inhibition studies were carried out with aminoguanidine and sodium borohydride. Aminoguanidine which has been shown to prevent the formation of advanced glycosylation endproducts on proteins *in vitro* and *in vivo* (Brownlee et al. 1986), can inhibit the formation of reactive intermediates only if it is present at the onset of the preincubation. Aminoguanidine is ineffective in preventing the reaction of the intermediate with added DNA, following the preincubation of glucose-6-phosphate and lysine. The addition of sodium borohydride to a preincubation solution, containing reactive intermediates or to already formed adducts, had no significant effect. These results suggest that the reactive intermediate has progressed past the Amadori product stage and no longer contains a reactive carbonyl group. We are currently attempting to isolate this reactive intermediate.

The potential importance of reducing sugars with genetic material is evidenced by the effects nonenzymatic glycosylation has on the biological integrity of phage and plasmid DNA (Bucala et al. 1984, 1985). When fl phage DNA was incubated *in vitro* with different concentrations of glucose or glucose-6-phosphate, the transfection efficiency of the reacted DNA was decreased dramatically. The decrease was more dramatic with glucose-6-phosphate than with an equal concentration of glucose (figure 1); a situation that is similar to the formation of advanced glycosylation endproducts on proteins.

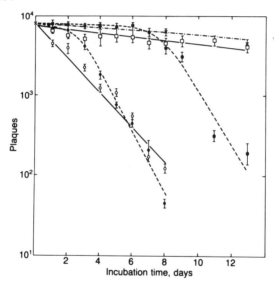

Figure 1. Rate of fl DNA inactivation by 25mM G-6-P (o), 25 mM glucose (□), 25mM G-6-P/5mM Boc-lysine(●), and 25mM glucose/5mM Boc-lysine (■). X, control DNA incubated with Boc-lysine alone for days indicated.

Experiments were designed to determine the effect of the reducing sugar, glucose-6-phosphate with double stranded DNA plasmid pBR322 (Bucala et al. 1985). Analogous to experiments using fl phage DNA, plasmid DNA showed an incubation time and sugar concentration dependent loss in transformation capacity. In addition to this decrease, those bacteria which had been transformed by plasmid DNA nonenzymatically glycosylated *in vitro* showed an increased plasmid mutation rate with exposure to increasing glucose-6-phosphate concentrations. Analysis of the recovered mutated plasmids showed the inactivation of the antibiotic markers was due to deletions or insertions of the DNA. In a preliminary experiment using a uvrC⁻ *E.coli* strain, no plasmid alterations were observed, indicating the possible role of the uvrABC pathway in generating the plasmid mutations.

These *in vitro* studies of DNA glycosylation were extended with a bacterial model that examined the mutation rate of plasmid DNA *in vivo* in bacteria that accumulated abnormally high levels of the reducing sugar, glucose-6-phosphate (Lee and Cerami, 1987). In these experiments, two mutant strains of *E.coli* were used, one of which had an inactive gene for the enzyme phosphoglucose isomerase (DF40), while the other had inactive genes for phosphoglucose isomerase and glucose-6-phosphate dehydrogenase (DF2000). When grown in minimal medium containing glucose and gluconate, the DF40 strain has a 20 fold increase in the intracellular concentration of glucose-6-phosphate, while the DF2000 strain has a 30 fold increase when compared to the control K10 strain (table 2). To investigate the effects of elevated glucose-6-phosphate level on DNA mutations *in vivo*, the three strains were transformed with the plasmid, pAMO06. This plasmid contains the selectable and screenable markers, ampicillin resistance and ß-galactosidase production respectively. The mutant strains were grown under conditions which were or were not conducive for glucose-6-phosphate accumulation. Following a 24 hour growth period, plasmid DNA was isolated and assayed for potential mutations of the ß-galactosidase gene in an ampicillin sensitive, lactose utilization deficient *E. coli* indicator strain. Colonies which were ampicillin resistant but exhibited a lac⁻ phenotype were scored as mutants. Plasmid DNA isolated from the DF40 strain which accumulated a 20 fold increase in glucose-6-phosphate under these growth conditions showed a 7 fold increase in plasmid mutation rate. Plasmid DNA isolated from the DF2000 strain which accumulated a 30 fold increase in glucose-6-phosphate under these conditions

TABLE 2. Glucose-6-phosphate levels found in cells grown in minimal medium containing glucose/gluconate or gluconate alone

Glucose-6-phosphate, μmoles per 5 x 10^9 cells		
strain	glucose/gluconate	gluconate
K10	0.028 ± 0.005	0.030 ± 0.003
DF40	0.553 ± 0.072	0.005 ± 0.002
DF2000	0.864 ± 0.011	0.004 ± 0.001

Overnight cultures of each strain grown in either gluconate or glucose/gluconate minimal medium were diluted to 10^8 cells per ml. Diluted culture (50ml) was extracted with perchloric acid then assayed for G-6-P content.

showed a 13 fold increase in plasmid mutation rate when compared to the control strain (table 3). When the three strains, K10, DF40 and DF2000 were grown in minimal medium containing gluconate alone, there was no significant increase in the intracellular glucose-6-phosphate levels or the plasmid mutation rate.

Analysis of the mutated plasmids from the DF2000 strain gave unexpected results. Mutated plasmids obtained from the DF2000 strain were mainly distributed between large insertions (>1Kb) and small plasmid size changes (<1Kb), whereas, mutated plasmids from the DF40 strain and the control K10 strain, showed a predominance of large plasmid size decreases (>1Kb). The reason behind the difference in the types of plasmid mutations found among these strains is still unknown at this time. Preliminary experiments investigating the role of RecA in these mutations failed to show any visible induction of RecA when the strains were grown under conditions which induced an increase in plasmid mutation rate.

Over the years, the hypothesis that DNA damage and mutations may contribute to the biological aging process has gained increased recognition. It has been hypothesized that differential gene expression, decline in DNA repair,

TABLE 3. Relative mutation rates of cells grown in gluconate alone or glucose/gluconate

Relative *lac⁻* mutagenesis per 10^5 transformants

strain	glucose/gluconate	gluconate
K10	0.67 ± 0.47	0.5 ± 0.5
DF40	4.84 ± 0.65	1.0 ± 1.0
DF2000	8.71 ± 1.24	1.5 ± 0.5

Plasmid DNA (50ng) isolated from cultures grown in gluconate or glucose/gluconate minimal medium was used to transform SB4288 competent cells. Colonies that were Amp^R but had a Lac⁻ phenotype were scored as mutants. Relative mutagenesis was determined by the ratio of mutants found in the mutant strains (DF40 or DF2000)/control strain (K10).

replication and transcription play major roles in the senescence and eventual death of a cell (Gensler and Berstein, 1981). Many age related changes in genetic material have been reported: increases in DNA strand breaks (Price, Modak and Makinodan, 1971) and the amount of DNA-histone complexes (Berdyshev and Zhelabovaskaya, 1972; Bojanovic et al. 1970); decreases in DNA replication (Petes et al. 1974; Collins and Chu, 1985), transcription (Berdyshev and Zhelabovaskaya, 1972) and repair (Niedermuller, Hofecker and Skalicky, 1985; Karran and Ormerod, 1973; Nette et al. 1984; Little, 1976). *In vitro* and *in vivo* models suggest that the nonenzymatic glycosylation of DNA could play a role in DNA strand breaks and intra- and interstrand crosslinks in mammalian cells. These types of DNA damage may contribute to some of the age related changes observed in genetic material with time.

REFERENCES

Berdyshev GD, Zhelabovaskaya SM (1972). Composition, template properties and thermostability of liver chromatin from rats of various age at deproteinization by NaCl solutions. Exp Geront 7:321-330.

Bojanovic JJ, Jevtovic AD, Pantic VS, Dugandzic SM, Jovanovic DS (1970) Thymus nucleoproteins. Thymus histones in young and adult rats. Gerontoligia 16:304-312.

Brownlee M, Vlassara H, Kooney A, Ulrich P, Cerami A (1986). Aminoguanidine prevents diabetes-induces arterial wall protein cross-linking. Science 232:1629-1632.

Brownlee M, Vlassara H, Cerami A (1984). Nonenzymatic glycosylation and the pathogenesis of diabetic complications. Ann Intern Med 101:527-537.

Bucala R, Model P, Russel M, Cerami A (1985). Modification of DNA by glucose-6-phosphate induces DNA rearrangements in an *Escherichia coli* plasmid. Proc Natl Acad Sci USA 82:8439-8442.

Bucala R, Model P, Cerami A (1984). Modification of DNA by reducing sugars: A possible mechanism for nucleic acid aging and age-related dysfunction in gene expression. Proc Natl Acad Sci USA 81:105-109.

Collins JM, Chu AK (1985). Reduction of DNA synthesis in aging but still proliferating cells. J Cell Phys 124:165-173.

Gensler HL, Berstein H (1981). DNA damage as the primary cause of aging. Quar Rev Bio 56:279-303.

Karran P, Ormerod MG (1973). Is the ability to repair damage to DNA related to the proliferative capacity of a cell? The rejoining of x-ray produced strand breaks. Biochim Biophys Acta 299:54-64.

Lee AT, Cerami A (1987a). Elevated glucose-6-phosphate levels are associated with plasmid mutations *in vivo*. Proc Natl Acad Sci USA 84:8311-8314.

Lee AT, Cerami A (1987b). The formation of reactive intermediate(s) of glucose-6-phosphate and lysine capable of rapidly reacting with DNA. Mut Res 179:151-158.

Little JB (1976). Relationship between DNA repair capacity and cellular aging. Gerontology 22:28-55.

Maillard LC (1912). Action des acides amines sur les sucres:formation des melanoidines par voie methodique. C.R. Seances Acad Sci 154:66-68.

Monnier VM, Kohn RR, Cerami A (1984). Accelerated age-related browning of human collagen in diabetes mellitus. Proc

Natl Acad Sci 81:583-587.

Monnier VM, Cerami A (1983). Nonenzymatic glycosylation and browning of proteins *in vivo*. J Am Chem Soc 215:431-449.

Monnier VM, Cerami A (1982). Nonenzymatic glycosylation and browning in diabetes and aging: studies on lens proteins. Diabetes 31, suppl 3 57-63.

Monnier VM, Cerami A (1981). Nonenzymatic browning *in vivo*: Possible process for aging of long-lived proteins. Science 211:491-493.

Monnier VM, Stevens VJ, Cerami A (1981). Maillard reactions involving proteins and carbohydrates *in vivo*: relevance to diabetes mellitus and aging. Prog Fd Nutr Sci 5:315-327.

Nette EG, Xi YP, Sun YK, Andrews AD, King DW (1984). A correlation between aging and DNA repair in human epidermal cells. Mech Ageing and Dev 24:283-292.

Niedermuller H, Hofecker G, Skalicky M (1985). Changes of DNA repair mechanisms during the aging of the rat. Mech Aging Dev 29:221-238.

Petes TD, Farber RA, Tarrant GM, Holliday R (1974). Altered rate of DNA replication an ageing human fibroblast cultures. Nature 251:434-436.

Price GB, Modak SP, Makinodan T (1971) Age-associated changes in the DNA of mouse tissue. Science 171:917-920.

The Maillard Reaction in Aging,
Diabetes, and Nutrition, pages 301–327
© 1989 Alan R. Liss, Inc.

THE MAILLARD REACTION IN FOODS

A. Kaanane and T. P. Labuza

Department of Food Science and Nutrition
University of Minnesota
St. Paul, MN   55108

ABSTRACT. The nonenzymatic browning (NEB)
reaction in food systems has been studied
extensively since its first discovery in 1912.
The reaction contributes both to positive and
negative effects on food quality and safety.
Of interest to the food industry is the control
of the browning reaction. Classic control
methods include elimination of reactable
substrate, lowering of pH, chelation of trace
minerals, limiting the water content, maintaining low temperatures and the use of
inhibitors like sulfite. Since 1986, when the
FDA banned the use of sulfite in certain
instances, there has been renewed interest in
browning inhibition studies. This paper will
review the classical methods used to inhibit
browning and then focus on the recent work on
acyclic formation rate of sugars and cysteine
inhibition.

INTRODUCTION

    The nonenzymatic browning reactions that occur in
foods have received much interest in the past fifty years.
These reactions which occur during both heat processing and
storage can have either desirable or undesirable effects
depending on the food type. In most cases, nonenzymatic
browning is undesirable because it results in deterioration
of flavor, a darkening and significant loss of nutrients in

particular protein quality. In addition it may result in
the formation of toxic substances, discussed elsewhere in
this book. Examples in which browning is desirable are
baked goods, beer, many breakfast foods and coffee.

In general, there are three basic types of nonenzymatic browning reactions that occur in food: (1) The
Maillard reaction which is a reaction between carbonyl
compounds and amino compounds; (2) caramelization which is
due to sugar degradation at high temperature and (3)
ascorbic acid degradation, the final steps of which include
the Maillard reaction. It is the Maillard reaction and
ascorbic acid degradation that causes serious losses of
quality of foods during processing and storage.

Nonenzymatic browning was first reported by Louis
Maillard in 1912. Maillard observed this reaction while
experimenting with sugars as the condensing agent for
formation of polypeptides. The chemistry of this reaction
in food systems has been extensively reviewed by Hodge
(1953), Ellis (1959), Labuza and Saltmarch (1981), Eriksson
(1981), Waller and Feather (1983) and Labuza and Schmidl
(1986).

The following is a general schematic for the reaction
including ascorbic acid degradation:

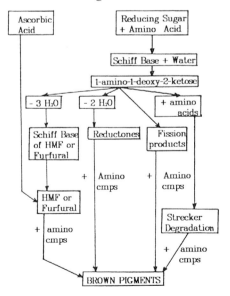

As can be seen, the reaction is a series of complex consecutive and interconnected processes. The complete reactions is far from being well understood at the present time. Even though the first step of the reaction is very simple as compared to the latter stages, no generally satisfactory procedure for controlling these reactions in foods and biological systems has been developed.

A long list of procedures have been suggested for control or prevention of the Maillard reaction (Feeney and Whitaker, 1982). Among these procedures are the following:

1. Removal of the offending carbohydrates by dialysis or by enzymatic action, a procedure not likely used for most foods.
2. Addition of chemical substances to block the carbonyl group on the sugars, such as sulfite, which is the common technique.
3. Addition of a chemical substance to compete with the amino group and to form covalent products with the carbonyl of the sugar, such as cysteine to form the thiozolidine. This is currently under investigation.
4. The blocking of amino groups, usually by covalent modification such as acylation or methylation and compart-mentalization (such as separating the carbonyl compounds and nitrogen compounds with starch).
5. Lowering the water activity (a_w) where a_w refers to the degree of binding of the water or availability of water. Generally at lower a_w the rate is less.
6. Lowering the pH.
7. Lowering the temperature.
8. Removing O_2 and metals especially in the case where ascorbic acid is present.

All of these methods present problems. The most widely used inhibitor in food as a means of controlling nonenzymatic browning as well as for other purposes are the sulfites. These inhibitors are also used currently in many commercial total parenteral nutrition solutions (TPN) to prevent the oxidation of amino acids (Schmidl et al.,1988).

The use of sulfite in TPN solutions may be question-able. Studies have shown that rapid breakdown of tryptophan occurs in amino acid solutions when sodium bisulfite is added (Kleinman et al., 1973). TPN solutions

containing bisulfite have been known to cause fatty liver
and raised serum liver enzyme levels in the human and in
rats (Grant et al., 1977). In addition, as of September
1985, 13 deaths and about 500 cases of adverse reactions
have been attributed to sulfites.

As a result, the Food and Drug Administration (FDA)
banned the use of sulfite preservatives in fresh vegetables
and fruits (FDA, 1986). Furthermore, FDA ruled that,
effective January 9, 1987, all packaged foods that contain
10 ppm or more of sulfur dioxide equivalents are required
to disclose on the label the presence of the sulfiting
agent. As a consequence, there has been renewed interest
in browning inhibition studies. This has been further
enhanced by the desire by drug companies to produce shelf
stable TPN solutions containing glucose and free amino
acids thereby eliminating patient hospital stay. Because
of the growing interest in the area of browning inhibition,
this paper will review the factors and the classical
methods used to inhibit nonenzymatic browning in foods and
then focus on the recent work on the determination of the
acyclic form (reducing form) of sugar using FTIR and on the
inhibition of the reaction by cysteine.

FACTORS AFFECTING NONENZYMATIC BROWNING AND METHODS FOR
PREVENTION

1. Temperature and Water Activity

Labuza and Saltmarch (1981a) in a review of the
literature found that under most storage conditions
(T<60°C), the extent of browning can be modeled as a zero
order reaction. On the other hand, loss of any reactive
reducing compounds or loss of available amines follows a
first order reaction. However at high temperatures,
(80°C) the plot of brown pigment against time will first
curve upward as in a first order reaction and reach a
maximum as substrate is used up.

Labuza (1984) has shown that, in general, for many
dehydrated foods, below about 32°C, lipid oxidation is the
factor that limits shelf-life, but because of the high
activation energy or Q_{10} for browning, browning pre-
dominates above this temperature. In general, the
temperature sensitivity (Q_{10}) or rate increase of browning

for a 10°C temperature increase ranges from about four to eight times.

Labuza and Schmidl (1986) reported that very few data exist on the level of browning needed to reach unacceptability as a function of food type or temperature. Nagy and Dinsmore (1974) found a relationship between furfural build up in orange juice, storage conditions and flavor change. Furfural is an intermediate compound in the browning reaction related to vitamin C degradation. Kaanane et al., (1988) studied the browning of Moroccan orange juice during storage and found higher furfural values than those of Nagy and Dinsmore (1974) at equivalent browning extents. They concluded that this is probably due to the differences existing between the intrinsic properties of the two juices used in these studies, especially the minerals and buffering capacity of the organic acids. As reported by Adrian (1982), the part played by temperature differs according to the chosen criterion i.e. browning pigment or amino acid loss. For example a glucose-glycine system heated for one hour at 90°C or 9 hr at 70°C has the same glycine loss, but the former has an UV absorbance twice as much as the latter (i.e. double the amount of browning). This indicates that the exact nature of the brown pigments produced is different at 70°C compared to 90°C.

Considerable data exists on the effect of storage temperature on loss of protein quality in foods (Labuza and Schmidl, 1986). It was pointed out that the problem with most of these studies however is that the investigators have used fairly high temperatures (>80°C) to produce significant losses of protein nutritive value in the food and this extent of loss never occurs in normal storage and has very rarely been tied to cause of protein malnutrition in humans or animals.

The browning reaction as a function of a_w follows the typical min-max pattern described by Labuza et al.,(1977) and Labuza and Saltmarch (1981b). Figure 1 shows the affect of a_w on the amount of browning of a glucose glycine model system held at 37°C (McWeeney 1973).

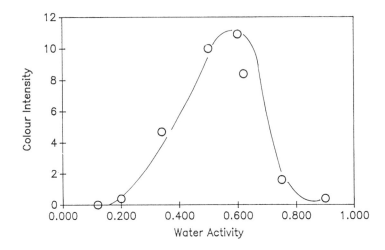

Figure 1. Effect of a_w on browning.

In general, the rate of browning increases from the dry state as water activity increases up to a maximum rate at an a_w of 0.5 to 0.8. Above that a_w, the rate decreases. The maximum stability for browning is achieved by adjusting the product to the monolayer moisture content or below and maintaining it there which of course is only applicable to dry foods. The basic physical principle is that solute mobility is severely limited below the monolayer value (Duckworth, 1981). Above this a_w, solutes become mobilized and will react. At higher a_ws, solutes are totally dissolved and thus any increase in a_w causes dilution with a decrease in reaction rates (Eickner and Karel, 1972)

Through multiple linear regression analysis Kaanane and Labuza (1985) developed statistical modes that related the rate constant of amino acid loss to both temperature and water activity (a_w). The model used was a variation of the Arrhenius relationship with a_w incorporated as:

$$\ln k = \ln k_o + c_1 \, a_w - (E_A + c_2 \, a_w) \, / \, RT$$

where:
    k = rate constant for any condition
    k_0 = the preexponential factor
    c_1 and c_2 = constants
    a_w = water activity
    E_A = general activation energy

Villota et al., (1980a) on the other hand developed a more empirical model for the extent of browning of foods again with both temperature and a_w factors. Their equation was based on an extensive analysis of literature data. Unfortunately neither the Kaanane and Labuza (1985) or Villota et al., (1980) models are used by the industry.

2. Effect of Sugar-Amine Ratio.

Wolfrom et al., (1974) reported that color development in D-glucose-glycine mixtures, containing 65% of water and stored at 65°C, showed a marked dependence on the relative proportion of the amino-acid to sugar ratio. Their data showed that the color production was relatively modest at a D-glucose/glycine ratio of 10:1 to 2:1, but that development of color rapidly accelerated at a ratio of 1:1 to 1:5. The results are shown in Figure 2.

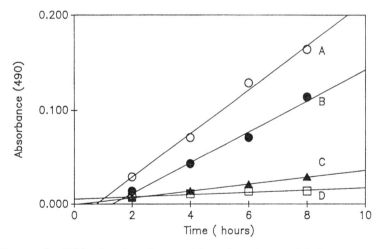

Figure 2. Effect of molar ratio of amino acid to sugar on the browning reaction. D-Glucose-glycine ratio: A 1:5; B 1:1; C 2:1; D 10:1, water content 65%, reaction temperature 65°C.

An opposite trend of the effect of the sugar-amino acid molar ratio on browning as shown in Figure 3 was reported by Warmebier et al (1976).

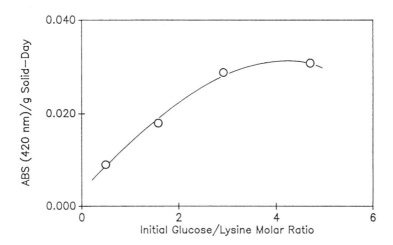

Figure 3. Zero order rate of brown pigment formation in a semimoist system (a_w=0.52) at 45°C and as a function of the glucose/lysine molar ratio.

As can be seen in Figure 3, the rate of pigment formation approaches a plateau at a glucose to lysine molar ratio of approximately three. This is similar to that found by Lea and Hannan (1950), for a casein model system humidified to a_w 0.7. The reason for these opposite effects are unclear but most likely is due to the lower a_w as compared to the other work done in solution.

3. Effect of Amino Acid Type

Wolfrom et al., (1974) studied the effect of amino acid type in a 1:1 D-glucose/amino acid mixture, on the extent of browning. A comparison was made between nine different amino acids that are known to exist freely in orange juice and other foods. Both, L-arginine and 4-aminobutyric acid gave the most intense and rapid color formation followed by glycine, alanine, serine and L-proline. Aspartic acid, L-glutamic acid and L-glutamine showed behavior similar to glycine.

Lysine is often reported as the most reactive amino acid in the Maillard reaction (Ashoor and Zent, 1984). This is hypothesized because lysine has two available amino groups on the molecule. Ashoor and Zent (1984) in a study on Maillard browning concluded that amino acids and amides may be classified into three groups according to the extent of Maillard browning produced when they are heated with common reducing sugars. The first group are the ones that produce a high extent of browning including lysine, glycine, tryptophan and tyrosine. The second group includes the intermediate browning producing ones which are proline, leucine, isoleucine, alanine, hydroxyproline, phenylalanine, methionine, valine and the amides glutamine and asparagine. The third group includes the low browning producing amino acids such as histidine, threonine, aspartic acid, arginine, glutamic acid, and cysteine. This is opposite to the result reported in a recent study in which Massaro and Labuza (1988) found that lysine produced the least brown color as compared to tryptophan and cysteine in a model system similar to TPN solutions at pH 5.5 - 5.7 and stored at $4^{\circ}C$ or $30^{\circ}C$. In another study on the formation of Maillard reaction products in parenteral alimentation solutions, Fry and Steglink (1982) found that proline and amino acids with hydrophobic side chains reacted more slowly than other amino acids. Of the 14 amino acids tested at $25^{\circ}C$ (the pH was not reported), tryptophan was the most reactive followed in order by serine and threonine. These conflicting results may be explained by the fact that the reactivity of different amino acids in the Maillard reaction also depends on pH. Thus it may be expected that amino acids that react similarly at some range of pH may not necessarily respond the same way and in the same order under other pH conditions.

4. Acylation and Methylation

The objective of acylation or methylation is to block the amino groups, usually by covalent modification. This makes the amino group of the amino acid unavailable for Maillard reaction. An example of this kind of modification is acetylation:

$$P\text{-}NH_2 + O \overset{C\text{-}CH_3}{\underset{C\text{-}CH_3}{\big\langle}} \xrightarrow[\text{pH} > 7]{} P\text{-}NH\text{-}\overset{O}{\overset{\|}{C}}\text{-}CH_3 + CH_3COOH$$

However these methods, in most cases, cannot be applied to foods to prevent the Maillard reaction because of the high pH needed for the reaction to occur. Lee et al., (1978) reported that limited methylation of food proteins would be particularly useful when they are incorporated as only part of the total protein of the food item for their particular functional attributes.

5. Effect of pH

Many investigators have studied the effect of pH on the rate of browning reaction (Underwood et al., 1959, Kato et al., 1969, Wolfrom et al., 1974, Feeney et al., 1975, Buera et al., 1987 and Ashoor and Zent, 1984). More detailed information on the effect of pH on the Maillard reaction can be found in a recent extensive review on the control of browning reaction in foods (Labuza and Schmidl, 1986).

In order to evaluate the effect of pH on the Maillard reaction, it is necessary to distinguish between two cases. The first is the effect of pH on color development in model systems containing free amino acids and reducing sugars. The second is the effect of pH when the system contains intact protein and reducing sugars. In the first case, the rate of color development due to browning shows a characteristic pH dependence that results in a bell-shaped curve. As an example, Ashoor and Zent (1984) studied the effect of pH on browning in the range of pH 6-12, using model systems containing different combinations of three amino acids and two reducing sugars. An example is shown in Figure 4.

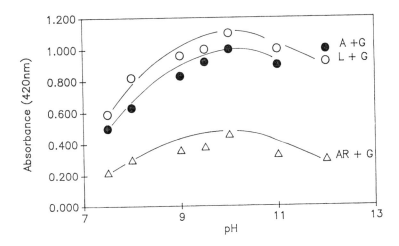

Figure 4. Effect of pH on the extent of browning of L-
lysine (L), L-alanine (A), and L-arginine (AR) in
solution with glucose (G) heated at 121°C for 10
mn.

They found that the Maillard browning intensity increased
as the pH of the system increased, with a maximum at a pH
value of about 10.0. It then decreased at higher pH
values. The increase in Maillard browning intensity when
pH goes up has also been reported by many researchers
(Schroeder et al., 1955, Underwood et al., 1959, Pomeranz
et al., 1962 and Wolfrom et al., 1974). The reason why
browning decreases at pHs higher then 10.0 is not clear.
Buera et al., (1987) used a model system containing 0.27M
sugars (fructose, glucose, lactose, maltose, sucrose and
xylose) and 0.067M glycine. The systems were adjusted to
a_w 0.9 and to different pHs (4-6). All the data showed an
increase in the rate of browning with an increase of pH.

In the literature available, in order to explain the
effect of pH on the rate of Maillard reaction, most of the
authors (Feeney et al., 1975, and Labuza and Schmidl, 1986)
implicated only the effect of pH on the equilibrium
reaction of the protonated and unprotonated forms of the
amino group which is:

$$-NH_3^+ \quad \xrightarrow{pH > 7} \quad -NH_2 + H^+$$

They stated that at the pKa of the amino group, 50% of the amine is in the protonated $-NH_3^+$ state and this protonated form prevents electron transfer. The extent of browning is minimal at a pH lower than the pKa of the amino acid. However we believe that there is another factor to explain this. As we will discuss later, the level of acyclic form or reducing form of sugar also affects the kinetics of browning. Canter and Peniston (1940) using a polarographic method of analysis determined the concentration of acyclic form of different reducing sugars in the pH range of 6.5-7.5. The results of this study are shown in Table 1.

TABLE 1.   Variation of acyclic form with pH at 25°C as % of the total concentration (0.1M)

	pH		
Sugar	6.5	7.0	7.5
D-Glucose	0.012	0.022	0.040
D-Galactose	0.070	0.085	0.140
D-Mannose	0.040	0.062	0.110
D-Xylose	0.100	0.130	0.360
D-Lyxose	0.150	0.180	0.360
L-Arabinose	0.130	0.220	0.400
D-Ribose	10.000	8.500	30.000
L-Allose	2.280	1.100	0.510

As it can be seen, as the pH increases the concentration of acyclic form also increased which in turn will affect the rate of browning. However the data presented in Table 1 are correct only with regard to order of magnitude since the validity of the method of analysis used is doubtful. The reason will be explained later in this review.

With respect to the effect of pH on browning when intact protein is used instead of free amino acids, the typical browning rate versus pH curve differs as show in Figure 5.

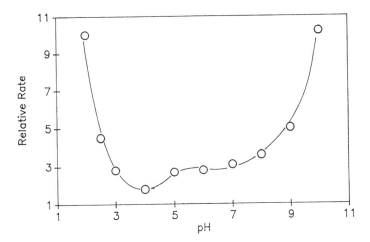

Figure 5. Effect of pH on relative rate of nonenzymatic
browning of an intact protein

In general, at pH 3, the rate is at a minimum. One
can see that below pH 3, the rate of browning increases
again. This is due probably to protein hydrolysis.
Finally as with amino acids the rate increases as pH rises
from 7 to 10.

6. Effect of Reducing Compounds

Many reducing species that participate in the browning
reaction can be found in most foods. These include several
sugars, vitamin C, orthophenols and various small molecular
weight flavor compounds naturally present, added or
produced from other reactions such as lipid oxidation
(Labuza and Schmidl, 1986). Vanillin is an example.

With respect to sugars, Labuza and Schmidl (1986)
stated that the key is whether or not the sugars are in a
reducing form. The reducing form of sugar is called the
acyclic or straight chain form. The mutarotation reaction
that takes place when crystalline reducing sugars are
dissolved in water or other suitable solvents is of
considerable theoretical and practical interest, and it is
a major determinant of the chemical and biochemical
behavior of sugars. For this reason, the kinetics of
mutarotation have been the subject of extensive studies

over a period of many years (Pigman and Isbell, 1968, Pigman and Anet 1972, and Franks et al., 1986). Sugars, when dissolved in water, undergo many transformations, particularly in the presence of acids and alkalies. These changes usually involve the carbon atom carrying the aldehyde or ketose groups. Most studies (Wertz et al., 1981, Pigman and Anet, 1972) concerning the mutarotation of sugar agreed that the interconversion of the cyclic anomers of sugar proceeds via a central intermediate which is the aldehydo or keto form of the sugar. This equilibrium reaction is as follows:

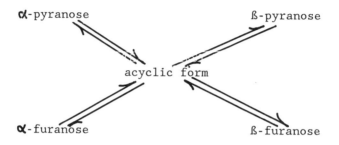

Early attempts to determine the composition of sugar solutions have resulted in a number of methods for estimating the proportions of the constituents and the rate of change from one form to another, but none of these methods was entirely satisfactory (Pigman and Anet, 1972). Canter and Peniston (1940) used the polarography technique to estimate the concentration of acyclic form of different sugars as a function of pH and total concentration of sugar (Table 1). Their measurement showed a polarographic wave, presumably arising from the reduction of the acyclic form at the dropping mercury cathode. However this method has been criticized. The height of the polarographic wave originally ascribed to the concentration of the acyclic form could be dependent on the rate of conversion of the ring forms into the acyclic form. Also any small impurities should affect the measurement. More recently, Hayward and Angyal (1977) used the circular dichroism technique to measure the acyclic form concentration for different solutions of sugars. The results obtained by these authors are presented in Table 2.

Table 2. Percentage of acyclic form of reducing sugars in aqueous solution at 20°C, pH 5.2-7.0.

Sugar	% Acyclic form
D-Fructose	0.700
D-Arabinose	0.030
L-Lyxose	0.030
D-Ribose	0.050
D-Xylose	0.020
D-Galactose	0.020
D-Glucose	0.002
D-Mannose	0.005

One problem with this method is that in order to be able to estimate the percentage of acyclic form, the author assumed that the molar dichroic - extinction coefficient (E^o) for the pure carbonyl form for all reducing sugars was equal to unity. This assumption may or may not be true. It can be seen that the results of Table 1 and Table 2 are quite different.

With respect to the relationship between the concentration of acyclic form of different sugars and the rate of browning, little work has been done. Burton and McWeeney (1963) reported that the higher the level of acyclic form in solution the faster the rate of browning. Recently, Bunn and Higgins (1981) using the results of Hayward and Angyal (1977) related the nonenzymatic glycosylation rate of hemoglobin to the concentration of acyclic form for different sugars. Some of their data are presented in Table 3 and plotted in Figure 6.

As can be seen the rate of condensation of various monosaccharides with hemoglobin varied over a 300-fold range and correlated well with the extent to which the sugar exists in the open form. This is true when aldose and ketose are considered separately. However if the two groups (aldose and ketose) are taken together, there is no clear relation between the rate of glycation of hemoglobin and the percent of acyclic form of sugar. The authors stated that their observations may be considered in terms

Table 3. Rates of condensation of monosaccharides with
          hemoglobin at 37°C.

Sugar	$K(10^{-3}mM^{-1}hr^{-1})$	% Carbonyl
Aldoses:		
D-Glucose	0.6	0.002
D-Mannose	3.6	0.005
Fucose	0.7	0.007
D-Allose	1.4	0.010
D-Galactose	2.8	0.020
D-Xylose	2.9	0.020
D-Talose	5.2	0.030
D-Ribose	10.0	0.040
D-Idose	55.0	0.200
Ketoses:		
L-Sorbose	1.0	0.200
D-Tagatose	0.3	0.600
D-Fructose	4.5	0.700
Xylulose	15.0	8.000

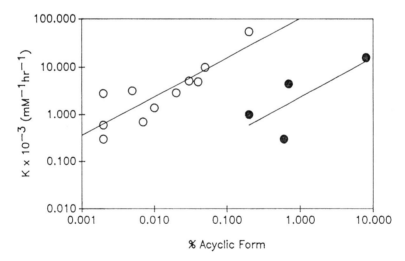

Figure 6. Rate of glycation of hemoglobin as a function of
          the % acyclic form of reducing sugar in solution.
          o-aldoses •-ketoses.

of biomolecular evolution. During the sequential development of anaerobic glycolysis, photosynthesis, and aerobic glycolysis, glucose rather than other stereoisomers has emerged as the universal metabolic fuel. This selectivity could be attributed to the stability of its ring structure.

The formation of the acyclic form involves the transfer of three electrons and three protons from the solvent which is usually water. Therefore it should be expected that the level of acyclic form in solutions will depend on such factors as pH, temperature, ions present in solution, and solvent type. Franks et al., (1986) studied the effect of cations on the anomeric equilibrium of D-glucose in aqueous solutions using Raman spectroscopy. This study showed the Ca^{2+} ion has a marked effect, shifting the equilibrium to favor the α-anomer. For other cations studied, the effect has been found to fall off in magnitude according to the series: $Ca^{2+} \sim La^{3+} > Cd^{2+} \sim Mg^{2+} \sim K^+$. It is interesting to note that the effect is largest for the Ca^{2+}, an important ion in biological systems. However no data exist on the effect of ions on the concentration of acyclic form of sugars in solution.

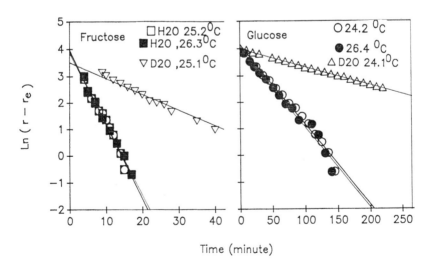

Figure 7. Effect of solvent type on mutarotation of glucose and fructose.

In general, data concerning the level of acyclic form of different sugars and how this level is affected by environmental factors are scarce in the literature. Recently our group started a project to investigate this area. The first experiment was designed to study the effect of solvent type. Figure 7 shows respectively the mutarotation kinetics of glucose and fructose in water and D_2O.

Results show that the mutarotation in both solvents follows first order kinetics. Assuming the following equilibrium:

$$\alpha\text{-pyranose} \underset{K_2}{\overset{K_1}{\rightleftharpoons}} \text{ß-pyranose}$$

The overall rate of mutarotation can be expressed as:

$$\ln[(\alpha - \alpha_{eq})/(\alpha_o - \alpha_{eq})] = -(k_1+k_2)t$$

where:

α = rotation angle at time t
α_{eq} = rotation angle at equilibrium
α_o = rotation angle at t=0
k_1 and k_2 = constant
t = time (mn)

The slope of a plot of $\ln(\alpha - \alpha_{eq})$ versus time gives (k_1+k_2).

The effect of the ions $FeCl_2$, $CaCl_2$, $CoCl_2$, KCl, and NaCl on the mutarotation of glucose and fructose in water was also studied. As an example, the effect of $CaCl_2$ on the mutarotation of glucose and fructose is shown in Figure 8. From these data it was concluded that the effect of solvent has a significant influence on the kinetics of mutarotation while the effect of the ions studied was not significant.

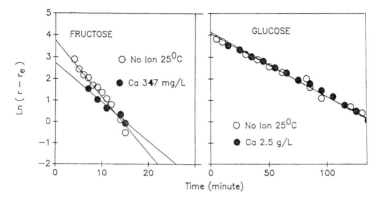

Figure 8. Effect of calcium ion on the mutarotation of glucose and fructose.

It is well known that the carbonyl group absorbs in the the Infra-Red region at about 1700-1750 cm^{-1}. Recently Fourier Transform Infra-Red (FTIR) spectroscopy has been developed as a consequence of the advance in computer science. This new technique is believed to be more time sensitive than the classical Infra-Red spectroscopy. For this reason, an investigation of the use of FTIR technique to determine the concentration of the acyclic form of different sugars is under investigation in our laboratory. The first step in developing this technique is to determine the minimum concentration of carbonyl group that can be detected by FTIR using butyraldehyde as a standard. A series of solutions of butyraldehyde in D_2O containing the following concentrations: $1.5 \ 10^{-5}$ moles/L, $2.8 \ 10^{-5}$ mole/L, $5.6 \ 10^{-5}$ moles/L, $1.1 \ 10^{-4}$ moles/L and $2.2 \ 10^{-4}$ moles/L were analyzes by FTIR. As an example Figure 9 shows the FTIR spectrogram of butyraldehyde at a concentration of $1.1 \ 10^{-4}$ mole/L.

It was found that the minimum concentration of carbonyl group that can be detected by FTIR technique is 1.6×10^{-5} moles/L. Assuming that the concetration of acyclic form in a 1 Molar solution of glucose is 0.002% as determined by Hayward and Angyal (1977) which corresponds to 2.0×10^{-5} moles/L, it was concluded that FTIR can be a useful tool to determine the acyclic form of different sugars and the effect of different factors such as pH, temperature and cations.

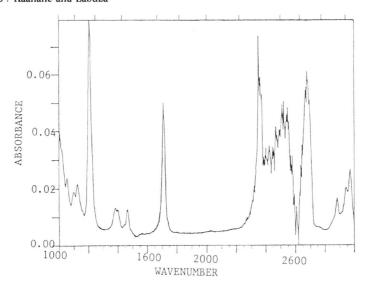

Figure 9. FTIR Spectrogram of butyraldehyde in D_2O
(Concentration 1.1 x 10^{-4} mole/L).

7. Cysteine Effect

Arnold (1969) studied the effect of L-cysteine and L-
cystine on the browning of milk. The result of this study
showed that L-cystine failed to inhibit browning, whereas
L-cysteine was effective at a concentration as low as
0.01%. This study also showed that L-cysteine (free base)
was preferred to L-Cysteine hydrochloride because this
latter produced an objectional sulfide flavor upon heating.
Yu et al., (1974) studied the effect of cysteine on the
browning due to ascorbic acid. It was found that cysteine
protected ascorbic acid degradation against the formation
of brown pigments. Montgomery (1983) used cysteine as an
inhibitor of browning in pear juice concentrate. The
results showed that cysteine treatment of pear juice
decreased the initial browning of pear juice concentrate
and decreased the rates of browning during storage at 1°C,
21°C and 38°C. The mechanism of action is that cysteine
reacts with the reducing compounds to produce colorless
complexes (Labuza and Schmidl, 1986). Recently, Massaro
and Labuza (1988) studied the effect of cysteine and
electrolytes on the kinetics of browning and amino acids
loss due to the Maillard reaction at 4 and 30°C in model
total parenteral nutrition (TPN) systems. Browning

developments in a commercial TPN solution (without sulfite) was also studied at the same temperature (4 and 30°C). The amino acid concentrations used in the model systems were the same as in the commercial solution and the pH was adjusted to 5.5 to 5.7. It should be noted that the systems have about 25% w/v of glucose present.

Table 4. Rate Constants for Brown Pigment Formation on a Molar Basis.

System[*]	Temperature (C)	Electrolytes	OD/Mole Day x 10^{-3}
A	4	+	5.50
(L)	4	-	3.50
	30	+	10.90
	30	-	8.20
B	4	+	35.80
(T)	4	-	42.40
	30	+	242.00
	30	-	259.00
C	4	+	32.70
(C)	4	-	21.30
	30	+	224.00
	30	-	264.00
D	4	+	6.92
(LT)	4	-	7.78
	30	+	48.40
	30	-	56.50
E	4	+	5.49
(LTC)	4	-	4.64
	30	+	51.50
	30	-	54.50
F	4	+	1.32
(Vamin N)	30	+	19.10

[*]L=Lysine, T=Tryptophan, C=Cysteine, F=Commercial TPN

The overall rate constants of the Maillard reaction on molar basis are presented in Table 4. The data for most of the systems exhibited pseudo-order kinetics except for the systems containing cysteine which followed a second order polynomial regression before reaching a plateau. As can be seen lysine alone showed the slowest browning rate while tryptophan was the highest. The combination of lysine/

tryptophan followed exactly the mole fraction rate constant; however in the presence of all three amino acids, the rate was decreased indicating an inhibition by cysteine. It was also noted that the presence of electrolytes including calcium was variable on the rate with single amino acids but slightly inhibitory for most combinations of amino acids.

8. Effect of Sulfites

Several reviews were published lately concerning the use and the status of sulfites as inhibitors of the Maillard reaction (Ann., 1986; Wedzicha, 1987; Modderman, 1987; Wedezicha and Kaputo, 1987; McWeeney et al., 1974; Song and Chichester, 1967 a and b). Sulfites are generally effective in the inhibition of browning. They are used in extending shelf-life of dehydrated food, fruit juices and wines. The effectiveness of sulfites in controlling this complex reaction probably lies in the number of quite distinct reactions in which it can participate with the carbonylic intermediates. However the amount that can be added is limited by governmental regulations and by taste considerations. In addition, because of the regulation adopted in 1986-1987 (FDA 1986) prohibiting its use in fresh fruits and vegetables and the labeling requirements, their use in foods is changing rapidly and new means of inhibition are being investigated.

9. Ion Effect

Labuza and Schmidl (1986) reported that little work has been done on the effect of minerals on the nonenzymatic browning reaction. Thomas (1969) reported that the use of calcium co-precipitate in processed cheese was very successful in controlling the browning reaction. Yu et al., (1974) studied the effect of $FeSO_4$, $CuSO_4$ and $CaCl_2$ on the browning reaction. They reported that at $72^{\circ}C$, color development caused by ascorbic acid and tryptophan was enhanced by the presence of $FeSO_4$, $CuSO_4$ and $NaHPO_4$ while $CaCl_2$ reduced the browning extent in model systems. Smith and Cline (1984) studied the relationship between calcium sources and browning in apple juice. It was found that when $CaCl_2$ was added to freshly pressed apple juice at a level of 0.2 mg/100ml, the browning reaction slowed significantly. Fry and Stegink (1982) studied the effect of electrolytes on the Maillard reaction in parenteral alimentation solutions at different temperatures. They used Na acetate, KCl, NaCl, $MgSO_4$, K_3PO_4 and Calcium gluconate. Their results showed that addition of electrolytes increased the extent of browning. Recently, Massaro and Labuza (1988) studied the effect of electrolyte on browning in total parenteral solution during a period of storage for up to six months. Using 95% confidence intervals, the authors concluded that the effect of electrolytes on the rate of brown color formation was not statistically significant except for the lysine plus tryptophan system. However the general trend was that the average rate constant was higher without addition of electrolytes.

ACKNOWLEDGEMENTS

Part of the information in the paper was conducted under a grant from the National Science Foundation (#NSF/CBT - 851 2914) and from the University of Minnesota Agricultural Experiment Station (18-78). One author (A. Kaanane) was supported for his studies by a joint US AID/Hassan II University Rabat, Morocco. We also wish to thank Dr. A. Moscowitz of the University of Minnesota Chemistry Department for help on the FTIR work.

REFERENCES

Adrian J (1982). The Maillard reaction. In Handbook of Nutritive Value of Processed Food, Volume I: Food for Human Use. CRC Press, Inc. Boca Raton, Florida, pp 529-609.

Ann. (1986). Sulfites as food ingredients. Food Technol. 40(6):47-52.

Arnold R (1969). Inhibition of heated-induced browning of milk by L-cysteine. J. Dairy Sci. 52(11):1857-1859.

Ashoor SH, Zent JB (1984). Maillard browning of common amino acids and sugars. J. Food Sci 49:1206-1207.

Buera Md, Chirife J, Resnik SL, Wetzler G (1987). Nonenzymatic browning in liquid model systems of high water activity: Kinetics of color changes due to Maillard's reaction between different single sugars and glycine and comparison with caramelization browning. J. Food Sci 42:1063-1067.

Bunn HF, Higgins PJ (1981). Reaction of monosaccharides

with proteins: possible evolutionary significance.
Science 213:222-224.

Burton HS, McWeeney DJ (1963). Nonenzymatic browning
reactions: Consideration of sugar stability. Nature
197:266-268.

Canter SM, Peniston QP (1940). The reduction of aldose at
the dropping mercury cathode: Estimation of the
aldehydo structure in aqueous solutions. JAOC 62:2113-
2121.

Duckworth RB (1981). Solute mobility in relation to water
content and water activity. In Rockland L (ed): "Water
Activity: Influence on Food Quality". Academic Press
New York 215-237.

Eichner K, Karel M (1972). The influence of water content
and water activity on the sugar - amino reaction inn
model systems under various conditions. J. Agr. Food
Chem. 20:218.

Ellis GP (1959). The Maillard reaction. Adv. Carb. Chem.
14:63-134.

Eriksson C (1981). Maillard reaction in foods. Pergamon
Press, New York.

FDA (1986). "Sulfiting agents: Revocation of GRAS status
for use on fruits and vegetables intended to be served
or sold raw to consumers". Federal Register 51:25021-
25198.

Feeney RE, Blankenhorn G, Dixon HBF (1975). Carbohydrate-
Amine reactions in protein chemistry. Adv. Protein
Chem. 29:135-203.

Feeney RE, Whitaker JR (1982). The Maillard reaction and
its prevention. In Cherry JP (ed)"Food Protein
Deterioration, Mechanisms and Functionality.". ACS
Symposium Series 206, ACS, Washington, D.C., pp 201-229.

Franks F, Hall JR, Irish DE, Norris K (1986). The effect
of cations on the anomeric equilibrium of D-glucose in
aqueous solution. A Raman-spectral study. Carbohydr.
Res. 157:53-64.

Fry LK, Stegink Ld (1982). Formation of Maillard reaction
products in parenteral alimentation solutions. J.
Nutr. 112:1631-1637.

Grant JP, Cox CE, Kleinman LM, Naher MM, Pittman MA,
Tangrea JA, Brown JH, Gross E, Beazley RM, Jones KS,
(1977). Serum hepatic enzyme and bilirubin elevation
during parenteral nutrition. Surg., Gyne., and obst.
145:573-580.

Hayward LD, Angyal SJ (1977). Asymmetry rule for the
circular dichroism of reducing sugars, and the

proportion of carbonyl forms in aqueous solutions thereof. Carbohydr. Res. 53:13-20.

Hodge JE (1953). Dehydrated foods. Chemistry of browning reactions in model systems. J. Arg. Food Chem. 1(15): 928-943.

Kaanane A, Labuza TP (1985). Change in available lysine loss reaction rate in fish flour due to an a_w change induced by a temperature shift. J. Food Sci. 50:582-584.

Kaanane A, Kane D, Labuza TP (1988). Time temperature effect on stability of Moroccan processed orange juice during storage. J. Food Sci. 53:1-4.

Kato H, Yamamoto M, Fujimaki M (1969). Mechanisms of browning degradation of D-fructose in special comparison with D-glucose glycine reaction. Agr. Biol. Chem. 33:939-940.

Kleinman LM, Tangrea JA, Gallelli JF, Brown JH, Gross E (1973). Stability of solutions of essential amino acids. Am. J. Hosp. Pharm. 30:1054-1057.

Labuza TP, Schmidl MK (1986). Advances in the control of browning reactions in foods. In Fennema O, Chang WH, Lii C (eds): "Role of Chemistry in the quality of Processed foods". Food and Nutrition Press, Wesport, Connecticut, pp 85-95.

Labuza TP, Warren K, Warmbier HC (1977). The physical aspect with respect to water and nonenzymatic browning. In "Nutritional Biochemical consequences of protein cross linking. Adv. Exp. Med. Biol. 86B:379.

Labuza TP, Saltmarch M (1981a). The nonenzymatic browning reaction as affected by water in foods. In Rockland L (ed): "Water activity: Influences on Food Quality," Academic Press, New York pp 605-650.

Labuza TP, Saltmarch M (1981b). Kinetics of browning and quality loss in whey powders during steady state and non-steady state storage conditions. J. Food Sci. 47:92-96.

Labuza TP (1984). Application of Chemical kinetics to the deterioration of foods. J. Chem. Ed. 61:348.

Lea CH, Hannan RS (1950). Studies on the reaction between proteins and reducing sugars in the "dry" state. 2. Further observations on the formation of the casein-glucose complex. Biochim. Biophys. Acta 4:518-531.

Lee HS, Sen LC, Clifford AJ, Whitaker JR, Feeney RE (1978). Effect of reductive alkylation of the Ë-amino group of lysyl residue of casein on its nutritive value in rats. J. Nutr. 180:687-696.

Maillard LC (1912). Action des acides, amines sur les

sucres: formation des melanodines par voie methodo-
logique. CR Acad. Sci. 154:66.

Massaro S, Labuza TP (1988). Browning and amino acid
losses in model total parenteral nutrition systems, with
specific reference to cysteine. Submitted for publication.

McWeeny DJ (1973). The role of carbohydrates in non-
enzymatic browning. In Birch G G, Green LF (eds):
"Molecular Structure and Function of Food Carbohydrate",
John Wiley and Sons. New York - Toronto, pp 21-32.

McWeeny DJ, Knowles ME, Hearne JF (1974). The chemistry of
non-enzymatic browning in foods and its control by
sulfites. J. Sci. Food Agric. 25:735-746

Modderman JP (1986). Technological aspects of use of
sulfiting agents in food. J. Assoc. off. Anal. Chem.
69(1):1-3.

Montgomery MW (1983). Cysteine as an inhibitor of browning
in pear juice concentrate. J. Food Sci. 48:951-952.

Nagy S, Dinsmore HL (1974). Relationship of furfural to
temperature abuse and flavor change in commercially
canned single-strength orange juice. J. Food Sci. 39:
1116-1119.

Pigman W, Isbell H (1968). Mutarotation of sugars
solution: part I. Adv. Carbohydr. chem. 23:11-20.

Pigman W, Anet EFLJ (1972). Mutarotation and actions of
acids and bases. In Pigman W, Horton D (eds): "The
Carbohydrates, Chemistry and Biochemistry", Academic
press, New York, San Francisco, London, pp 165-194.

Pomeranz Y, Johnson JA, Schellenberger JA (1962). Effect
of various sugars on browning. J. Food Sci. 29:350.

Schemidl MK, Massaro SS, Labuza TP (1988). Parenteral and
enteral food systems. Food Technol. 42:77-87.

Schroeder LJ, Iacobellis M, Smith AH (1955). The influence
of water and pH on the reaction between amino compounds
and carbohydrates. J. Biol. Chem 212:973-983.

Smith RB, Cline RA (1984). A laboratory and field study on
the relationship between calcium sources and browning
in apple juice. J. Food Sci. 49:1419-1421.

Song PS, Chichester CO (1967a). Kinetics behavior and
mechanism of inhibition in the Maillard reaction. IV.
Mechanism of inhibitors. J. Food Sci. 32:107-115.

Song PS, Chichester CO (1967b). Kinetic behavior and
mechanism of inhibition in the Maillard reaction. III.
Kinetic behavior and the inhibition in the reaction
between D-glucose and glycine. J. Food Sci. 32:98-106.

Thomas MA (1969). Browning reaction in cheddar cheese.

Aust. J. Dairy Technol. Dec:185-189.

Underwood JC, Lento Jr HG, Willits CO (1959). Browning of sugar solutions. Effect of pH on the color produced in dilute glucose solutions containing amino acids with the amino group in different positions in the molecule. Food Res. 24:181-184.

Villota, R, Saguy I, Karel M (1980). Storage stability of dehydrated food: Evaluation of literature data. J. Food Quality 3:123-216.

Waller G,, Feather M (1983). The maillard reaction in foods and nutrition. ACS Symposium Series 215.

Warmbier HC, Schnickels RA, Labuza TP (1976). Nonenzymatic browning kinetics in an intermediate moisture model system: Effect of glucose to lysine ration. J. Food Sci. 41:981-983.

Wedzicha BL (1987). Review: Chemistry of Sulfur Dioxide in vegetable dehydration. Int. J. Food Sci. Technol. 22:433-450.

Wedzicha BL, Kaputo MT (1987). Reaction of melanoidins with sulfur dioxide: stoichiometry of the reaction. Int. J. Food Sci. Technol. 22:643-651.

Wertz PW, Garver JC, Anderson L (1981). Anatomy of a complex mutarotation. Kinetics of tautomerization of -D-galactopyranose and ß-D-galactopyranose in water. J. Am Chem. Soc. 103:3916-3922.

Wolfrom ML, Kashimura N, Horton D (1974). Factors affecting the Maillard browning reaction between sugars and amino acids. Studies on the nonenzymatic browning of de-hydrated orange juice. J. Agr. Food Chem. 22:796-800.

Yu MH, Wu MT, Wang DJ, Salunkhe DK (1974). Nonenzymatic browning in synthetic systems containing ascorbic acid, amino acids, organic acids, and inorganic salts. J. Inst. CAN Sci. Technol. Aliment. 7:279-282.

The Maillard Reaction in Aging,
Diabetes, and Nutrition, pages 329–342
© 1989 Alan R. Liss, Inc.

EFFECT OF MAILLARD REACTION PRODUCTS ON PROTEIN DIGESTION

Rickard Öste

Department of Nutrition, Chemical Center, University of
Lund, P.O. Box 124, 221 00 Lund, Sweden.

ABSTRACT. A summary is given of experiments
performed to study the effects of Maillard
reaction products on protein digestion and
uptake. A double-isotope technique was used to
evaluate the impact of compounds formed in the
Maillard reaction on the intestinal uptake of
dietary proteins in rats. It was found that
low-molecular weight compounds from a glucose-
lysine reaction mixture reduced the plasma
level of dietary protein-derived lysine. The
reaction mixture inhibited in vitro carboxypeptidase A (E.C. 3.4.17.1) and the brush
border enzyme aminopeptidase N (E.C.
3.4.11.2). A glucose-lysine reaction compound,
2-formyl-5-(hydroxymethyl)pyrrole-1-norleucine
was found to be a strong competitive inhibitor
of aminopeptidase N (Ki = 0.2mM) in vitro.
When given to rats (3 mg/g diet), it reduced
the plasma level of lysine derived from both
dietary free and protein-bound lysine. This
compound also inhibited carboxypeptidase A, as
did a number of substituted furans and pyrroles.

INTRODUCTION

The inherent nutritive value of a protein is characterized by its amino acid composition and the in vivo digestibility, as outlined in the FAO/WHO report on protein and
energy requirements (1985). Food processing may alter the
protein nutritive value from both these points of view.
Heating may increase or decrease the protein digestibility
(Hung et al, 1984; Fapojuwo et al, 1987; Semino and Cerletti, 1987; Hamaker, 1986; Chung et al, 1986) and may alter
the content of essential amino acid (review: Mauron, 1982).

During conditions favoring the Maillard reaction, loss
of biological availability of the essential amino acid,
lysine, is likely to occur as the result of the early reaction steps. This nutritional effect of the Maillard reaction
has been the subject of extensive reviews by Adrian (1982),
and Mauron (1981). Lysine may be lost especially in foodstuffs with a high content of reducing carbohydrates such as
milk (Finot, 1981) and, particularly, lactose hydrolyzed
milk (Burvall et al., 1977). The nutritional disadvantage of
the reduction in available lysine in a foodstuff will depend
on the overall amino acid composition of the diet and, in
practice, also on who the consumer is, because the need of
essential amino acids varies with age (FAO/WHO, 1985). This
means that, from the point of view of amino acid composition, a certain reduction of lysine availability, i.e, a
certain degree of Maillard reaction, may be tolerable as
long as there is no other adverse effect resulting from the
heating. However, the severe Maillard reaction may also
reduce the overall protein digestibility (Chung et al.,
1986, Kneipfel, 1981; Sgarbieri et al., 1973) leading to a
generally lowered protein utilization that may not be com-
pensated for by the addition of lysine or protein complemen-
tation.

The reason for the reduced protein digestibility may be
attributed to changes in protein solubility and the formation of cross-links, which may follow the Maillard reaction
(Kato et al, 1987, 1986). Indirect effects of the Maillard
reaction on protein utilization have been suggested by
Adrian (1974), who claims that water-soluble "premelanoidins" reduce the protein digestibility and also affect the
utilization of absorbed amino acids. Valle-Riestra and
Barnes (1970) attributed the reduced uptake of a severely
heated glucose-egg albumen mixture to a decreased pancreatic

enzyme secretion. However, no direct evidence for the responsible mechanisms has been presented.

Experiments will be summarized that were performed to increase the understanding of how the Maillard reaction may affect the protein nutritive value of foods. Studies were made with a glucose-lysine reaction mixture and with pure compounds and both in vivo on rats and in vitro with proteolytic enzymes. The detailed methodology and the results have been published (Öste et al., 1987; Öste et al. 1986; Öste and Sjödin, 1984).

METHODS

To manufacture a model Maillard reaction mixture, equimolar amounts of glucose and lysine were boiled at pH 6.5 for 24 hours. The mixture was separated into a low-molecular weight (MW < 6,000-8,000 daltons) and a high-molecular weight fraction. Pure Maillard reaction compounds were synthesized, essentially according to the literature, or when available, purchased.

To specifically study the digestion of exogenous protein in rats, a methodology was developed as follows: A solution of a radioactive amino acid (U-^{14}C-lysine, 3,4-^{3}H-lysine or ^{35}S-cystine) was injected into the wing vein of a laying hen. The eggs were recovered, the egg white separated and dialyzed and then lyophilized. Autoradiographic studies on TLC-separated acid hydrolyzates of the egg white showed that the ^{14}C- or ^{3}H-radioactivity present was almost exclusively derived from protein-bound lysine. These labeled proteins were then used to prepare nutritionally balanced diets with a protein content of 10%, containing differently labelled free lysine or protein-bound lysine, or, on one occasion, protein-bound ^{35}S-cystine and protein-bound ^{3}H-lysine. A portion of the diet, with or without the addition of Maillard reaction compounds, was given to fasting, growing rats (weight 100-120g) early in the morning to be consumed *ad libitum*. Only rats that consumed the portion within 15 min were included in the study. Radioactivity was measured in the plasma of blood samples obtained after feeding. In particular, the ratio between different typse of labeling was determined.

The effects of added Maillard reaction products on the activities of pepsin, trypsin, chymotrypsin and carboxypeptidases A and B were measured with commercially obtained enzymes. The effects on the activities of brush border and cytosolic peptidases were studied with crude preparations of the enzymes from pig intestine (Sjöström et al., 1978) using enzyme specific substrates. Kinetic experiments on aminopeptidase N were performed with the purified enzyme, prepared as described by Sjöström et al. (1978).

STUDIES ON A GLUCOSE-LYSINE REACTION MIXTURE

Totally, 1.5% (w/w) of the low molecular weight fraction from the glucose-lysine reaction mixture was added to the diet containing free ^{3}H-lysine and protein-bound ^{14}C-lysine. This resulted in a statistically significant reduction (13%) of the ratio of ^{14}C to ^{3}H in plasma two hours after feeding compared with the control diet (no addition) (Table 1; Öste and Sjödin, 1984). In a second experiment, 1.5% of the low-molecular weight fraction was added to a diet containing protein-bound radiolabelled lysine (^{3}H) and cysteine (^{35}S). The ratio between these two labels in plasma was not different from that obtained with the control diet without Maillard compounds (Table 1).

TABLE 1. Ratio of radioactivity (dpm) in the plasma of rats two hours after ingestion of radiolabeled free lysine or protein-bound cystine and protein-bound lysine.

Radioisotope diet	Ratio of labels in plasma
Free ^{3}H-lysine mixed with ^{14}C-lysine labeled egg white	^{14}C/^{3}H
+ 1.5% LMW fraction (7)	0.102* r=9.8
Control (6)	0.117 r=12.0
^{3}H-lysine- and ^{35}S-cystein-labeled egg white	^{35}S/^{3}H
+ 1.5% LMW fraction (8)	0.233 r=4.7
Control (7)	0.235 r=6.4

*Value significantly different from control (p<0.05, Student's t-test). r=coefficient of variation. Within parenthesis: number of rats. LMW: Low-molecular weight Maillard reaction products. From Öste and Sjödin, (1984).

The design of the double-isotope study of dietary effects on the digestion of exogenous protein was based on the assumption that any change in the ratio of the level of radioactivity in the plasma arising from respectively dietary free and protein-bound lysine reflects a change in the rate or degree of protein digestion. Because all the other factors that may affect the level of amino acids in the plasma (see Eggum, 1973; Young and Scrimshaw, 1972) apparently were identical in both the experimental and the control group, this should be a reasonable supposition. Further , it is reasonable to assume that the recorded radioactivity in the plasma originates from the presence of free amino acids. Although this may not be a requirement for the validity of the assay, studies by Dawson and Porter (1962) indicate this to be a fact. They performed experiments with rats fed ^{14}C-labeled protein and found that the radioactivity of portal and systemic plasmas were almost exclusively due to free amino acids even 3 hours after feeding. The results were thus interpreted as an interference by the Maillard reaction products with the intestinal digestion of dietary protein and/or the absorption of liberated peptides.

Experiments were performed to examine whether the low molecular weight glucose-lysine reaction mixture inhibited enzymes of the gastrointestinal proteolysis. Activity measurements in the presence of this mixture (0.25-1.0 mg/mL) revealed that the pancreatic enzyme carboxypeptidase A and the brush border membrane enzyme aminopeptidase N (EC 3.4.11.2) were strongly inhibited. The activities of pepsin, trypsin, chymotrypsin, carboxypeptidase B, aminopeptidase A (EC 3.4.11.7), dipeptidylpeptidase IV (EC 3.4.14.5) as well as the cytosolic glycylleucine dipeptidase (EC 3.4.13.11) and alanylproline dipeptidase (E.C. 3.4.13.9) were unaffected by these concentrations of the glucose-lysine reaction mixture (Öste et al, 1986). Inhibition of aminopeptidase N was of the mixed type, whereas inhibition of carboxypeptidase A did not follow classical enzyme kinetics (Fig. 1).

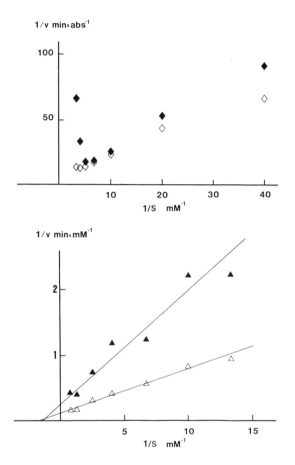

Figure 1. Effect of the low-molecular weight fraction of the glucose-lysine reaction mixture on enzyme kinetics. Reciprocal plots of velocity (v) versus substrate concentration (S). Upper figure: Hydrolysis of N-hippuryl-L-phenylalanine by carboxypeptidase A (in 0.1 M Na-borate, 0.3 M NaCl, pH 7.6 at 30 °C). Filled symbols: Addition of 0.5 mg/mL of the glucose-lysine reaction mixture. Open symbols: No addition. Lower figure: Hydrolysis of L-alanyl-p-nitroanilide by aminopeptidase N (in 0.05 M Tris-HCl, pH 7.3 at 37 °C). Filled symbols: Addition of 0.25 mg/mL of the glucose-lysine reaction mixture (Km 0.7 mM, Vmax 40 mMxmin^{-1}). Open symbols: No addition (Km 0.5 mM, Vmax 80 mMxmin^{-1}). From Öste et al. (1986).

The significant finding of the *in vitro* experiments in relation to the *in vivo* observations may perhaps be the inhibition of aminopeptidase N. The present view of protein digestion focuses attention on the role of peptidases of the small intestine in protein digestion (Kim and Erickson, 1986), recognizing that perhaps 50% of the amino acids that escape the action of pancreatic enzymes are still peptide-bound (Chung, 1979). Of the brush border membrane peptidases, aminopeptidase N is found in highest concentration (Sjöström et al., 1978), and this enzyme has been shown to play a central role in the final peptide digestion in rats (Friedrich et al., 1980a,b).

Further studies on fractions of the low-molecular weight glucose-lysine reaction mixture revealed that a number of compounds present in the mixture inhibited carboxypeptidase A and aminopeptidase N. 2-formyl-5(hydroxymethyl)pyrrole-1-norleucine, a compound that had been isolated from a glucose-lysine reaction mixture by Miller et al. (1980), was identified as the major component in one strongly inhibiting fraction.

STUDIES ON SINGLE MAILLARD REACTION COMPOUNDS

Synthetic 2-formyl-5(hydroxymethyl)pyrrole-1-norleucine was found to be a strong inhibitor of both carboxypeptidase A and aminopeptidase N. A number of chemically related compounds were then assayed to uncover typical features of Maillard reaction products that may possess inhibitory properties (Fig.2; Öste et al., 1987).

Various substituted furans and pyrroles inhibited carboxypeptidase A. Because the inhibition did not accord with classical theory of enzyme kinetics (Dixon and Webb, 1966), the relative strength of the inhibitors was subjectively evaluated from the shape of the initial velocity/substrate concentration curves (Fig. 2 and Fig. 3). The strongest inhibitors were furans with a carboxylic group as a substituent, and the addition of 0.1 mM 5-(hydroxymethyl)-2-furoic acid or 2-furoic acid abolished the activity of carboxypeptidase A at high substrate concentrations. These two compounds may be formed through oxidation of the well-known Maillard reaction products 5-(hydroxymethyl)-2-furaldehyde (HMF) and 2-furaldehyde (Pernemalm, 1978). In addition, some pyrroles were found to be potent inhibitors of carboxypeptidase A (compounds 1,3 and 6 in Fig.2).

Structure a (pyrrole/furan), structure b (pyridine), and structure 20:

$$H_3N^+-CH-CO_2^-$$ with $(CH_2)_4$ chain linked to $N-CH_2-CH(OH)$ and furanose ring bearing OH groups — **20**

| | | | structure a | | | inhibition (K_i, mM) | |
compd	X	R_1	R_2	name		carboxy-peptidase A	amino-peptidase N
1	N(CH$_2$)$_4$CH(NH$_2$)CO$_2$H	CHO	CH$_2$OH	DL-2-formyl-5-(hydroxymethyl)pyrrole-1-norleucine		**	competitive (0.2)
2	NH	CHO	CH$_2$OH	5-(hydroxymethyl)pyrrole-2-carboxaldehyde		**	–
3	NH	CHO	H	pyrrole-2-carboxaldehyde		*	–
4	NH	CHO	CHO	pyrrole-2,5-dicarboxaldehyde		*	–
5	NH	CHO	CH$_3$	5-methylpyrrole-2-carboxaldehyde		**	–
6	NH	COCH$_3$	H	2-acetylpyrrole		*	–
7	NCH$_2$CO$_2$H	CH$_3$	CH$_3$	2,5-dimethylpyrrole-1-acetic acid		*	competitive (0.6)
8	NCH$_2$CO$_2$H	H	H	pyrrole-1-acetic acid		–	competitive (4)
9	O	CHO	CH$_2$OH	5-(hydroxymethyl)-2-furaldehyde		*	–
10	O	CHO	H	2-furaldehyde		**	–
11	O	CO$_2$H	H	2-furoic acid		***	weak
12	O	CO$_2$H	CH$_3$	5-methyl-2-furoic acid		***	weak
13	O	CO$_2$H	CH$_2$OH	5-(hydroxymethyl)-2-furoic acid		***	–

| | | | structure b | | inhibition | |
compd	R_1	R_2	R_3	name	carboxypeptidase A	aminopeptidase N
14	H	CH$_3$	OH	2-methyl-3-pyridinol	–	–
15	CH$_3$	H	OH	6-methyl-3-pyridinol	*	–
16	H	CH$_3$	H	2-methylpyridine	*	NA

| | | inhibition | |
compd	name	carboxy-peptidase A	amino-peptidase N
17	levulic acid	*	–
18	propionic acid	–	NA

| | | inhibition | |
compd	name	carboxy-peptidase A	amino-peptidase N
19	α-hydroxypropionic acid	NA	weak
20	1-deoxy-1-2-N-(L-lysino)-D-fructose	–	–

Figure 2. Inhibition of carboxypeptidase A (strenght propotional to number of asterisks) and aminopeptidase N by compounds formed in, or similar to those formed in the Maillard reaction. No inhibition: – , not assayed: NA. From Öste et al. (1987).

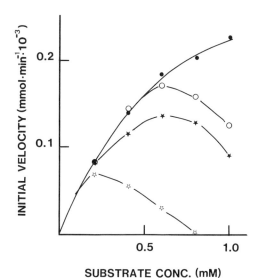

Figure 3. Effect of additions of 2-furaldehyde (0.4 mM, ✶), 5-(hydroxymethyl)-2-furoic acid (0.1mM, ✩), or 6-methyl-3-pyridinol (0.4 mM, ○), on the velocity of hydrolysis of N-hippuryl-L-phenylalanine by carboxypeptidase A (in 0.1 M Na-borate, 0.3 M NaCl, pH 7.6 at 30 °C). ●: no addition. From Öste et al. (1987).

Six of the examined compounds exhibited inhibitory properties when assayed with aminopeptidase N. Three of these were N-substituted pyrroles. The most notable inhibition was observed with the originally identified 2-formyl-5(hydroxymethyl)pyrrole-1-norleucine (K_i = 0.2 mM). The inhibition was competitive. Because the glucose-lysine reaction mixture was a mixed-type inhibitor of aminopeptidase N, assays were made to identify a noncompetitive or mixed type inhibitor. In spite of the considerable efforts put into this, such compounds could not be detected in fractions from a glucose-lysine reaction mixture that was examined for new Maillard reaction products (Miller et al., 1984).

The question that now arose was whether Maillard compounds with known in vitro enzyme inhibitory capacities in fact would affect the in vivo utilization of protein. To study this, a small amount of 2-formyl-5(hydroxymethyl)pyrrole-1-norleucine (3 mg/g diet) was added to the experimental diet containing radiolabeled free and protein-bound lysine (see above).

The results (Table 2) showed a small (10%), but statistically significant, reduction of the absolute levels of
both isotopes in the plasma after feeding, but no difference
in the ratio of the labels, as compared with the control. An
explanation of this observation would be an effect on the
absorption of lysine by the added compound. Because neutral
amino acids are known to act as competitive inhibitors of
the active lysine transport (Hellier and Holdsworth, 1975),
2-formyl-5(hydroxymethyl)pyrrole-1-norleucine, being also a
neutral amino acid, may act in the same way.

Addition of a strong inhibitor of carboxypeptidase A,
2-furoic acid, to the diet did not significantly affect the
plasma levels of radioactivity.

TABLE 2. The radioactivity in plasma of rats three hours
from feeding an experimental diet containing radiolabeled
free (^{3}H)- and protein bound (^{14}C)-lysine with or without
the addition of single Maillard reaction compounds.

	(^{3}H)		(^{14}C)		(^{14}C/^{3}H)	
	Mean	SD	Mean	SD	Mean ratio	SD
Control diet (7)	29,057	1365	12,646	940	0.438	0.020
Addition of compound 1 (7)	26,307*	2186	11,589*	819	0.427	0.037
Addition of compound 11 (7)	27,877	1871	11,860	720	0.442	0.031

*Significantly different from control (P<0.05, Student's
t-test). Values are dpm/mL. SD: standard deviation. Within
parenthesis: number of rats. Names and structures of compounds 1 and 11 in Figure 2. From Öste et al. (1987).

The enzyme inhibitory compounds that were identified,
substituted furans and pyrroles, are commonly found Maillard
reaction products. Furans are formed also in the caveiza-
tion reaction of carbohydrates, although the presence of

amines catalyze their formation (Feeney et al., 1975). N-un-substituted pyrroles are assumed to be formed via a reaction pathway that includes Strecker degradation of free amino acids (Nyhammar et al., 1983). In food, protein-bound amino groups are more likely to be the dominant amino reactant in the Maillard reaction. This would favor the formation of N-substituted pyrroles, as indicated by studies of Olsson et al. (1977, 1978) on glucose reactions with glycine or methylamine.

It is thus to be expected that compounds such as the inhibitor 2-formyl-5(hydroxymethyl)pyrrole-1-norleucine may be present in heated foodstuffs. Direct measurements of the concentration of this compound in foods have in fact recent-ly been performed (Chiang, 1988). Levels varied between 1 and 200 ppm in nonheated and heated food samples to be com-pared with the concentration of 3,000 ppm in the diet of the in vivo experiment performed by us. Chiang made the analysis on warm-water extracts of the food samples, i.e., the analy-ses were performed on the free compound. It is reasonable to assume that additional 2-formyl-5(hydroxymethyl)pyrrole-1-norleucine may be formed with protein bound lysine and that the total content in the food may have been considerably higher. Nevertheless, it is likely that the concentration of any specific pyrrole or furan formed in heated foodstuffs is very low compared with reactant concentrations, as indicated by the yields from model reactions mixtures (Olsson et al., 1977, 1978, Miller et al., 1984). The amount of any single, inhibiting Maillard reaction product in foods is probably insufficient to bring about an effect on digestion *in vivo*. However, the combined effect of a number of various inhibi-tors formed in a severely heated foodstuff may be sufficient to affect the dietary protein utilization.

CONCLUSIONS

Compounds formed in the Maillard reaction may influence the utilization of dietary proteins in rats. This effect may be the result of an inhibition of enzymes involved in the digestion and uptake of proteins in the intestine, especial-ly aminopeptidase N of the brush border. The concentrations of identified inhibitors are, however, probably low in heated foodstuffs, and it is unclear to what extent they would, in fact, contribute to a reduced protein uptake from such products.

REFERENCES

Adrian J, (1982). The Maillard reaction. In Rechcigl M Jr, (ed): "Handbook of Nutritive Value of Processed Food," Vol 1, Boca Raton, FL: CRC Press, pp 529-608.

Adrian J, (1974). Nutritional and physiological consequences of the Maillard reaction. Wld Rev Nutr Diet 19: 71-122.

Burvall A, Asp NG, Dahlqvist A, Öste R (1977). Nutritional value of lactose-hydrolysed milk: protein quality after some industrial processes. J Dairy Res 44: 549-553.

Chiang GH (1988). High-Performance Liquid Chromatographic Determination of -Pyrrole-lysine in Processed Food. J Agric Food Chem 36: 506-509.

Chung YC, Kim YS, Shadcher A, Garrido A, Mac Gregor IL, Sleisenger MH (1979). Protein digestion and absorption in human small intestine. Gastroent 76:1415-1421.

Chung SY, Swaisgood HE, Castignani GL (1986). Effects of Alkali Treatment and Heat Treatment in the Presence of Fructose on Digestibility of Foof Proteins as Determined by an Immobilized Digestive Enzyme Assay (IDEA). J Agric Food Chem 34:579-584.

Dawson R, Porter JWG (1962). An investigation into protein digestion with ^{14}C-labelled protein. 2. The transport of ^{14}C-labelled nitrogenous compounds in the rat and cat. Br J Nutr 16:27-38.

Dixon M, Webb EC (1966). "Enzymes". London: Longmans, Green and Co.

Eggum BO (1973). The Levels of Blood Amino Acids and Blood Urea as Indicators of Protein Quality. In Porter JWG, Rolls BA (eds): "Protein in Human Nutrition," London: Academic Press, pp 317-327.

FAO/WHO/UNU (1985) "Energy and protein requirements" WHO Technical Report Series, Geneva: WHO.

Fapojuwo OO, Maga JA, Jansen GR (1987). Effect of Extrusion Cooking on in vitro Protein Digestibility of Sorghum. J Food Science 52:218-219.

Feeney RE, Blankenhorn G, Dixon HBF (1975). Carbonyl-amine reactions in protein chemistry. Adv Prot Chem 29: 135-203.

Finot PA, Deutsch R, Bujard E (1981). The Extent of the Maillard Reaction during the Processing of Milk. In Eriksson C (ed):"Maillard Reactions in Food," Progress in Food and Nutrition Science Vol 5(1-6), Oxford: Pergamon Press, pp 345-356.

Friedrich M, Schenk G, Noack R (1980a). Studies on the physiological importance of the microvilli-bound leucine arylamidase in the final digestion of protein. Part I. Nahrung 24:727-734.

Friedrich M, Uhlig J, Schenk G, Noack R (1980b). Studies on the physiological importance of the microvilli-bound leucine arylamidase in the final digestion of protein. Part II. Nahrung 24:735-740.

Hamaker BR, Kirleis AW, Mertz ET, Axtell JD (1986). Effect of Cooking on the Protein Profiles and in Vitro Diestibility of Sorghum and Maize. J Agric Food Chem 34:647-649.

Hellier MD, Holdsworth CD (1975). Digestion and Absorption of Proteins. In McColl I, Sladen GEG (eds): "Intestinal Absorption in Man," London: Academic Press, pp 143-186.

Hung ND, Cseke E, Vas M, Szabolcsi G (1984). Processed Protein Foods Characterized by In Vitro Digestion Rates. J Food Science 49:1535-1542.

Kato H, Cho RK, Okitani A, Hayase F (1987). Responsibility of 3-Deoxyglucosone for the Glucose-Induced Polymerization of Proteins. Agric Biol Chem 51:683-689.

Kato Y, Matsuda T, Kato N, Watanabe K, Nakamura R (1986). Browning and Insolubilization of Ovalbumin by the Maillard Reaction with Some Aldohexoses. J Agric Food Chem 34: 351-355.

Kim YS, Erickson RH (1985). Role of Peptidases of the Human Small Intestine in Protein Digestion. Gastroent 88: 1071-1073.

Kenipfel JE (1981). Nitrogen and Energy Availabilities in Foods and Feeds Subjected to Heating. In Eriksson C (ed):"Maillard Reactions in Food," Prog Food Nutr Sci Vol 5(1-6), Oxford: Pergamon Press, pp 177-192.

Mauron J (1982) Effect of processing on nutritive value of food:protein. In Rechcigl M Jr, (ed): "Handbook of Nutritive Value of Processed Food," Vol 1, Boca Raton, FL: CRC Press, pp 429-471.

Mauron J (1981) The Maillard Reaction in Food; A Critical Review from the Nutritional Standpoint. In Eriksson C (ed):"Maillard Reactions in Food," Progress in Food and Nutrition Science Vol 5(1-6), Oxford: Pergamon Press, pp 5-36.

Miller R, Olsson K, Pernemalm PÅ (1984). Formation of Aromatic Compounds from Carbohydrates.IX. Reaction of d-Glucose and l-Lysine in Slightly Acidic, Aqueous Solution. Acta Chem Scand B38:689-694.

Miller R, Olsson K, Pernemalm PÅ, Theander O, (1980). Studies on the Maillard Reaction. In Marshall J, (ed): "Mechanisms of Saccharide Polymerization/Depolymerization," New York: Academic Press, pp 421-430.

Nyhammar T, Olsson K, Pernemalm PÅ (1983) On the formation of 2-Acylpyrroles and 3-pyridinols in the Maillard Reaction through Strecker Degradation. Acta Chem Scand B37: 879-889.

Olsson K, Pernemalm, PÅ, Popoff T, Theander O (1977). Formation of Aromatic Compounds from Carbohydrates. V. Reaction of D-glucose and Methylamine in Slightly Acidic, Aqueous Solution. Acta Chem Scand B31:469-474.

Olsson K, Pernemalm PÅ, Theander O (1978). Formation of Aromatic Compounds from Carbohydrates. VII. Reaction of D-glucose and Glycine in Slightly Acidic, Aqueous Solution. Acta Chem Scand B32: 249-256.

Öste RE, Dahlqvist A, Sjöström H, Noren O, Miller R (1986). Effect of Maillard Reaction Products on Protein Digestion. In Vitro Studies. J Agric Food Chem 34:355-358.

Öste RE, Miller R, Sjöström H, Noren O (1987). Effect of Maillard Reaction Products on Protein Digestion. Studies on Pure Compounds. J Agric Food Chem 35:938-942.

Öste RE, Sjödin P (1984). Effect of Maillard Reaction Products on Protein Digestion. In Vivo Studies on Rats. J Nutr 114:2228-2234.

Pernemalm PÅ (1978). Studies on the Maillard Reaction. PhD thesis. Swedish University of Agricultural Sciences, Uppsala.

Semino GA, Cerletti P (1987). Effect of Preliminary Thermal Treatment on the Digestion by Trypsin of Lupin Seed Protein. J Agric Food Chem 35:656-660.

Sgarbieri VC, Amaya J, Tanaka M, Chichester CO (1973). Response of rats to amino acid supplementation of brown egg albumin. J Nutr 103:1731-1738.

Sjöström H, Noren O, Jeppesen L, Staun M, Svensson B, Christensen L (1978). Purification of Different Amphifilic Forms of a Microvillus Aminopeptidase from Pig Small Intestine Using Immuno-adsorbent Chromatography. Eur J Biochem 88:503-511.

Valle-Riestra J and Barnes RH (1970). Digestion of heat-damaged egg albumin by the rat. J Nutr 100:873-882.

Young V, Scrimshaw NS (1972). The Nutritional Significance of Plasma and Urinary Amino Acids. In Bigwood EJ (ed): "Protein and Amino Acid Functions," Oxford: Pergamon Press pp 541-569.

The Maillard Reaction in Aging,
Diabetes, and Nutrition, pages 343–358
© 1989 Alan R. Liss, Inc.

METABOLIC TRANSIT AND TOXICITY OF MAILLARD REACTION
PRODUCTS

Paul-André Finot and Diane E. Furniss

Nestec Ltd., Nestlé Research Centre, Vers-
chez-les-Blanc, CH-1000 Lausanne 26,
Switzerland.

ABSTRACT

The feeding of Maillard reaction products (MRP) has
been reported to lead to a variety of effects on metabolism
which may be classed as "anti-nutritional" or "anti-
physiological", depending on whether they are due to the
loss of essential nutrients or to the presence of the MRP
per se. This paper describes the sensitivity of essential
nutrients in the "early" and "advanced" stages of the
Maillard reaction, the metabolic transit of Amadori
compounds, premelanoidins, melanoidins, hydroxymethylfurfural, carboxymethyl-lysine, as well as the effects of
MRP on pancreatic amylase and on urinary zinc excretion.

INTRODUCTION

Maillard reactions in food proteins occur during
industrial processing and storage, but also during various
home-cooking procedures (Mauron, 1981). The formation of
amino-sugar condensation products and their derivatives may
alter the chemical profile of a food and decrease its
nutritional value. In many cases, and when only the early
stages of the reaction have occurred, the decreased
nutritional value may stem entirely from the loss of the
essential amino acid lysine, the most reactive of the amino
acids (Mauron, 1981; Hurrell, 1984). However, when the
reaction has proceeded to the advanced stages other amino
acids and nutrients may be lost.

The feeding of Maillard reaction products (MRP) to experimental animals has been reported to lead to a variety of effects on metabolism which have been classed as "anti-nutritional" or "anti-physiological" (Adrian, 1974). The word "toxic" is commonly misused for both effects. Experimentally these two types of effects are not easy to distinguish. This task may, however, be facilitated by the feeding of quantifiable levels of purified MRP, or of MRP formed under well-controlled reaction conditions in nutritionally adequate diets. A knowledge of the metabolic transit of the various categories of MRP may also be an invaluable aid to the interpretation of the experimental data.

The following paper will firstly review the major nutrient losses resulting from the Maillard reaction and secondly the absorption and metabolism of MRP. Finally, some experimental data which may help to understand the origin of the effect of MRP on pancreatic enzyme activity and on Zn metabolism will be discussed.

NUTRIENT LOSSES ACCOMPANYING THE MAILLARD REACTION

Lysine

The most important nutritional consequences of the Maillard reaction during the industrial processing of milk and milk-based products concern lysine (Finot, 1983; Hurrell, 1984). The participation of this amino acid in the so-called "early" and "advanced" stages of the Maillard reaction is summarised in Figure 1.

In practise it is important to note that high levels of the Amadori compound may be formed in the early Maillard reaction without any noticeable browning of the product. This is the case when milk powders are spray-dried. However, lysine is destroyed during the chemical degradation of the Amadori compounds in the advanced Maillard reaction and the food darkens. This is true when products are sterilised "in-can".

Figure 2a illustrates the two major stages of the Maillard reaction in a milk powder heated at 70°C. In the early stage the reactive lysine content decreases and the Amadori compound, lactose-lysine is formed but there is no destruction of lysine. In the later stages, lysine is destroyed as the Amadori compound degrades, and reacts further. The participation of lysine in the early, and the advanced stages of the Maillard reaction may be estimated by measurement of lysine, and of furosine, a derivative formed from the Amadori compound upon acid hydrolysis (Finot et al. 1981; Finot, 1983).

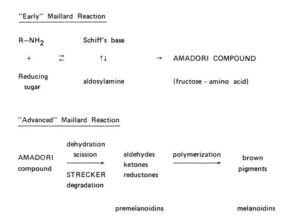

Figure 1 : "Early" and "Advanced" Maillard reaction stages in food systems

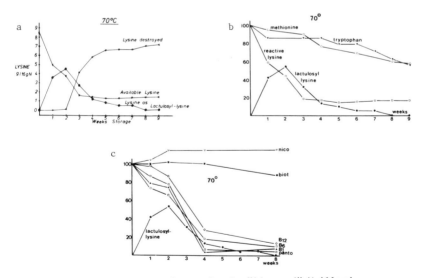

Figure 2 : Nutrient losses in the "Advanced" Maillard stage (a) Lysine, (b) Other amino acids, (c) vitamins

Advanced Maillard Derivatives

Model system melanoidins: The absorption and metabolism of the melanoidin fractions isolated from protein-sugar, or amino-acid-sugar model systems have been studied respectively by Finot and Magnenat (1981) and Nair et al (1981). The derivatives of low molecular-weight were partly absorbed at around 23-30% of the ingested dose. In contrast, the higher molecular-weight fractions were virtually unabsorbed.

Carboxymethyl lysine (CML): CML was first detected in the urine of human infants and is a normal constituent of human urine in small amounts (Wadman et al. 1975). This compound was later reported to be produced on incubation of proteins with glucose in the presence of oxygen (Baynes et al. 1986). Our own studies have demonstrated the presence of CML in the urine of rats fed heat-processed proteins containing either fructose-lysine (FL) or lysinoalanine (LAL) (Table 1) (Liardon et al. 1987).

Sample	Ingested protein
Whey protein	12 ± 3
Alkali-treated whey protein	250 ± 25
Casein control	7 ± 2
Casein + free LAL	12 ± 3
Casein control	12 ± 1
Maillardized casein (21% blocked lysine)	84 ± 13

Table 1 : Urinary excretion of carboxymethyl lysine

In theory both FL and LAL could be precursors of CML (Fig. 3); FL following its chemical and biological oxidation, and LAL upon in vivo deamination and decarboxylation. However, the detection of significant amounts of CML in the dietary protein, and the relatively low amounts of CML detected in the urine of rats fed LAL-rich diets led to the conclusion that dietary CML is the principle source of the urinary compound (Liardon et al. 1987).

Other amino acids

In the heated milk powder model (Fig. 2b) methionine and tryptophan were the first amino acids to react after lysine. These amino acids were stable in the early Maillard reaction but appeared to react with the degradation products of lysine formed in the advanced stages (Finot, 1983).

The B vitamins and pantothenic acid

The B vitamins (B1, B6 and B12), pantothenic acid and folic acid were progressively reduced with time of heating the heated milk powder (Fig. 2c). In contrast, nicotinic acid and biotin were found to be relatively insensitive to the heat treatment.

METABOLISM OF MAILLARD COMPOUNDS

Most of the data on the absorption and metabolic transit of MRP has been obtained from feeding experiments in the rat. Early and advanced Maillard derivatives have been studied either individually as the purified compounds, or as a group of substances formed in a model system and separated according to molecular-weight.

Early Maillard derivatives

Free Amadori compounds : Fructose-lysine, fructose-tryptophan, fructose-phenylalanine and fructose-methionine are well absorbed (20-70%) by the rat, and are excreted in the urine essentially non-modified (Finot and Magnenat, 1981; Tanaka et al. 1975; Perkins et al. 1981; Horn et al, 1968).

Protein-bound Amadori compounds : The metabolic transit of the protein-bound Amadori compounds, fructose-lysine and lactose-lysine has been studied in the rat (Finot and Magnenat, 1981). Around 12% of the ingested dose was absorbed. The unabsorbed fraction was found to be almost completely metabolised by the intestinal flora. The absorption of protein-bound Amadori compounds by the human infant has also been studied. Niederwieser et al. (1975) reported that around 16% and 55% of the dose ingested from a glucose-containing infant formula were excreted in the urine and faeces respectively.

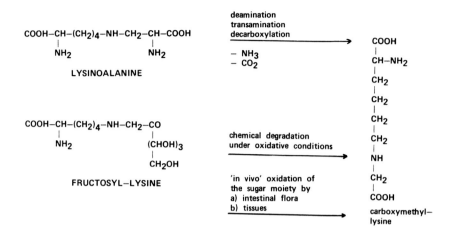

Figure 3 : Possible origin of carboxymethyl lysine

Hydroxymethyl fufural (HMF): HMF, one of the major products of the advanced Maillard reaction, may be formed upon 1-2 enolisation of the Amadori compound, or by the heat treatment of sugars (Feather, 1981). This derivative is present in numerous processed foods, particularly in sterilized milks (Mulchandani, et al, 1979) and glucose-containing parenteral nutrition solutions (Jellum et al. 1973).

Metabolic transit studies with ^{14}C-HMF have shown that this compound, irrespective of its mode of administration, is rapidly and almost completely excreted in the urine as one of two metabolites, hydroxymethyl furoic acid and its glycine conjugate hydroxymethyl furoyl glycine (Fig. 4) (Germond et al. 1987). This result was somewhat unexpected since in an earlier human study around 50% of an intra-venous dose of HMF was reported to be retained (Jellum et al. 1973). Germond et al. (1987) explain this difference by the fact that the glycine conjugate of HMF was not extractable by the procedure used by Jellum et al. (1973).

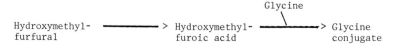

Figure 4 : Metabolism of hydroxymethyl furfural

EFFECTS OF MAILLARD COMPOUNDS ON METABOLISM

The major effects of the MRP on metabolism are outlined in table 2, along with current ideas on the origin of the effect, i.e. nutritional or specific.

		Origin, Nutritional + (N) or specific ‡ (S)
1.	Reduced growth	N
2.	Inhibition of proteases (intestinal and pancreatic)	N + S
3.	Inhibition of disaccharidases	N + S
4.	Organ hypertrophy	N
5.	Altered blood chemistry	N
6.	Altered mineral metabolism (Zn, Ca)	S
7.	Cellular changes in kidney	S

+ Nutritional; may be corrected by amino acid supplementation or increased dietary protein.

‡ Specific; proven effect of purified MRP or MRP in nutritionally adequate diets.

Table 2 : Overview of effects of Maillard reaction products on metabolism (Animal studies)

Effects of nutritional origin

The literature contains numerous reports of "anti-physiological" or toxic effects of MRP based on animal experiments in which severely browned protein of poor biological value was fed. These effects were in many cases of nutritional origin and could be corrected by an appropriate supplement of the amino acid(s) destroyed in the Maillard reaction, or by increasing the dietary protein level (Pintauro et al. 1983). Thus the reported effects of the MRP on relative organ weight and blood biochemistry (Adrian, 1974; Lee et al. 1974, 1982) all appear to be of nutritional origin and a secondary result of the reduction in growth rate (Table 2).

Mixed Effects

Other effects, such as the stimulation or inhibition of pancreatic and intestinal enzymes (Adrian, 1973; Lee et al. 1977; Oste and Sjodin, 1984; Schneeman and Dunaif,

1984), appear in some cases to be of nutritional origin, and in some cases specific (Table 2). Our studies indicate that the pancreatic response to MRP may be nutritional. This will be discussed in the next section. In contrast the studies of Oste and co-workers have demonstrated specific effects of various low molecular-weight furan and pyrrole Maillard derivatives on certain enzymes of the intestinal mucosa (Oste et al. 1986, 1987).

Effects of the MRP 'per se' (Specific Effects)

Finally, rat feeding studies, in which well-defined model systems of the Maillard reaction have been employed, have indicated that certain MRP may have an effect on the kidney (Table 2). Von Wangenheim et al (1979) first reported cytological modifications in the proximal tubule of the rat kidney on feeding MRP from heated casein-glucose model systems. Our own studies, also using casein-glucose model systems have confirmed this finding, although the nature of the cytological changes differed (Furniss, 1988).

Recently, we have reported an effect of MRP on urinary zinc (Zn) excretion which also appears to be specific (Furniss et al. 1986). This will be discussed later.

EXPERIMENTAL APPROACH USED TO DEFINE THE EFFECTS

The following two rat studies illustrate the type of experimental approach we have used to separate the effects on metabolism of nutritional origin from the effects of the MRP per se. In each study, the MRP were quantified by the furosine technique (Finot et al. 1981; Finot, 1983).

A.   The Effect of MRP on Pancreatic Enzymes

Metabolic transit studies have shown that the early Maillard derivative, fructose-lysine (FL) enters the pancreas (Figure 5)(Finot and Magnenat, 1981). We therefore considered the possibility that FL itself may be responsible for the alteration of pancreatic amylase, trypsin and chymotrypsin activity reported on feeding Maillard protein (Adrian, 1973; Lee et al. 1982; Schneeman and Dunaif, 1984).

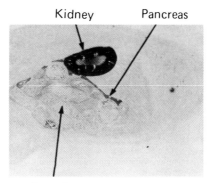

Figure 5 : Autoradioagraphy of rats 8h after i.v.
infusion of ε-fructose-14C-lysine

The pancreatic response to the feeding of free
protein-bound FL was investigated. Casein was incubated
with glucose in the presence of 15% H_2O (w/v) at 37°C.
Under these conditions lysine was the only amino acid to
react, and FL was the almost exclusive MRP formed. Minimal
levels of the advanced MRP were present. Maillard casein
(MC) was fed alone, or with a supplement of lysine to
compensate for the analytically determined loss of reactive
lysine. MC was also fed with a supplement of free FL. All
diets contained around 18% protein and were fed for a
period of 14 days. Pancreatic amylase, trypsin and
chymotrypsin activities were determined after sacrifice as
described by Temler et al. (1984)(Table 3).

Diet	Reactive Lysine	Lysine as Fructose-Lysine		Pancreatic Amylase
		Bound	Free	
	%	%	%	U/mg
Casein	1.46			37.6
Maillard Casein	0.75	0.71		15.7[a]
Maillard Casein + Lysine	1.46	0.71		27.4[a]
Maillard Casein + Fructose-lysine	0.75	0.71	0.286	12.2[a]

[a] Significantly different from the control

Table 3 : Effect of fructose-lysine on
pancreatic amylase

The results clearly show that the unsupplemented MC containing protein-bound FL reduced pancreatic amylase considerably, but that this effect was partially reversed by the supplementation of lysine. FL as the free compound had no effect on pancreatic amylase. MC had no effect on pancreatic trypsin or chymotrypsin activities (data not shown).

It was thus evident that the response of pancreatic amylase to Maillard protein is principally due to the inadequate level of biologically available lysine. It also remained possible that the origin was totally nutritional if the level of lysine supplementation was inadequate. This would be true if free and protein-bound lysine did not have equivalent effects on amylase and/or if the lysine supplement which was calculated to replace the chemically estimated loss, was insufficient.

B.   The Effect of MRP on Zn Metabolism

Several studies have indicated that there may be an effect of orally or parenterally administered MRP on Zn metabolism (Stegink et al. 1975, 1981; Johnson et al. 1983; Furniss et al. 1986; Lykken et al. 1986). In these studies the MRP were suggested to chelate Zn, and to increase its loss via the urinary or faecal pathway. However, the nature of the MRP with chelating properties was not identified. Our own studies in the rat indicated a strong positive correlation between the urinary levels of FL and the urinary loss of Zn (Figure 6)(Furniss 1988). The hyperzinc-uria associated with the ingestion of MRP is interesting from a clinical perspective since this condition is also found in the diabetic state (Kinlaw et al. 1983).

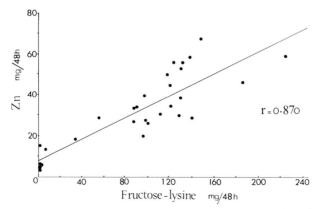

Figure 6 : Correlation between urinary Zn and urinary
           fructose-lysine

Two further rat studies were performed with the objective of determining whether the MRP which induce hyperzincuria were of the early, or the advanced type. In the first study MRP formed in casein-sugar model systems were fed. In the second study the effect of feeding purified FL was investigated.

Experiment 1. Casein was incubated with either glucose or lactose under controlled reaction conditions. Two different levels of MRP were obtained for each sugar type. The first level contained predominantly early MRP, whereas the second level contained both early and advanced-type MRP.

MAILLARD MODEL	LYSINE % BLOCKAGE (early)	LYSINE % DESTRUCTION (advanced)
CASEIN/GLUCOSE :		
SPRAY–DRIED	40·1	8·9
HEATED 3d, 60°	51·4	26·2
CASEIN/LACTOSE :		
HEATED 1d, 50°	36·8	5·5
HEATED 3d, 60°	42·3	33·9

Table 4 :   Casein/glucose and Casein/lactose model systems

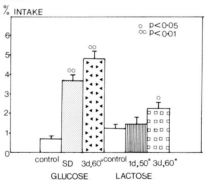

Figure 7 :   Urinary zinc excretion in rats fed casein/ glucose and casein/lactose model systems

The casein-sugar model systems were incorporated into nutritionally adequate diets containing 20mg/Kg Zn and fed to rats for 21 days. Urinary Zn excretion was measured over 9-14 days of feeding.

The results are shown in Figure 7. The first and second levels of MRP from casein-glucose increased urinary Zn excretion (expressed as a percent of the dietary Zn intake), by respectively 5-fold and 7-fold the control level. However, the feeding of lactose MRP had a smaller effect and was not significant at the first level.

Experiment 2: Free FL was added to the rat diets at a level of 5.0g/Kg. Urinary Zn was measured over the initial 14 days of feeding. Otherwise, the experimental design was as described in Experiment 1.

Daily urinary excretion was found to be $2.4 \pm 0.4 \mu$ g for the control group and $3.0 \pm 0.5 \mu$ g for the group fed the FL supplement, implying that this MRP does not have chelating properties for Zn.

These experimental results suggest that the hyperzincuria of feeding MRP from casein-glucose was probably induced by degradation products of FL, rather than FL itself. It is also clear that MRP formed from lactose are less potent inducers of hyperzincuria.

CONCLUSIONS

Animal studies have indicated that the ingestion of foods containing MRP may lead to a variety of effects on metabolism. However, most of these effects are of nutritional origin and result from the loss of essential nutrients, particularly lysine. The close interrelationship between the loss of nutrients during the Maillard reaction and the formation of new compounds makes it difficult to attribute specific "anti-physiological" effects to the MRP. However, an evaluation of the quantity of MRP absorbed and excreted in metabolic transit studies with purified MRP constitutes an excellent experimental approach to this problem. In this way the MRP, FL and HMF, which may occur at relatively high levels in processed foods, and are partly absorbed, have been found to be completely and rapidly excreted.

In the food industry the technologies used in processing are almost inevitably accompanied by the Maillard reaction. However, the quantification of the MRP and the appropriate modification of the processing technologies helps avoid nutrient losses in the product which could be critical to the consumer (e.g. premature and full-term infants, enterally-fed patients).

REFERENCES

ADRIAN, J. (1974) Nutritional and physiological consequences of the Maillard reaction. World Rev. Nutr. Diet. 19:71-122

BAYNES, J.W., AHMED, M.U., FISHER, C.I., HULL, C.I., LEHMAN, T.A., WATKINS, N.G. and THORPE, S.R. (1986) Studies on glycation of proteins and Maillard reaction of glycated proteins under physiological conditions. In: M. FUJIMAKI, M. NAMIKI and H. KATO (Eds): Developments in food science. 13. Tokyo: Kodansha Ltd, Elsevier, pp. 421-432.

FEATHER, M.S. (1981) Amine-assisted sugar dehydration reactions. In C. ERIKSSON (Eds): "Progress in food and nutrition science". Vol. 5. Oxford, Pergamon Press, pp. 37-45.

FINOT, P.A., DEUTSCH, R. and BUJARD, E. (1981) The extent of the Maillard reaction during the processing of milk. Prog. Fd. Nutr. Sci. 5:345-55.

FINOT, P.A. and MAGNENAT, E. (1981) Metabolic transit of early and advanced Maillard products. Prog. Fd. Nutr. Sci. 5:193-207.

FINOT, P.A. (1983) Chemical modifications of the milk proteins during processing and storage. Nutritional, metabolic and physiological consequences. In KAUFMANN, W. (Eds) Gelsenkirchen-Buer, F.R. Germany: Verlag Th. Mann KG, pp. 357-369

FURNISS, D.E., HURRELL, R.F. and FINOT P.A. (1986) Modification of urinary zinc excretion in the rat associated with the feeding of Maillard reaction products. pp 544-546 Acta Pharmacol. Toxicol. 59:S7 188-90

FURNISS, D.E. (1988) The effect of Maillard reaction products and lysinoanaline on zinc metabolism. PhD. Thesis No. 950, University of Fribourg, Switzerland

GERMOND, J.E., PHILIPPOSSIAN, G., RICHLI, U., BRACCO, I. and ARNAUD, M.J. (1987) Rapid and complete urinary elimination of (14-C)-5-hydroxymethyl-2-furaldehyde administered orally or intravenously to rats. J. Toxicol. Env. Health 22:79-89.

HORN, M.J., LICHTENSTEIN, H. and WOMACK, M. (1968) Availability of amino acids. A methionine-fructose compound and its availability to micro-organisms and rats. J. Agric. Fd Chem. 16:741-745.
HURRELL, R.F. (1984) Reactions of food proteins during processing and storage and their nutritional consequences. In : Development in food proteins. HUDSON, B.J.F. (Eds) Elsevier Applied Science Publishers, London 3:213-244

KINLAW, W.B., LEVINE, A.S., MORLEY, J.E., SILVIS, S.E. and McCLAIN C.I. (1983) Abnormal zinc metabolism in type II diabetis mellitus. Am. J. Medic. 75:273-277

JELLUM, E., BORRESON, H.C. and ELDJARN, L. (1973) The presence of furan derivatives in patients receiving fructose-containing solutions intravenously. Clin. Chim. Acta 47:191-201.

JOHNSON, P.E., LYKKEN, G., MAHALKO, J., MILNE, D., INMAN, L., SANDSTEAD, H.H., GARCIA, W.J. and INGLETT, G.E. (1983) The effect of browned and unbrowned corn products on absorption of zinc, iron and copper in humans. In: The Maillard reaction in food and nutrition WALLER, G.R. and FEATHER, M.S. (Eds) American Chemical Society, Washington D.C. pp 349-360.

LEE, C.M., LEE, T.-C. and CHICHESTER, C.O. (1974) Physiological consequences of browned food products. Proc. IX Int. Cong. Food Science and Technology, Madrid, Spain.

LEE, C.M., LEE, T.-C. and CHICHESTER, C.O. (1977) The effect of Maillard reaction products on disaccharidase activities in the rat. J. Agr. Food Chem. 25:775-78

LEE, T.-C., PINTAURO, S.J. and CHICHESTER, C.O. (1982) Nutritional and Toxicological effects of nonenzymatic Maillard browning. Diabetes 31:37-46.

LIARDON, R., de WECK-GAUDARD, D., PHILIPPOSSIAN, G. and FINOT, P.A. (1987) Identification of H $^\xi$ carboxymethyl-lysine : a new Maillard reaction product, in rat urine. J.

Agric. Food Chem. 35:427-431.

LYKKEN, G.IO., MAHALKO, J., JOHNSON,. P.E., MILNE, D., SANDSTEAD, H.H., GARCIA, W.J., DINITZIS, F.R. and INGLETT, G.E. (1986) Effect of browned and unbrowned corn products intrinsically labelled with 65-Zn on absorption of 65-Zn in humans. J. Nutr. 116:795-801.

MAURON, J. (1981) The Maillard reaction in food; a critical review from the nutritional standpoint. Prog. Fd. Nutr. Sci. 5:5-35.

MULCHANDANI, R.P., JOSEPHSON, R.V. and HARPER, W. (1979) Effect of processing on liquid infant milk formulas. 1. Freshly processed products. J. Dairy Sci. 62:1527-36

NAIR, B.M., OSTE, R., ASP, N.G. and PERNEMALM, P.-A. (1981) Absorption and distribution of a C-14-glucose lysine reaction mixture in the rat. Prog. Fd Nutr. Sci. 5:217-22

NIEDERWIESER, A., GILIBERTI, P. and MATASOVIC. (1975) N-e-(1-deoxyfructosyl)-lysine in urine after ingestion of a lactose-free, glucose-containing milk formula. European Society for Paediatric Research, Budapest.

OSTE, R.E., DAHLQVIST, A., SJOESTROEM, H., NOROEN, O. and MILLER, R. (1986) Effect of Maillard reaction products on protein digestion. In vitro studies. J. Agr. Food Chem. 34:355-58.

OSTE, R.E., MILLER, R., SJOESTROEM, H. and NOROEN, O. (1987) Effect of Maillard reaction products on protein digestion. Studies on pure compounds. J. agr. Food Chem. 35:938-42.

OSTE, R.E. and SJOEDIN, P. (1984) Effect of Maillard reaction products on protein digestion. In vivo studies on rats. J. Nutr. 114:2228-34.

PERKINS, E.G., BAKER, D.H., JOHNSON, G.H. and MAKOWSKI, E. (1981) The metabolism of fructose-phenylalanine in the rat. Prog. Fd Nutr. Sci. 5:229-42.

PINTAURO, S.J., LEE, T-C., and CHICHESTER, C.O. (1983)

Nutritional and toxicological effects of Maillard browned protein ingestion in the rat. In: The Maillard reaction in foods and nutrition (Eds) WALLER, R., and FEATHER, M.S. American Chemical Society pp 467-83.

SCHNEEMAN, B.O. and DUNAIF, G. (1984) Nutritional and gastrointestinal response to ehated non-fat dry milk. J. Agr. Food Chem. 32:477-80.

STEGINK, L.D., FREEMAN, J.B., DEN BESTEN, L. and FILER, L.J. (1981) Maillard reaction products in parenteral nutrition. Prog. Fd Nutr. Sci. 5:265-78

STEGINK, L.D., FREEMAN, J.B., MEYER, P.D., FILER, L.K. and DEN BESTEN, L. (1975) Excessive trace metal ion excretion due to sugar-amino acid complexes during total parenteral nutrition. Fed. Proc. 34:931.

TANAKA, M., LEE, T-C. and CHICHESTER, C.O. (1975) Nutritional consequences of the Maillard reaction. The absorption of fructose-L-tryptophan in the large intestine of the rat. J. Nutr. 105:989-94.

TEMLER, R.S., DORMOND, C.A., SIMON, E., MOREL, B. and METTRAUX, C. (1984) Response of rat pancreatic proteases to dietary proteins, their hydrolysates and soybean trypsin inhibitor. J. Nutr. 114:270-278.

VON WANGENHEIM, B. (1979) Unterzuchung über die Wirkung von Fructoselysin auf die Tubulusepithelzelle der Rattenniere. Inaugural Dissertation, Ludwig-Maximilians University, Munich.

WADMAN, S.K., DE BREE, P.K., VAN SPRANG, F.J., KAMERLING, J.P., HAVERKAMP, J. and VLIEGENTHART, J.F.G. (1975) H $^\xi$ - (Carboxymethyl)-lysine, a constituant of human urine. Clin. Chim. Acta 59:313-320.

The Maillard Reaction in Aging,
Diabetes, and Nutrition, pages 359–376
© 1989 Alan R. Liss, Inc.

GENOTOXICITY TESTING OF MAILLARD REACTION PRODUCTS

Takayuki Shibamoto

Department of Environmental Toxicology,
University of California, Davis, CA 95616

ABSTRACT

Since the development of short-term genotoxicity tests such as the Ames assay, the mutagenicity
of Maillard reaction products has been tested
extensively. Some products have exhibited strong
activity. For example, one of the earliest studies
demonstrated some mutagenic activity in a dichloromethane extract of a D-glucose/ammonia Maillard
model system. Many researchers have attempted to
pinpoint the principal chemical(s) of mutagenicity
of the Maillard products using various sugar-amino
acid browning model systems over last two decades.
However, no mutagenic individual Maillard product
has been isolated and identified. Nitrite has
been also used as a reactant in browning reaction
model systems, primarily to investigate the
formation of potentially mutagenic or carcinogenic
N-nitroso compounds. Recently some potent mutagens
isolated from pyrolyzed amino acids or proteins
have begun to receive attention as Maillard
reaction products.

INTRODUCTION

Food is a mixture of large numbers of chemicals such as
proteins, amino acids, carbohydrates, lipids, vitamins, and
minerals. These chemicals undergo complex reactions when

they are heated. Among the reactions occurring in food during heat treatment, the browning or Maillard, reaction, plays the most important role in the formation of chemicals, including mutagens and possible carcinogens. In 1912, Maillard advanced the hypothesis that non-enzymatic browning reactions occur when an amino group of an amino acid and a carbonyl group of a sugar react in the presence of heat (Maillard, 1912). Since Hodge (1953) indicated that simple model systems consisting of a sugar and an amino acid could be used to learn about complex food systems, many investigations of the products formed by the Maillard reaction have been conducted. One of the earliest works was focused on brown color formation. Song and Chichester (1967) studied kinetic behavior and the mechanism of biological activity of Maillard products using a glycine/glucose model system. Jemmali (1969) obtained substances which had effects on the cellular metabolism of certain bacteria from a casein/glucose model system. Yamaguchi and Fujimaki (1970) reported some antioxidative activity in the products obtained from a glycine/D-xylose model system.

Spingarn and Garvie (1979) reported mutagenic activity in an extract obtained from a heated D-glucose/ammonia model system using the Ames *Salmonella*/microsome test. Since then, many other workers have tested the mutagenicity of browning products formed in various other model systems using same test systems (Mihara and Shibamoto, 1980; Shibamoto et al., 1981). Around the same time, the isolation and identification of Maillard products was stimulated by the development of advanced analytical instrumentation such as gas chromatography/mass spectroscopy (GC/MS). For example, nearly one hundred volatile chemicals were identified in a simple browning model system consisting of L-rhamnose and ammonia (Shibamoto and Bernhard, 1978). Many researchers attempted to pinpoint the principle(s) of mutagenic Maillard reaction products. However, no individual chemical having mutagenic activity has been isolated and identified in the Maillard reaction systems.

The mutagenicity of heat-treated foods has received much attention since the 1970s. Sugimura et al. (1977) found strong mutagens in tryptophan and phenylalanine pyrolysis products which were subsequently proved to be carcinogenic in tests with animals such as hamsters, rats, and mice (Sugimura, 1980). It is obvious that the Maillard reaction occurring in food produces some genotoxic chemicals. Therefore, the effects of Maillard reaction products upon our health must be thoroughly understood.

SUGAR-AMINO ACID SYSTEMS

In 1980s, extensive mutagenicity testing on the products of Maillard browning model systems has been conducted. For example, the reaction mixture obtained from a cysteamine/D-glucose/water browning model system was separated into eleven fractions. Seven fractions were isolated from a dichloromethane extract by HPLC, and four more fractions from the residual aqueous solution by ion-exchange column chromatography. Each fraction was tested for mutagenicity using *S. typhimurium* strains TA98 and TA100, with or without S9 mix. The results of the mutagenicity testing are shown in Figure 1. The reaction mixtures obtained from cysteamine/D-glucose/NaNO$_2$ model systems were also examined for mutagenicity, with positive results (Mihara and Shibamoto, 1980). The presence of the nitrite ion in the browning reaction appears to enhance formation of mutagenic materials. Later, some N-nitroso compounds (N-nitrosothiazolidines) were isolated and identified from the reaction mixture of the above model system. These mutagenic chemicals formed by the Maillard reaction will be discussed later.

Gazzani et al. (1987) tested mutagenic activity of the Maillard reaction products of ribose or glucose with 17 different amino acids using *S. typhimurium* strains TA98 and TA100. Mutagenic compounds were formed in the Maillard reactions with both ribose and glucose for 14 of the amino acids tested (alanine, aspargine, aspartic acid, cysteine, cystine, glycine, leucine, methionine, phenylalanine, pro-line, hydroxyproline, serine, threonine, valine). Arginine, glutamic acid, and isoleucine did not yield any mutagenic products. The mutagenic activity in the ribose reactions was generally higher than that in the glucose reactions. The same authors tested the DNA-damaging activity of the Maillard products of glucose- or ribose-amino acids in the "rec-assay" system of *B. subtilis* and obtained positive results from histidine, proline, hydroxyproline and valine Maillard model systems. They suggested that ribose may be involved in the potential carcinogenicity of cooked meat.

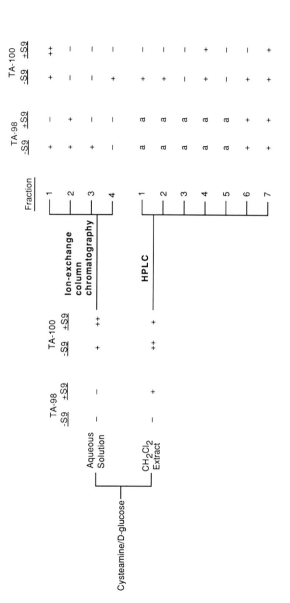

Figure 1. Results of mutagenicity tests on cysteamine/D-glucose model system. a: Not tested

Powrie et al. (1981) tested the genotoxicity of various sugar-amino acid Maillard reaction systems using three short-term bioassays; a chromosome aberration test, the *Saccharomyces cerevisiae* test, and *Salmonella* mutagenesis assay. They observed that all of the Maillard reaction solutions induced significant increases in chromosome aberrations in Chinese hamster ovary cells with no S9 activation. Mitotic recombination and mutation occurred in *Saccharomyces cerevisiae* strain D5 cells when exposed to all Maillard reaction solutions. The Maillard reaction mixtures also exhibited mutagenicity toward *S. typhimurium* strain TA100. These workers also reported that mutagen concentration in the browning reaction solution was dependent on initial pH.

The participation of creatine and creatinine and Maillard reaction products in developing mutagenic activity was studied in model systems by Jagerstad et al. (1982; 1983). Considerable mutagenic activity was exhibited when creatinine was heated with typical Maillard reactants such as glucose and glycine or alanine. They concluded that the high boiling point (ca. 130°C) of the solvent was important for the production of mutagenic activity. Boiling all reactants in water only produced no mutagenic activity. Also essential for the production of mutagenicity was the combination of all three reactants. Combining any two of these reactants produced no mutagenic activity. Jagerstad et al. (1983) also tested the role of the Maillard reaction products in the mutagenicity of model mixtures. Addition of 2-methylpyridine and 2,5-dimethylpyrazine to the model system consisting of glucose and glycine or alanine increased the mutagenic activity by between 50 and 80%. Later Nes (1987) found that the most potent stimulation of mutagen formation by creatine was in the glycine-glucose system at pH 9.0. While no mutagenic activity was detectable without creatine, a substantial level of mutagen activity was found even in the presence of the lowest dose of creatine (0.1M).

SUGAR AND AMMONIA SYSTEMS

In order to investigate the role of a simple precursors of the Maillard reaction in mutagen formation, reactants such as ammonia and hydrogen sulfide were used in some studies. As mentioned above, a model system consisted of a simple amine and a carbonyl compound is commonly used to study complex food systems. Maillard reaction products obtained from various model systems of this type have been tested for mutagenicity. Spingarn and Garvie (1979) found some mutagenic activity of reaction products extracted from sugar-ammonia model systems heated at 100°C. They concluded that mutagen production in a model system is linked to the formation of pyrazine, a major product of the browning reaction. In fact, the degree of mutagenicity of browning products increases with the extent of browning (Shinohara, 1983).

Dichloromethane extracts obtained from the reaction of rhamnose, ammonia, and hydrogen sulfide in an aqueous solution exhibited mutagenic activity in the Ames assay (Toda et al., 1981). When this dichloromethane extract was fractionated by column chromatography, the resulting fractions showed considerably reduced mutagenicity. This reduction in mutagenicity may be due to the loss of co-mutagens or primary mutagens from the system during chromatographic separation. The chemicals identified in the mutagenic fractions were imidazole derivatives. However, neither authentic alkylimidazoles nor any mixtures of them exhibited mutagenicity. An outline of the results obtained from this Maillard model system is shown in Figure 2.

When maltol was heated with ammonia in an aqueous solution, mutagenic reaction products were formed (Shibamoto et al., 1981). The main components of the mutagenic fraction obtained by TLC and HPLC were 2-ethyl-3-hydroxy-6-methylpyridine and acetamide. However, both compounds were found to be nonmutagenic. An outline of the results obtained from a maltol/ammonia Maillard model system is shown in Figure 3.

1,5(or 7)-Dimethyl-2,3,6,7-tetrahydro-1H,5H-biscyclo-pentapyrazine isolated from the reaction of 2-hydroxy-3-methyl-2-cyclopenten-1-one (cyclotene) and ammonia under simulated cooking conditions was reportedly mutagenic toward *S. typhimurium* strain TA 1538 and TA98 (Shibamoto, 1980). A Maillard reaction model system consisting of diacetyl and ammonia produced frameshift and base-pair substitution mutagens when heated for 20 min and 120 min (Shibamoto, 1984). This simple system produced several interesting products which are listed in Table 1. The major product was 2,4,5-trimethylimidazole, which showed no mutagenicity

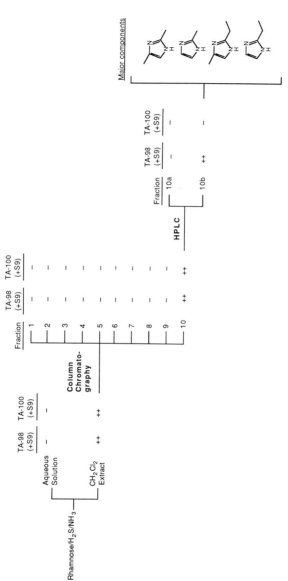

Figure 2. Results of mutagenicity tests on rhamnose/H₂S/NH₃ model systems.

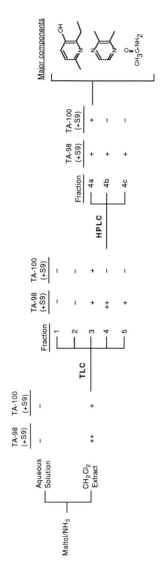

Figure 3. Results of mutagenicity tests on maltol/NH₃ model system.

toward *S. typhimurium* strains TA98 and TA100 with or without metabolic activation. Diacetyl alone was reportedly mutagenic towards *S. typhimurium* strain TA100 with metabolic activation (Bjeldanes and Chew, 1979).

TABLE 1. Compounds Identified in the Ether Extract Obtained from Diacetyl-Ammonia Reaction Mixture

Compound	Proportion of total gas chromatographic peak area%
Acetic acid	2.3
Tetramethylpyrazine	1.0
Acetamide	1.8
2,4,5-Trimethylimidazole	91.6

Pyrazines and imidazoles were major volatile Maillard reaction products. For example, 51 pyrazines and 9 imidazoles were identified in a rhamnose/ammonia Maillard reaction system (Shibamoto and Bernhard, 1980). They comprised 79.8% and 7.5% of the total organic solvent extract, respectively. Pyrazines identified in the Maillard model systems have not all been tested for mutagenicity. Stich et al. (1980) reported that four alkylpyrazines, 2-methyl-, 2-ethyl-, 2,5-dimethyl-, and 2,6-dimethylpyrazine, did not exhibit mutagenicity toward *S. typhimurium* strains TA98, TA1537, or TA100 with or without microsomal activation. However, these compounds gave positive reactions with *Saccharomyces cerevisiae* strain D5 and induced a significant increase in the frequency of chromosome aberrations in Chinese hamster ovary cells.

SUGAR-AMINE-NITRITE SYSTEMS

Numerous studies have utilized nitrite as a reactant in browning reaction model systems, primarily to investigate the formation of potentially mutagenic or carcinogenic N-nitroso compounds. An extensive worldwide research effort has been underway for the past 20 years on the chemistry, occurrence, toxicity, carcinogenicity and control of N-nitroso compounds in foods, beverages, tobacco and the environment (National Research Council, 1981). Low ppb levels of volatile N-nitroso compounds have been reported in many foodstuffs which undergo sugar-amino acid Maillard reactions during processing or cooking, including fried bacon, beer, scotch whiskey, malt, coffee and dried milk powder. In some of these foods such as bacon nitrite is added during processing, while in others the suspected nitrosating agents are either naturally occurring nitrite, nitrite from nitrate reduction or oxides of nitrogen from open-flame drying of the products. In fact, Shibamoto (1983) found that soy sauce treated with 2000 ppm nitrite was mutagenic and suggested that N-nitrosodimethylamine, N-nitrosodiethylamine and N-nitrosoproline as possible mutagenic products in nitrite-treated soy sauce. The Maillard reaction products, (-)-(1S,3S)-1-methyl-1,2,3,4-tetrahydro-β-carboline-3-carboxylic acid [(-)-(1S,3S)-MTCA] and its stereoisomer (-)-(1R,3S)-MTCA, were found to form mutagens with nitrite (Wakabayashi et al., 1983, Ochiai et al., 1984).

The detection of thiazoles and thiazolines in cooked foods (Shibamoto, 1980) and in browning model systems prompted recent investigations of the N-nitrosation of thiazolidine and its 2-alkyl derivatives. Sakaguchi and Shibamoto (1979) isolated N-nitroso-2-methylthiazolidine as a major volatile product from the reaction of cysteamine, acetaldehyde, and nitrite in an aqueous solution. N-Nitrosothiazolidine has recently been reported in fried bacon at levels up to about 5 ppb (Gray et al., 1982; Kimoto, 1982). Sekizawa and Shibamoto (1980) tested several purified N-nitrosothiazolidines for mutagenicity in the Ames assay. Umano et al. (1984) reported mutagenicity of 2-hydroxyalkyl-N-nitrosothiazolidines. N-nitrosothiazolidine showed positive responses in a microbial system and in a hepatocellular system, exhibiting weak mutagenicity at the lowest level tested (1 mg/plate) in the rec assay in *Bacillus subtilis*, and induced statistically significant levels of DNA repair in primary hepatocyte cultures at concentrations ranging from 2×10^{-4} to 2×10^{-3} M (Loury et al., 1984). Rosenkranz and Klopman (1987) suggested that N-nitrosothiazolidine had a high probability of being a moderately potent carcinogen. However, a recent study by Lijinsky and coworkers (1988) showed this prediction to be incorrect. Twenty rats exposed to a large dose of approximately 410 mg/kg N-nitrosothiazolidine showed no significant increase in cancer during an average life span of 110 weeks.

HEATED FOOD SYSTEMS

In contrast to simple Maillard model systems, more complex systems which are closer to actual foodstuffs have also been used to investigate the formation of mutagenic compounds in the Maillard reaction. A charred sample prepared from potato starch heated with ammonium carbonate at 600°C exhibited strong mutagenicity in the Ames assay (Shibamoto, 1984). The basic fraction of this sample was the most mutagenic. Starch and a mixture of starch and glycine were heated without water at 290°C and volatile chemicals produced were tested for mutagenicity by the Ames assay (Wei et al., 1981). The samples from the starch and glycine system showed distinct dose-related mutagenic activities towards *S. typhimurium* strain TA98 with metabolic activation both in agar-incorporation and preincubation assays. Samples from the starch alone did not show any mutagenic activity towards *S. typhimurium* strains TA98 or TA100 with or without S9 mix. These results suggest that mutagen formation requires a complete Maillard system rather than starch alone. The chemical analysis of the above samples (Tables 2 and 3) indicated major differences in the products formed from starch alone and starch with glycine. Starch alone produced more furan derivatives and starch with glycine produced more nitrogen-containing heterocyclic compounds (Umano and Shibamoto, 1984). Furans are known to undergo secondary Maillard reactions to form heterocyclic compounds (Shibamoto, 1977). It is difficult to pinpoint the principle(s) of mutagenicity in the products identified. It seems that a high temperature treatment is crucial for mutagen formation in the Maillard reaction. Also, nitrogen-containing compounds seem to play an important role in the mutagenicity of the Maillard products.

The Maillard reaction products prepared from model systems consisting of major milk components were tested for mutagenicity in the Ames assay (Rogers and Shibamoto, 1982). Samples obtained by heating aqueous solutions of casein and/or lactose and non-fat dried milk under either neutral or basic conditions exhibited no significant mutagenic activity. On the other hand, the tar samples prepared by heating the same milk components in the dry state exhibited

TABLE 2. Major Compounds Identified in Starch Heated Alone or with Glycine

Compound	GC Peak area%	
	Starch alone	Starch with glycine
3-Hydroxy-2-methyl-1,4-pyrone (maltol)	0.24	-
3-Hydroxy-2-ethyl-tetrahydro-1,4-pyrone	11.86	-
3,5-Dihydroxy-1,4-naphthoquinone	-	10.75
2-Methoxyphenol	-	12.36
2-Ethoxyphenol	-	26.18
Furfural	38.96	0.08
2-Methylfurfural	11.96	-
2-Acetylfuran	5.85	1.81
4-Methyl-2-propylfuran	26.59	-

TABLE 3. Major Nitrogen-Containing Compounds Identified in Starch Heated with Glycine

Compounds	GC peak area %
Pyrazine	11.25
Pyridine	7.64
Pyrrole	2.08
3-Methylpyridine	2.78
2,4-Dimethylpyrrole	5.00
2,5-Dimethylpyrrole	13.89
N-Methylacetamide	0.01
2-Hydroxymethylimidazole	2.23
2-Acetylpyrrole	0.42
2-Ethyl-4,5-dimethylimidazole	6.60
2-Methylbenzimidazole	1.01

strong mutagenicity, primarily to *S. typhimurium* strain TA98, but only with S9 mix. A casein/lactose mixture and non-fat dried milk were also heated with baking soda in the dry state. The presence of the baking soda increased the mutagenicity of the browning products; the tar from the non-fat dried milk heated with baking soda was the most potently mutagenic of all the samples towards strain TA98 and also produced a positive response in strain TA100 in the presence of S9 mix. When whole milk was heated under conditions simulating commercial heat-sterilization (65°C for 30 min), none of the samples from the above milk exhibited mutagenicity in the Ames assay (Sekizawa and Shibamoto, 1986). It was concluded that heat treatment in the temperature range from 100 to 150°C, even for long periods (5 h), does not produce mutagens in milk.

HEATED FOODS AND BEVERAGES

Dichloromethane extracts of distillates obtained from coffee heated to 150 or 300°C exhibited mutagenicity towards *S. typhimurium* strain TA98 with S9 mix (Blair and Shibamoto, 1984). Only the basic fraction obtained from this sample exhibited mutagenicity (Sasaki et al., 1987). Chemical analysis of this fraction identified many nitrogen containing heterocyclic compounds (Table 4). Caffeine is known to have a synergistic effect on some mutagens. However, caffeine does not exhibit any potentiating effect in coffee. Decaffeinated instant coffee both with and without added caffeine gave results similar to those obtained with ordinary instant coffee in the Ames test (Aeschbacher and Wurzner, 1980).

Tryptophan heated alone at a high temperature produced a mutagenic tar (Nagao et al., 1977). These researchers later isolated the well-known food pyrolysate mutagens Trp-P-1 (3-amino-1,4-dimethyl-5H-pyrido[4,3-b]indole) and Try-P-2 (3-amino-1-methyl-5H-pyrido[4,3-b]indole) from a basic fraction of the tryptophan pyrolysate. It is, however, difficult to classify these compounds as Maillard reaction products according to the definition given above because these chemicals form in the absence of a carbonyl compound. Recently, such chemicals have begun to receive attention in the field of research of the Maillard reaction. Details of these mutagens are described in Nagao et al. (1983).

TABLE 4. Major Compounds Identified in the Over Heated Brewed Coffee

Compound	GC peak area %
Pyridine	12.85
2-Methylpyridine	0.21
3-Methylpyridine	2.73
3-Ethylpyridine	2.15
3-Acetylpyridine	0.10
2,2'-Bipyridine	0.27
2-Methylpyrazine	0.32
2,5-Dimethylpyrazine	0.57
2,6-Dimethylpyrazine	0.08
2-Ethyl-5(or 6)-methylpyrazine	1.16
5,6,7,8-Tetrahydroquinoxaline	0.21
2-Methyl-6,7-dihydro-5H-cyclopentapyrazine	0.21
Pyrrolo[1,2-a]pyrazine	0.01
5 (or 6)-Methylpyrrolo[1,2-a]pyrazine	0.01
2-Methyl-5,6,7,8-tetrahydroquinoxaline	0.49
5-Methylquinoxaline	0.01
2-Methylpyrrolo[1,2-a]pyrazine	0.13
2-Methylquinoline	0.01
4-Methyl-2(1H)-quinolinone	0.14
Caffeine	3.12

CONCLUSION

As L.C. Maillard proposed in 1912, the reaction between amines and carbonyls implicated *in vivo* damages, the Maillard reaction has been proved to initiate certain damages in biological systems. Some products formed by this reaction in processed foods exhibited strong mutagenicity, suggesting possible formation of carcinogens. Further studies on the Maillard reaction from the biological viewpoint are in order to assess our health.

ACKNOWLEDGMENT

The effort and assistance of P. Fitch and H. Yeo for preparation of this manuscript is gratefully acknowledged.

REFERENCES

Aeschbacer HU, Wurzner HP (1980). An evaluation of instant and regular coffee in the Ames mutagenicity test. Toxicology Lett 5:139-142.

Bjeldanes LF, Chew H (1979). Mutagenicity of 1,2-dicarbonyl compounds: maltol, kojic acid, diacetyl and related substances. Mutation Res 67:367-371.

Blair CA, Shibamoto T (1984). Ames mutagenicity tests of overheated brewed coffee. Food Chem Toxicol 22:971-975.

Gazzani G, Vagnarelli P, Cuzzoni MT, Mazza PG (1987). Mutagenic activity of the Maillard reaction products of ribose with different amino acids. J Food Chem 52:757-760.

Gray JI, Reddy SK, Price JF, Mandagere A, Wilkens WF (1982). Inhibition of N-nitrosamines in bacon. Food Tech 36:39-45.

Hodge JE (1953). Chemistry of browning reactions in model systems. J Agric Food Chem 1:928-943.

Jagerstad M, Laser Reutersward A, Olsson R, Grivas S, Nyhammar T, Olsson K, Dahlqvist A (1983). Creatin(in)e and Maillard reaction products as precursors of mutagenic compounds: effects of various amino acids. Food Chem 12:255-264.

Jennali M (1969). Influence of the Maillard reaction products on some bacteria of the intestinal flora. J Appl Bact 32:151-155.

Kimoto WI, Pensabene JW, Fiddler W (1982). Isolation and identification of N-nitrosothiazolidine in fried bacon. J Agric Food Chem 30:757-760.

Lijinsky W, Kovatch RM, Keefer LD, Saavedra JE, Hansen TJ, Miller AJ, Fiddler W (1988). Carcinogenesis in rats by cyclic N-nitrosamines containing sulphur. Food Chem Toxicol 26:3-7.

Loury DJ, Byard JL, Shibamoto T (1984). Genotoxicity of N-nitrosothiazolidine in microbial and hepatocellular test systems. Food Chem Toxicol 22:1013-1014.

Maillard LC (1912). Action of amino acids on sugars. Compt Rend 154:66-68.

Mihara S, Shibamoto T (1980). Mutagenicity of products obtained from cysteamine-glucose browning model systems. J Agric Food Chem 28:62-66.

Nagao M, Sato S, Sugimura T (1983). Mutagens produced by heating foods. In "The Maillard Reaction in Foods and

Nutrition," ACS Symposium series 215, Washington DC, pp 521-536.

Nagao M, Yahagi T, Kawauchi T, Seino Y, Honda M, Matsukura N, Sugimura T, Wakabayashi K, Tsuji K, Kosuge T (1977). Mutagens in foods and especially pyrolysis products of protein. In Scott D, Bridges BA, Sobels FH (Eds): "Progress in Genetic Toxicology," Elsevier, Amsterdam, pp 259-264.

National Research Council (1981). The health effects of nitrate, nitrite, and N-nitroso compounds. Part 1. National Academy Press, Washington, DC, p 538.

Nes IF (1987). Formation of mutagens in an amino acid-glucose model system and the effect of creatine. Food Chem 24:137-146.

Ochiai M, Wakabayashi K, Nagao M, Sugimura T (1984). Tyramine is a major mutagen precursor in soy sauce, being convertible to a mutagen by nitrite. Gann 75:1-3.

Powrie WD, Wu CH, Rosin MP, Stich HF (1981). Clastogenic and mutagenic activities of Maillard reaction model systems. J Food Sci 46:1433-1438.

Rogers AM, Shibamoto T (1982). Mutagenicity of the products obtained from heated milk systems. Food Chem Toxicol 20:259-263.

Rosendranz HS, Klopman G (1987). Computer automated structure evaluation of the carcinogenicity of N-nitrosothiazolidine and N-nitrosothiazolidine-4-carboxylic acid. Food Chem Toxicol 25:253-256.

Sakaguchi M, Shibamoto T (1979). Isolation of N-nitroso-2-methylthiazolidine from a cysteamine-acetaldehyde-sodium nitrite model system. Agric Biol Chem 43:667-669.

Sasaki Y, Shibamoto T, Wei CI, Fernando S (1987). Biological and chemical studies on overheated brewed coffee. Food Chem Toxicol 25:225-228.

Sekizawa J, Shibamoto T (1980). Mutagenicity of 2-alkyl-N-nitrosothiazolidines. J Agric Food Chem 28:781-783.

Sekizawa J, Shibamoto T (1986). Salmonella/microsome mutagenicity tests of heat-processed milk samples. Food Chem Toxicol 24:987-988.

Shibamoto T (1977). Formation of sulfur- and nitrogen-containing compounds from the reaction of furfural with hydrogen sulfide and ammonia. J Agric Food Chem 25:206-208.

Shibamoto T (1980). Heterocyclic compounds found in cooked meats. J Agric Food Chem 28:237-243.

Shibamoto T (1980). Mutagenicity of 1,5(or 7)-dimethyl-2,3,6,7-tetrahydro-1H,5H-bicyclopentapyrazine obtained from a cyclotene/NH3 browning model system. J Agric Food Chem 28:883-884.

Shibamoto T (1983). Possible mutagenic constituents in nitrite-treated soy sauce. Food Chem Toxicol 21:745-747.

Shibamoto T (1984). Ames mutagenicity tests of products from a heated potato-starch system. Food Chem Toxicol 22:119-122.

Shibamoto T (1984). Mutagen formation in browning model systems. J Appl Toxicol 4:97-100.

Shibamoto T, Bernhard RA (1978). Formation of heterocyclic compounds from the reaction of L-rhamnose with ammonia. J Agric Food Chem 26:183-187.

Shibamoto T, Bernhard RA (1978). Formation of heterocyclic compounds from the reaction of L-rhamnose with ammonia. J Agric Food Chem 26:183-187.

Shibamoto T, Nishimura O, Mihara S (1981). Mutagenicity of products obtained from a maltol-ammonia browning model system. J Agric food Chem 29:643-646.

Shinohara K, Jahan N, Janaka M, Yamamoto K, Wu R-T, Murakami H, Omura H (1983). Formation of mutagens by amino-carbonyl reactions. Mutation Res 122:279-286.

Song PS, Chichester CO (1967). Kinetic behavior and mechanism of inhibition in the Maillard reaction. J Food Sci 32:107-115.

Spingarn NE, Garvie CT (1979). Formation of mutagens in sugar-ammonia medel systems. J Agric Food Chem 27:1319-1321.

Stich HF, Stich W, Rosin MP, Powrie WD (1980). Mutagenic acitivity of pyrazine derivatives: a comparative study with *Salmonella typhimurium, Saccharomyces cerevisiae* and Chinese hamster ovary cells. Food Cosmet Toxicol 18:581-584.

Sugimura T (1980). Mutagenicity and carcinogens produced during cooking processes. 9th Short Conference on Mutagens and Carcinogens in the Diet and Digestive Tract, p 11.

Sugimura T, Nagao M, Kawachi T, Honda M, Yahagi T, Seino Y, Sato S, Matsukura N, Shirai A, Sawamura M, and Matsumoto H (1977). Mutagen-carcinogens in food with special reference to highly mutagenic pyrolytic product in broiled foods. Cell Prolif 4:1561-1577.

Toda H, Sekizawa J, Shibamoto T (1981). Mutagenicity of the L-rhamnose-ammonia-hydrogen sulfide browning reaction mixture. J Agric Food Chem 29:381-384.

Umano K, Shibamoto T (1984). Chemical studies on heated starch/glycine model systems. Agric Biol Chem 48:1387-1393.

Umano K, Shibamoto T, Fernando SY, Wei CI (1984). Mutagenicity of 2-hydroxyalkyl-N-nitrosothiazolidines. Food Chem Toxicol 22:253-259.

Wakabayashi K, Ochiai M, Saito H, Tsuda M, Suwa Y, Nagao M, Sugimura T (1983). Presence of 1-methyl-1,2,3,4-tetrahydro-b-carboline-3-carboxylic acid, a precursor of a mutagenic nitroso compound, in soy sauce. Proc Natl Aca Sci USA 80:2912-2916.

Wei CI, Kitamura K, Shibamoto T (1981). Mutagenicity of Maillard browning products obtained from a starch-glycine model system. Food Cosmet Toxicol 19:749-751.

Yamaguchi N, Fujimaki M (1970). Studies on browning reaction products from reducing sugars and amino acid. Nippon Shokuhin Kogyo Gakkaishi 4:136-144.

The Maillard Reaction in Aging,
Diabetes, and Nutrition, pages 377–390
© 1989 Alan R. Liss, Inc.

NUTRITIONAL TOXICOLOGY: ON THE MECHANISMS OF INHIBITION
OF FORMATION OF POTENT CARCINOGENS DURING COOKING.

J.H. Weisburger and R.C. Jones

American Health Foundation, Valhalla, New York,
10595 USA

ABSTRACT.   Frying or broiling of meat or fish yields
powerful genotoxic carcinogens such as 2-amino-3-
methylimidazo[4,5-f]quinoline (IQ) and related amino-
imidazo azaarene carcinogens. We have explored the
mode of formation and inhibition of production of
these carcinogens. Maillard reactions from precursor
amino acids, hydroxyamino acids, and simple carbohydrates appear to yield reactive aldehydes that interact with creatinine to produce specific mutagens/car-
cinogens. The simplest such IQ-like mutagen, 2-amino-
5-ethylidene-1-methylimidazol-4-one, was prepared from
acetaldehyde and creatinine. The formation of mutagens in laboratory models and during realistic frying
of meat was effectively blocked by L-tryptophan,
L-proline, and mixtures thereof. The underlying mechanism rests on competition, between the inhibitors
containing an indole ring and creatinine, for interme-
diary reactive aldehydes produced during Maillard type
reactions. The inhibition by L-tryptophan, L-proline,
and other indoles is effective and can also be implemented practically.

Maillard reactions have traditionally been studied
because many of the flavors and odors associated with desirable foods arise directly from such reactions during
storage or cooking (Mauron, 1981; Waller and Feather, 1983;
Fujimaki et al., 1987). With the advent of improved knowledge in cancer research that a key element in the change
of normal cells to neoplastic cells is the transformation

of DNA by exogenous reactive chemicals, now termed genotoxic, and the development of the concept that cancer is the result of a somatic mutation, tests have been developed to readily detect and measure such genotoxic chemicals. One widely used test was developed by Ames and involves the use of reverse mutations in Salmonella typhimurium. Another test of carcinogencity, developed by Williams, is based on the occurrence of DNA repair in freshly explanted liver cells. Although a number of other rapid, in vitro and in vivo bioassays exist, a combination or battery of the Ames test and the Williams test, which avoids false positives and false negatives more than other combinations, is beginning to be accepted as a reliable means of detecting genotoxic agents (Williams and Weisburger, 1986).

Using the Ames test, the group of Sugimura et al. (1977) discovered over 10 years ago that the surface of fried meat and fried fish displayed powerful mutagenic activity. Previously, Kuratsune's group and Lijinsky and Shubik (see Fazio and Howard, 1983) found the known carcinogen benzpyrene and related polycyclic aromatic hydrocarbons at the surface of fried meat. Sugimura et al. (1977) reported that, when the mutagenic activity in fried meat was measured, it contained much more such activity than could be accounted for by the presence of polycyclic aromatic hydrocarbons. Extraction of the mutagenic components and chromatographic separation into individual compounds identified them as belonging to a totally new class of mutagen, heterocyclic amines, typified by 2-amino-3-methyl-imidazo[4,5-f]quinoline (IQ) and related quinoxalines (MeIQx; 4,8-diMeIQx, etc.) (Vuolo and Schuessler, 1985; Felton et al., 1986; Hatch et al., 1986; Knudsen, 1986; Shibamoto, this volume).

These chemicals proved to be among the most mutagenic, when expressed as revertants per mmol, of any compound known thus far. They were also quite active in the DNA repair test of Williams, and indeed in virtually all tests measuring genotoxicity (Loury and Byard, 1985; Wild et al., 1985; Terada et al., 1986; Yoshimi et al., 1988). Thus, these chemicals can be reliably classified as genotoxic. As could be expected from such a classification, animal bioassays revealed them to be toxic and carcinogenic for several specific target organs including the liver, urinary bladder, pancreas, intestinal tract with emphasis on colon, and mammary gland (See Bird and Bruce, 1984; Tanaka et al., 1985; Sugimura, 1988).

A number of investigators, including members of this Institute, have documented that the amount and type of dietary fat can exert powerful, promoting effects in the colon, mammary gland, and pancreas, organs affected by nutritional carcinogenesis in the Western World (Rose, 1985). On the other hand, fat may have little enhancing effect on carcinogenesis in the liver and urinary bladder, perhaps accounting for the fact that neoplasms in these organs are at low incidence in the West. The mutagens formed during cooking are easily detected because of high specific mutagenic activity, but the amount present and thence consumed per day by meat-eating populations is relatively small (Felton et al., 1984; Sugimura, 1988). However, such foods are consumed daily from childhood onwards. It has been suggested that the occurrence of colon, breast, and perhaps pancreas cancer (in the latter case carcinogens from tobacco smoke may also be involved) may stem from the daily intake of small amounts of such genotoxic carcinogens, together with continuing, powerful promotion provided by the customary intake of fats from a high-fat diet of 35-45% of daily calories in fat (Weisburger, 1986). The effect of fat is reasonably well established, and therefore, recommendations have been made to limit the daily fat intake to 20-25% of calories, which might reduce the promoting potential (Rose, 1987).

Another approach to cancer prevention at these important target organs is to study the possibility of avoiding the formation of these mutagens and carcinogens during cooking. One such method applicable to ground meat is to add about 10% or more of soy protein that has been shown to inhibit the formation of mutagens (Wang et al.,1982). Another advantage of soy protein/meat mixtures is that total fat is reduced by dilution with good quality protein in the final product. Antioxidants also lowered the formation of mutagens during cooking.

We discovered the addition of L-tryptophan and related indoles to be a more specific means of lowering the formation of mutagens. This method is based on the following background information (Jones and Weisburger, 1988a; 1988b). The laboratory of Jägerstad (1983) first demonstrated that the formation of mutagens during cooking requires creatinine as the essential component. She and others (Matsushima, 1982; Nes 1986, 1987; Reuterswärd et al. 1987a; 1987b) have demonstrated that the higher the creatinine level in model systems or in fried foods, the greater the formation of these mutagens. The overall mechanism of Maillard reactions in forming IQ-type mutagens, including the determination of the reactive intermediates that interact with creatinine, is as yet obscure. We have observed, however, that the addition of L-trp to in vitro reflux systems such as that of Jägerstad (See pp. 155–167, in Knudsen, 1986) yielded a dose-related inhibition of the formation of mutagens.

Table 1. Inhibition of the Formation of IQ-type Mutagens by L-Trp in Liquid-Reflux Models[a]

mM L-trp added	TA98 + S9 Avg.rev.col./pl. per 0.1 ml reflux sample		% Inhibition	
	Study 1	Study 2	Study 1	Study 2
Complete Model[b]				
0 (control)	545[c] ± 77	1170[c] ± 58	control	
1.75	460[c] ± 70 ($p>0.05$)	–	20	–
3.5	235[c] ± 17 ($p<0.05$)	–	70	–
17	230[c] ± 5 ($p<0.05$)	–	70	–
70	–	250[c] ± 8 ($p<0.05$)	–	90
105	–	140[c]± 16 ($p<0.05$)	–	100
DEG negative control	50	70	–	–
IQ (5 ng/pl) (positive control)	960[b]	1130[b]	–	–

[a] From: Jones and Weisburger (1988a)

[b] A solution of 35 mM glucose, 70 mM glycine, and 70 mM creatinine in 57 ml diethylene glycol (DEG) and 3 ml distilled water was refluxed for 2 hrs at 150°C for 2 hrs. After cooling, 100 ul aliquots were tested for mutagenicity in _Salmonella_ _typhimurium_ TA98 + induced rat S9 liver fraction. Where used, L-trp was added to

the solution prior to reflux. Comparisons are made between groups and DEG vehicle control. The positive control was 2-amino-3-methylimidazo[4,5-f]quinoline.

c   Significant value (2x background) with data given as mean ± standard error from triplicate plates.

Mixtures of L-trp and L-proline are also effective inhibitors.

Table 2. Inhibition of the Formation of IQ-type Mutagens by L-Proline and L-Tryptophan in Liquid-Reflux Models.[a,b]

(mM) Ingredients	TA98+S9 Avg.rev.col/plate			Percent Inhibition		
	Exp.1	Exp.2	Exp.3	Exp.1	Exp.2	Exp.3
Control (gluc+gly+cr)	1590[c]	1665[c]	590[c]			
Pro(7)	1460[c]			8		
Pro(35)	1330[c]			16		
Trp(7)	1015[c]			35		
Pro(7)+Trp(7)	820[c]			50		
Pro(35)+Trp(7)	460[c]			75		
Pro(35)+Trp(14)		245[c]			90	
Pro(35)+Trp(35)			160[c]			80
Pro(70)		720[c]			60	
Trp(70)			160[c]			80
Pro(105)		740[c]			55	
Pro(140)		1045[c]			40	
DEG neg control	60	45	60			
5 ng IQ-plate (positive control)	915[c]	950[c]	830[c]			

a   From Jones and Weisburger (1988c)
b   Conditions were the same as those in footnote b, Table 1.
c   Significant value (2x background) with data given as mean ± standard error from triplicate plates.

The role of tryptophan may be to compete with creatinine for the reactive intermediates. For example, the usual system leading to this class of mutagens involves heating a solution of a carbohydrate, such as glucose or fructose, an amino acid such as glycine or alanine, and creatinine.

Depending on conditions and reactants, such mixtures typically produce carcinogens such as 2-amino-3,8-dimethyl [4,5-f]quinoxaline, or the 3,4,8-trimethyl analog (Jägerstad et al., 1983; Knudsen, 1986).

Heating a solution of hydroxyamino acid threonine leads to intermediates that react with creatinine and yield two mutagenic products that have been characterized (Fig. 1). The major product (2-amino-5-ethylidene-1-methylimadazol-4-one) can also be formed directly by the reaction between acetaldehyde and creatinine, thus, 1. proving by synthesis the structure of the adduct formed from threonine, and 2. demonstrating that aldehydes can react with creatinine (Jones and Weisburger, 1988c). Threonine and creatinine in the presence of L-trp, do not form significant amounts of the mutagens noted above; rather the intermediate reacts with L-trp to yield 2-carboxy-8-(1'-hydroxyethyl)pyrrolo(2,3-b)indole, product of the reaction of acetaldehyde with a cyclisation complex derived from L-tryptophan (Jones and Weisburger, 1988, unpublished). This finding directs attention to the likelihood that reactive aldehydes are the key intermediates in the Maillard reactions during frying or broiling of meat or fish leading to IQ or IQ_x carcinogens (Fig. 2). Indeed, it has been discovered that the formation of powerful mutagens and carcinogens during frying or broiling of fish or meat can be lowered, most likely through similar mechanisms, by the addition of relatively small amounts of L-trp and other indoles (Table 3). We have formulated practical means of performing this by adding L-trp to meat sauce applied to meat prior to cooking (Jones and Weisburger, 1988a,b).

Lowering individual fat intake is likely effective at anytime in reducing the risk of cancer development because the underlying mechanism involves promotion, which is a highly dose-dependent and reversible phenomenon (Rose, 1987). For example, the Western intake of fat of 40% of calories yields a concentration of about 12 mg/g of stool of bile acids, with demonstrated promoting potential for colon cancer. In contrast, the traditional low fat intake in Japan (15-20% of calories) yields a bile acid concentration of 4 mg/g. Likewise Western populations switching from a high to a low fat level lower the effective concentration of bile acids within days (Hill, 1971). Thus, the recommendation for lower risk is likely to be effective almost immediately upon changing lifestyle. This approach

Mechanism of Inhibition of Aminoimidazol-4-one Mutagen Formation by L-Tryptophan

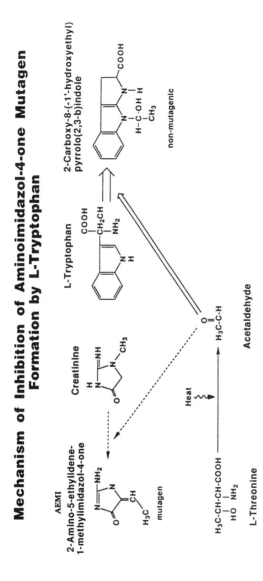

Figure 1. Mechanism of inhibition of formation of IQ-like mutagens, 2-amino-5-ethylidene-1-methylimidazol-4-one during refluxing of 70 mM L-threonine and 70 mM creatinine in 57 ml DEG and 3 ml water at 150°C for 2 hr. (From: Jones and Weisburger, 1988d).

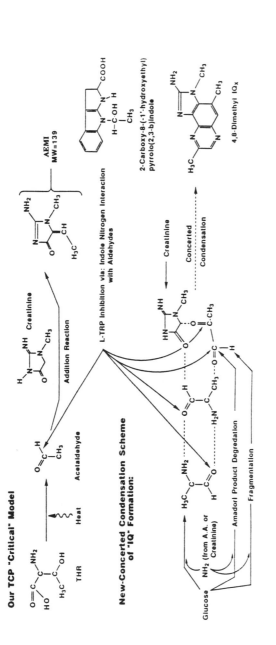

Figure 2. Possible mechanism of inhibition of formation of IQ-like and IQ-type mutagens by competition between L-tryptophan, through the indole nitrogen, and creatinine (From: Jones and Weisburger, 1988d).

Table 3. Inhibition of the formation of IQ-Type Mutagens by L-Tryptophan During Broiling or Frying of Lean Beef[a]

Sample	Broiled beef model Avg.Rev. Col./Plate			Fried beef model	
	Study 1.	Study 2.	% Inhibition	Avg.Rev. Col./Pl.	% Inhibition
Plain patty control	515[c] ± 15			–	
SS[b] patty control	450[c] ± 28 (p>0.05)	280[c] ± 28		360[c] ± 21	–
50 mg L-trp/side (0.69 mg/cm²)	–	270[c] ± 13 (p>0.05)	6	–	
60 mg L-trp/side (0.83 mg/cm²)	–	–		280[c] ± 20 (p<0.05)	33
75 mg L-trp/side (1.04 mg/cm²)	–	120[c] ± 22 (p<0.05)	100[c]	150[c] ± 8 (p<0.05)	88
100 mg L-trp/side (1.38 mg/cm²)	–	110 ± 5 (p<0.05)		–	
150 mg L-trp/side (2.07 mg/cm²)	115[c] ± 7 (p<0.05)	–	99	–	
DMSO control	55	60		60	
IQ (5 ng/plate)	635[c]	1265[c]		1025[c]	

a From Jones and Weisburger (1988a)

b The amount of L-Trp shown was dissolved in steak sauce (SS) and applied in 2.5 ml per side to both sides prior to oven broiling (temperature 235°C) or frying in a pan (220°C) for 5 min per side. A series of solvent extractions and partitions yielded samples that were tested for mutagenicity as a solution in dimethylsulfoxide.

c Significant value (2x background) with data given as mean ± std. error from triplicate plates.

has been proposed for patients having the usual medical management including surgical removal of a primary colon or breast cancer to delay or avoid future recurrence (Wynder et al., 1986).

On the other hand, with genotoxic carcinogens, knowledge of the underlying mechanisms suggests that exposure to such agents leads to a permanent increase in risk. For example, gastric cancer stems from exposure to genotoxic agents without much influence of promoters (Correa, 1983; Mirvish, 1983; Howson et al, 1986; Weisburger, 1986). This neoplastic disease was prevalent in traditional Japan. However, migrants from high-risk Japan to much lower risk U.S.A. have maintained their risk for disease (Haenszel, 1975). Likewise, Japanese used to have a lower risk for colon cancer, albeit they consumed fried fish containing IQ-type carcinogens, but in the presence of a low-fat diet, the disease was not expressed. However, when individuals migrate from Japan and acquire Western high fat traditions they acquire the high risk for colon cancer in the same generation (Haenszel, 1975; Stemmerman et al., 1987). The cell duplication rate of intestinal mucosa is a main factor to lock in abnormal expression of the genotoxic carcinogen-DNA reaction. This cell turnover is fairly constant; albeit, it is modulated by intestinal pH, calcium ions, or bile acid concentration, in turn, controlled by dietary fat (Lipkin, 1988, Sorenson et al, 1988). However, migrants from Japan continue at a relatively low risk for breast cancer (Locke and King, 1980; Tominaga, 1985). A possible explanation for this difference between colon and breast cancer risk in migrants may stem from the fact that during sexual maturation, mammary tissue displays a burst of high level DNA synthesis and cell duplication, conditions favoring the transformation of normal to early neoplastic cells in the presence of a carcinogen. Thus, the group aged 10-15 at the time of the single high radiation exposure from the atomic bomb in Hiroshima led to a 4 X higher breast cancer rate than in individuals who were older and the breast fully developed (Boyce and Hoover, 1981). Perhaps the food-derived genotoxic carcinogens affecting mammary tissue yield a relatively lower exposure in Japan than in the U.S., and the required metabolism to a reactive carcinogen may also be fat-dependent.

In summary, the combined results presented suggest that avoidance of the nutritionally-linked genotoxic carcinogens, affecting breast, intestinal tract, and also other tissues such as pancreas, early in life may be a significant means to decrease the risk of later cancer development in these organs. The approach proposed, the addition of small amounts of L-tryptophan and L-proline, prior to cooking of meats and fish, is effective and can be readily implemented practically.

REFERENCES

Bird RP, Bruce WR (1984). Damaging effect of dietary components to colon epithelial cells in vivo: effect of mutagenic heterocyclic amines. JNCI 73:237-240.

Boyce JD, Hoover RN (1981). Radiogenic breast cancer: age effects and implications for models of human carcinogenesis. In Burchenal JH, Oettgen HF (eds): "Cancer: Achievements, Challenges, and Prospects for the 1980s," Vol 1, New York: Grune and Stratton, pp 209-221.

Correa P (1983). The gastric precancerous process. Cancer Surv 2:437-450.

Fazio T, Howard JW (1983). Polycyclic aromatic hydrocarbons in foods. In Bjorseth A (ed): "Handbook of Polycyclic Aromatic Hydrocarbons," New York: Marcel Dekker, pp. 461-505.

Felton JS, Knize MG, Wood C, Wuebbles BJ, Healy SK, Stuermer DH, Bjeldanes LF, Kimble BJ, Hatch FT (1984). Isolation and characterization of new mutagens from fried ground beef. Carcinogenesis 5:95-102.

Felton JS, Knize MG, Shen NH, Lewis PR, Andresen BD, Happe J, Hatch FT (1986). The isolation and identification of a new mutagen from fried ground beef: 2-amino-1-methyl-6-phenylimidazo[4,5-b]pyridine (PhIP). Carcinogenesis 7:1081-1086.

Fujimaki M, Namiki M, Kato H (eds) (1987). Amino-Carbonyl Reactions in Food and Biological Systems. New York-Amsterdam: Elsevier.

Haenszel W (1975). Migrant studies. In Fraumeni Jr JF (ed): "Persons at High Risk of Cancer: An Approach to Cancer Etiology and Control," New York: Academic Press, pp 361-371.

Hatch FT, Nishimura S, Powrie WD, Kolonel LN (eds) (1986). Formation of mutagens during cooking and heat processing of food. Environ Health Perspect 67:3-157.

Howson CP, Hiyama T, Wynder EL (1986). The decline in gastric cancer: epidemiology of an unplanned triumph. Epidemiol Rev 8:1-27.

Jägerstad M, Reuterswärd AL, Olsson R, Grivas S, Nyhammar T, Olsson K, Dahlqvist A (1983). Creatin(in)e and Maillard reaction products as precursors of mutagenic compounds: effects of various amino acids. Food Chemistry 12:255-264.

Jones RC, Weisburger JH (1988a). L-Tryptophan inhibits formation of mutagens during cooking of meat and in laboratory models. Mutat Res 206:343-349.

Jones RC, Weisburger JH (1988b). Characterization of aminoalkylimidazol-4-one mutagens from liquid-reflux models. Mutat Res 222:43-51.

Jones RC, Weisburger JH (1988c). Inhibition of aminoimidazoquinoxaline-type and aminoimidazol-4-one type mutagen formation in liquid-reflux models by the amino acids L-proline and/or L-tryptophan. Environ Molec Mutagen 11, 509-514.

Jones RC, Weisburger JH (1988d). Inhibition of aminoimidazoquinoxaline-type and aminoimidazol-4-one type mutagen formation in liquid reflux models by L-tryptophan and other selected indoles. Jpn. J. Cancer Res (Gann) 79, 222-230.

Knudsen I (ed) (1986). "Genetic Toxicology of the Diet." New York, Alan R. Liss.

Locke FB, King H (1980). Cancer mortality risk among Japanese in the United States. JNCI 65:1149-1156.

Loury DJ, Byard JL (1985). Genotoxicity of the cooked-food mutagens IQ and MeIQ in primary cultures of rat, hamster, and guinea pig hepatocytes. Environ Mutagen 7:245-254.

Matsushima T (1982). Mechanisms of conversion of food components to mutagens and carcinogens. In Arnott MS, van Eys J, Wang Y-M (eds): "Molecular Interrelations of Nutrition and Cancer," New York: Raven Press, pp 35-42.

Mauron J (1981). The Maillard reaction in food; a critical review from the nutritional standpoint. Prog Fd Nutr Sci 5:5-35.

Mirvish SS (1983). The etiology of gastric cancer. Intragastric nitrosamide formation and other theories. JNCI 71:629-647.

Nes IF (1986). Mutagen formation in fried meat emulsion containing various amounts of creatine. Mutat. Res. 175:145-148.

Nes IF (1987). Formation of mutagens in an amino acid-glucose model system and the effect of creatine. Food Chem 24:137-146.

Reuterswärd AL, Skog K, Jägerstad M (1987a). Effects of creatine and creatinine content on the mutagenic activity of meat extracts, bouillons and gravies from different sources. Fd Chem Toxic 25:747-754.

Reuterswärd AL, Skog K, Jägerstad M (1987b). Mutagenicity of pan-fried bovine tissues in relation to their content of creatine, creatinine, monosaccharides and free amino acids. Fd Chem Toxic 25:755-762.

Rose, D.P. (ed) (1987). Proceedings: Workshop on new developments on dietary fat and fiber in carcinogenesis. Prev. Med. 16, 449-595.

Sorenson AW, Slattery ML, Ford MH (1988). Calcium and colon cancer: a review. Nutr Cancer 11:135-145.

Stemmermann GN, Nomura AMY, Kolonel LN (1987). Cancer among Japanese-Americans in Hawaii. Gann Monogr Cancer Res 33, 99-108.

Sugimura T (1988). New environmental carcinogens in daily life. Trends Pharmacol Sci 9:205-209.

Sugimura T, Nagao M, Kawachi T, Honda M, Yahagi T, Seino Y, Sato S, Matsukura N, Matsushima T, Shirai A, Sawamura M, Matsumoto H (1977). Mutagen-carcinogens in food, with special reference to highly mutagenic pyrolytic products in broiled foods. In Hiatt HH, Watson JD, Winsten JA (eds): "Origins of Human Cancer," Cold Spring Harbor, NY: Cold Spring Harbor Lab, pp 1561-1577.

Terada M, Nagao M, Nakayasu M, Sakamoto H, Nakasato F, Sugimura T (1986). Mutagenic activities of heterocyclic amines in Chinese hamster lung cells in culture. Environ Health Perspect 67:117-119.

Tominaga S (1985). Cancer incidence in Japanese in Japan, Hawaii, and Western United States. Natl Cancer Inst Monogr 69:83-92.

Vuolo LL, Schuessler GJ (1985). Review: Putative mutagens and carcinogens in foods. Environ Mutagenesis 7:577-598.

Waller GR, Feather MS (eds) (1983). "The Maillard Reaction in Foods and Nutrition," ACS Symposium Series 215. Washington DC: American Chemical Society.

Wang YY, Vuolo LL, Spingarn NE, Weisburger JH (1982). Formation of mutagens in cooked foods. V. The mutagen reducing effect of soy protein concentrates and antioxidants during frying of beef. Cancer Letts 16, 179-189.

Weisburger JH (1986). Application of the mechanisms of nutritional carcinogenesies to the prevention of cancer. In Y Hayashi, M Nagao, T Sugimura, S Takayama, L Tomatis, LW Wattenberg, GN Wogan (eds) "Diet, Nutrition and Cancer," Tokyo: Japan Sci Societies Press, pp 11-26.

Wild D, Gocke E, Harnasch D, Kaiser G, King M-T (1985). Differential mutagenic activity of IQ (2-amino-3-methyl-imidazo[4,5-f]quinoline) in <u>Salmonella typhimurium</u> strains in vitro and in vivo, in <u>Drosophila</u>, and in mice. Mutat Res 156:93-102.

Wynder EL, Rose DP, Cohen LA (1986). Diet and breast cancer in causation and therapy. Cancer 58, 1804-1813.

Yoshimi N, Sugie S, Iwata H, Mori H, Williams GM (1988). Species and sex differences in genotoxicity of heterocyclic aminopyrolysis and cooking products in the hepatocyte primary culture/DNA repair test using rat, mouse, and hamster hepatocytes. Environ Molec Mutagenesis 12:53-64.

AN EPILOGUE

THE MAILLARD REACTION *in vivo: QUO VADIS*

The Maillard reaction is older than man himself, making its debut in the formation of the primordial soup. The modern era of the reaction dates from the time of Louis Maillard, starting in the second decade of this century. Progress in understanding the chemistry of the Maillard reaction has been steady throughout the last 75 years, but in the last 15 years, following evidence that the reaction proceeds *in vivo*, there has been surge of interest in the relevance of the reaction to physiological and pathological processes. Even since the Third International Symposium on the Maillard Reaction in 1985, a number of critical observations have been made, and new and exciting avenues of research have been opened up. Most of these observations and ideas have been presented and discussed at this meeting which was oriented largely toward discussions of the Maillard reaction in living systems.

Several central themes were recurrent in our discussions. First, there was a strong consensus that rigorous chemical approaches will be essential to further progress in characterizing the pathways and products of the Maillard reaction *in vivo*. While the focus on defining the reaction chemistry is clear, the scope of this task has become less well defined as a result of the recent evidence for autoxidative pathways of glycation of protein. Although products of this pathway have not yet been identified, studies in model systems suggest an interplay between glycation and oxidation of proteins and argue for a role of the Maillard reaction in age-related oxidative damage to proteins. Although there are uncertainties regarding the mechanisms involved, there is now convincing evidence for a number of post-glycation or Advanced Glycosylation End-products (AGE products) in tissue proteins, and several laboratories are active in the identification and quantitation of both fluorescent and non-fluorescent Maillard products which have been detected *in vivo*. Some of these products appear to increase both in diabetes and during normal aging, and it may soon be possible to address at a chemical level the role of the Maillard reaction in aging and diabetes and the relationship between the pathogenesis of complications in these processes.

A second theme was the relationship between the sorbitol pathway and the Maillard reaction in the development of complications in diabetes. Increased sorbitol pathway activity and nonenzymatic glycosylation of protein have often been presented as alternative hypotheses for the development of insulin-dependent pathophysiology in diabetes. However it now appears that the two pathways may be interrelated and their impact in diabetes compounded. This viewpoint was developed from evidence for fructosylation of protein *in vivo* and the rapid rate of browning of fructose adducts to protein and from new information on the effects of glycation on the kinetic properties of aldose reductase. Further studies on the effects of aldose reductase inhibitors on the glycation and browning of protein will undoubtedly be forthcoming. The results of these studies may reshape our current thinking on the central mechanisms by which the Maillard reaction exerts its impact in diabetes and aging.

A third focus of discussion was on the mechanisms by which the body deals with Maillard products following their formation *in vivo*. There is growing evidence that glycation is not a transparent modification of proteins, that glycated proteins are recognized differently from non-glycated proteins, and that there are physiological mechanisms for eliminating glycated and browned proteins from the body. Understanding the role of these scavenger pathways for turnover of glycated and AGEd proteins and the interplay between protein catabolism and remodeling of tissues emerges as an important avenue for future research. The results of these studies may be relevant not only for understanding the turnover of browned proteins, but should also provide insight into the metabolism of proteins damaged by other chemical processes, including oxidative modification via autoxidative glycosylation or other mechanisms. Methods for pharmacological modulation of the Maillard reaction were also discussed, but clearly this is an area where research and development should progress hand-in-hand, where there is much potential for growth and discovery.

While the focus of the meeting was on the Maillard reaction *in vivo*, the presentations by food scientists on aspects of the reaction *in vitro* provided an important perspective, directly because of their relevance to nutrition and toxicology, but also indirectly as models for studies on the Maillard reaction *in vivo*. Some of the products originally detected in Maillard reactions in foods have now been detected *in vivo*, and certainly more will be discovered with time. These products alter the digestion and metabolism of proteins and have a pathological impact because of their toxicology and genotoxicity. Understanding the mechanisms of toxicity of Maillard products found in foods may yield insight into the mechanisms by which these same products formed *in vivo* could affect cellular and physiological processes. Similarly, methods for limiting the Maillard reaction during food processing and storage may suggest pharmacological approaches to modulating the reaction *in vivo*.

Our goals in assembling the many participants for this conference were broad, and perhaps over-ambitious: to place the developments of the last several years in a clearer perspective, to develop camaraderie and foster collaborative interactions among the principle researchers in the field, to attract new scientists with different backgrounds, talents and perspectives, and, perhaps most important, to develop a consensus map for the direction of future research. That map is undoubtedly as inaccurate as a medieval map of the world, but we hope that the exchange of ideas at our meeting in Bethesda and the written summaries presented here provide a general direction for the future. It was refreshing at this meeting to realize how much has happened over the past few years, awe-inspiring to realize how much remains to be done, and tantalizing to imagine the advances that will take place during the next few years.

John W. Baynes

Vincent M. Monnier

Index

C. S. Tsai
Dept. of Chem.
Carleton Univ.